Drug Testing

Drug Testing

John Fay

Butterworth–Heinemann
Boston   London   Singapore   Sydney   Toronto   Wellington

Recognizing the importance of preserving what has been written, it is the policy of Butterworth–Heinemann to have the books it publishes printed on acid-free paper, and we exert our best efforts to that end.

Library of Congress Cataloging-in-Publication Data
Fay, John, 1934–
  Drug testing / John Fay.
    p. cm.
  Includes bibliographical references (p.).
  ISBN 0-409-90239-X
    1. Employees—Drug testing. I. Title.
HF5549.5.D7F38   1990
658.3'822—dc20   90-32616

British Library Cataloguing in Publication Data
Fay, John
  Drug testing.
  1. Drugs. Testing
  I. Title
  615.19

  ISBN 0-409-90239-X

Butterworth–Heinemann
80 Montvale Avenue
Stoneham, MA 02180

10 9 8 7 6 5 4 3 2 1

Printed in the United States of America

This book is dedicated to Calvina.

Contents

Preface

Drug abuse and the crime and social problems that flow from it constitute one of the United States' most serious and frustrating challenges. The challenge is serious because of the social and economic costs imposed by drug abuse, and it is frustrating because we have not yet found a way to deal with it effectively.

Many people in our society, particularly the young, use drugs such as alcohol, marijuana, hallucinogens, opiates, and cocaine. New drugs such as crack, fentanyl, and designer drugs (drugs that are slightly different chemically from controlled drugs but that have the same effects) have spread rapidly through all segments of society. Hospitals are reporting increased rates of drug-related emergency cases, and citizens everywhere rank drugs and crime as major concerns.

Considerable evidence exists to show that drug abuse contributes to the frequency and intensity of many types of crime, from white-collar offenses and political corruption to property offenses and violence. Similar evidence exists to show that safety in the workplace and the profitability of businesses are directly affected by substance abuse.

Improving our understanding of the factors that influence abuse both on and off the job is important in developing interventions and strategies to reduce drug-related problems. Although we have not found the right answer to eradicating or even reducing drug abuse, some progress has been made in defining the many facets of the problem. But much more still needs to be done.

Finding a solution to this problem will be very difficult. We know that drugs interact with other complex social, psychological, and pharmacological factors to influence the behavior of abusing individuals. We also know that some people who do not use illicit drugs profit from the demand for them.

The federal government has adopted a policy of making illicit drug use unacceptable either socially or in the workplace. This strategy is aimed at reversing the present levels of drug abuse and the losses that flow from it. This policy has garnered much support in Congress, the state legislatures, the business community, and a broad cross-section of the public. It is not a total answer but is definitely a step in the right direction.

When gathering material for this book, I was struck by the fact that much research gives the impression that drug abuse in the workplace is a recent phenomenon. The truth is that drug abuse, especially the abuse of alcohol, which is a drug in every sense of the word, has always been present in the workplace. Similarly, employers have tried to curb such abuse throughout history. The problem has gone uncorrected not so much because business has failed to address it but because society in general has been unable to understand the dimensions of drug abuse, find a cure, and, above all else, set up preventive measures.

Some members of the business community developed and applied some of the earliest programs for ridding the workplace of drugs. Many of the testing programs recently adopted by the criminal justice system to identify drug-abusing criminals and prisoners are based on programs conceived in the business sector. Now is not the time to rest on laurels, however, but to work even harder to apply effective antidrug programs.

While the examination of employees to determine their fitness for work is not new, the techniques for examination are. For instance, the technology on which urinalysis is based has advanced almost to the point of 100 percent accuracy. In addition, drug testing is a double-edged tool. One edge deters and the other detects. Drug-abusing employees who know they will be discharged or disciplined if identified through testing are motivated to stop drug use. The identification of employees with drug problems is the first step toward treatment and possible cure. Drug testing is only one of several tools available to help management eliminate drug abuse in the workplace. Others are education, training, discipline, counseling, and rehabilitation.

This book was written for organizational leaders who recognize that drug testing is an effective tool but that it, like all tools, works best when skillfully applied. The issue today is not whether drug testing can be used but the manner of its use. In the near future, courts and legislatures will no doubt continue to consider legal challenges to drug testing, and through the evolution of case and statutory law, a body of fair and effective practices will emerge to guide employers in the use of this valuable tool.

Chapter 1

An Overview

Today's business leaders are learning that an organization's natural drive for productivity and quality, and even the ability to compete and survive, are threatened by workplace drug abuse. Company executives are also starting to worry that the patterns of abuse now occurring among the young will be carried into the work forces of the future.

The issue has implications beyond companies or even industries. Drug abuse by workers is a matter for national concern, since the major business activities of today, and to a greater extent tomorrow, take place in a global arena where competitors are strong and the stakes high. American businesses will not be in the running if they are hobbled by drug abuse.

The business community has a great deal of leverage in deterring illegal drug use in society. Business leaders are ideally positioned to discourage drug use and to promote preventive efforts within the community. When antidrug programs emanate from business leaders, a strong message is sent to workers and their families: The workplace is off-limits to drug users.

More and more companies are beginning to use urinalysis to detect employee drug use. In the past, many companies believed that an employee's drug use did not affect his or her performance in the workplace. Today, that view is no longer popular, as most employers believe that drug use that detracts from an employee's performance is a legitimate concern.

What do employees think about urinalysis? Surprisingly, there appears to be a solid core of employees who dislike working alongside drug users. Workers who are opposed to drug testing tend to fall into two camps: those who believe that it is a violation of workers' constitutional rights, and those who respect an employer's right to test for drugs but question the methods used.

The issue of drug testing is a continuation of the long-standing conflict between management's prerogative to control conditions in the workplace and the employee's right to personal privacy. To date, the employer's position has pretty much prevailed in administrative and court proceedings concerning the issue.

It can be argued that business has an obligation to help create and maintain a drug-free society. No longer can business deny the seriousness of illegal drug use or look the other way when such use affects employee performance.

There is no argument that the roots of our nation's drug problem lie within the individual as well as the social fabric of our society. The strength and determination needed to rid our nation of its drug problem also reside in these places, and business is clearly a key factor in effecting a positive change.

Without a demand for illegal drugs, there would be no supply of them. The government has shifted its focus of attack to include users as well as suppliers and is now concerned with preventing people from becoming involved in the use of illegal drugs. Prevention of illegal drug use in the workplace has tremendous potential for suppressing the demand.

Prevention begins in the home and extends to work, education, religion, and other extrafamilial systems. A positive mental attitude and strong character flow from the support and values obtained within the family unit, but prevention of illegal drug use cannot be achieved without an enduring commitment from businesspeople, educators, religious leaders, medical practitioners, and criminal justice officials.

Unions and employee associations can also play a key role in curbing illegal drug use. The leaders of unions and associations are in general agreement that they must provide direction to their members in this area. While some disagreement exists as to what that direction should be, there is a genuine concern among labor leaders that unchecked drug use endangers the health and safety of workers and beyond that generally causes damage to the image of labor organizations. The capacity of a labor organization to supply a competent work force and to represent that work force in regard to safety, health, benefits, and wages can be undermined by a minority of drug-abusing members. Although union and employee association leaders share the same concerns as ownership and management, the two sides differ in respect to a remedy.

Employers have found urinalysis to be an effective remedy, but labor leaders oppose the use of this without approval by union members. The matter has come up before the National Labor Relations Board (NLRB), and its general counsel (legal department) has ruled that unionized employers are required under the National Labor Relations Act to bargain collectively and in good faith regarding the implementation of drug or alcohol testing of both employees and applicants. The general counsel advises that the start-up of a drug- and alcohol-testing program constitutes a substantial change in the terms and conditions of employment, thereby triggering the requirement for mandatory bargaining. The advice holds even when the employer already has rules prohibiting drug and alcohol use and has a program of mandatory physical evaluations to determine fitness for duty. If, however, the right to bargain collectively on this issue has been clearly waived in a preexisting agreement, the employer is not required to bargain with employees again.

This advice was ignored when the NLRB subsequently decided that it was the employer's prerogative to test job candidates for drug use without union approval. The case involved a newspaper and a union local that represented some of the employees. Newspaper management wanted to test applicants for drug use before offering them jobs, and the union claimed that the procedure should be part of a bargaining agreement. In deciding that the employer could conduct preemployment drug testing without union involvement, the NLRB essentially said that businesses in all industry sectors can conduct preemployment drug tests.

A DRUG-TESTING POLICY

A drug-testing policy must seek to strike a balance between the need to maintain a safe and productive workplace and the need to respect the personal privacy and dignity of workers. The first step for management is to document the necessity for such a program. Management must ask itself the following questions: To what extent is abuse present, and what are its dimensions? Where should testing be targeted, and who will be subject to it?

The next step is to define the policy violations and corresponding enforcement and disciplinary measures. The policy also should discuss the consequences of a positive drug test and define the opportunities for an employee to explain why a test showed positive and to file an appeal and/or a grievance.

Prevention of potential civil rights violations requires a well-thought-out policy that is based on unbiased, accurate, and legally defensible drug testing for the job in question. Common sense will go a long way in the prevention of legal challenges. Examples of common-sense approaches include developing reasonable procedures, seeking the support of union leaders, and making employees aware of the need for the policy.

The frequency of drug testing is usually based on the risk factors associated with safety, security, and health. The least intrusive policy requires testing only after an accident occurs or other reasonable cause is shown. High-risk occupations in which the public safety is of special concern may require routine testing. In these cases, testing is often tied to evaluation of fitness for duty or to annual physical examinations. Extremely hazardous and very high risk occupations may require periodic unannounced or random testing to ensure the health and safety of employees and the general public. Pilots, nuclear plant operators, and hazardous cargo transporters might fall into this category.

The process of drafting and implementing a drug-testing policy can be enhanced enormously when there is cooperation between labor and management. Zero tolerance of drugs and uniform application to all employees are two points on which both sides usually agree. Acceptance of a policy also can be facilitated if the policy is presented as a means for protecting the health and safety of users and nonusers alike. Not to be ignored are the negative economic consequences of drug use, which include lower efficiency, productivity, and profits; increased absenteeism and crime; more accidents; and high workmen's compensation and medical claims.

Policies vary depending on factors such as company size, operating location, nature of the business, culture of the industry and work force, laws and regulations, and management philosophy. Despite these differences, policies contain several common elements.

Prohibited Activities

At minimum, a policy should state that on-the-job use, possession, and distribution of illegal drugs is forbidden. More controversially, the prohibition might extend to off-the-job use. An employer may claim an interest in an employee's drug use away from work because of the harm such use can do to the employer's business reputation. A supporting point is the fact that the use of illegal drugs is against the law, and the employer, as a law-abiding corporate citizen, cannot tolerate having criminals in the work force.

Another compelling reason exists for prohibiting off-duty use of drugs. A number of scientific studies indicate that drug use has a lingering effect and can cause impairment even if the user exhibits no perceptible signs of such use. This might compromise the user's fitness for duty, especially if he or she performs safety-sensitive functions. George W. Moody, M.D., chief of the Substance Abuse Treatment Unit at the Philadelphia Veterans Administration Medical Center, has described the mental disorders produced by prolonged use of stimulants and hallucinogens, as well as the depression caused by sedatives. He notes that a drug use pattern that appears casual and controlled may change rapidly:

> Although a person might initially use a substance of abuse in off-duty hours and demonstrate little or no impairment on the job, the mere fact that the person uses the drug carries a significant danger that this controlled, sporadic pattern will change to an uncontrolled, abusive pattern in which he or she is unable to check their impulses to use the drug. The result is more frequent use and a greater likelihood of becoming impaired while at work.

Residual effects from marijuana use also appear to be supported by recent research. These are of particular concern because they can occur unexpectedly while the user is at work.

In addition, an off-duty user of drugs may be reluctant to turn in a fellow worker who is impaired on the job. In some cases, coworkers may be unaware of a problem until they witness an accident or unsafe action that threatens their safety. Under pressure from coworkers, some users will stop using drugs, but others will take special care to conceal their use or will respond negatively to expressions of concern from coworkers.

An off-duty user's anxieties about how he or she will obtain and pay for drugs also might be a distraction at work. For a worker engaged in hazardous duties, any distraction is dangerous for the worker as well as those around him or her.

An employer who prohibits off-duty drug use is making the statement that safety can be adequately protected only if employees, especially those engaged in safety-sensitive functions, are free from the effects of drugs used without proper medical supervision. The employer is concluding that it is not responsible to permit a risk to exist by taking no action or by attempting to address the drug problem only when overt manifestations are present in the workplace. Indeed, the detection of drug abuse by a worker seeking to hide his or her habit is usually not possible until the advanced stages of dependence, and even then indications of abuse are not always clear. By the time the problem is identified, the worker is likely to have been responsible for minor accidents, waste, and decreased productivity.

Even drug use accompanied by a pronounced decline in performance can go unnoticed. The failure of supervisors to detect and report impairment is a strong argument for random and unannounced drug testing. In defense of supervisors, it should be noted that the behavioral signals of drug abuse are often identical or similar to symptoms of medical problems such as allergies and are thus easily explained away by the user.

The diagnostic criteria used by medical professionals to detect drug abuse are not easily applied by those outside the medical profession. For instance, marijuana and cocaine primarily affect the higher brain functions of judgment, decision making, reaction time, and other psychomotor skills. These drugs also affect motivation and the desire to achieve established work goals. It would be very difficult for a supervisor to reliably detect impairment in these areas.

Some labor organizations continue to maintain that what an employee does on his or her own time is beyond the legitimate interest of the employer. This belief is gradually giving way to a realization that it is not possible to separate drug use off the job from fitness on the job. Some labor-management agreements acknowledge that safety is compromised when an employee tests positive for drug use, whether or not on-duty use or impairment can be demonstrated.

Surveillance of employees during off-duty time is unreasonable, but it is not unreasonable to require that employees take medication only as prescribed and that they not use substances that are unlawful to possess or use. Voluntary compliance with a prohibition against off-duty drug use is feasible, provided that noncompliance is made susceptible to detection by on-duty drug testing.

Policy Sanctions

A policy must specify the actions that the employer intends to take against employees who engage in prohibited activities. The disciplinary options for each type of violation must be spelled out clearly. Penalties should vary based on the severity of the violation. For example, selling drugs would call for the most severe sanction, whereas testing positive for drug use would merit a less severe disciplinary action.

The most important considerations in administering discipline are fairness and uniformity. A key task of management is to communicate the policy to all employees and to inform them, either in the policy or other written materials, of the consequences of noncompliance. This task also involves telling employees of any inquiry and appeals processes that are in place to guard against unfairness. When the policy has been explained in detail, the stage is set for careful and deliberate application of it.

The manager responsible for administering discipline must weigh the employee's interests against those of the organization. Maintaining this balance is easier said than done. Even well-intentioned efforts to administer discipline according to what is best for the employee are likely to lead to charges of favoritism, while discipline that is based on zero tolerance of illegal drug use may be decried as overly harsh. The manager must focus on the offense itself and the circumstances under which it occurred. An employee's past record or future promise should be less important considerations. In some situations, such as violations involving the sale of drugs, a manager will have no choice but to terminate the offending employee.

An appeal process must be available to employees who fail a drug test. This can take the form of a confidential meeting between an employee and his or her supervisor or review by a physician or other professional who is knowledgeable about substance abuse. The appeal process also might include a physical examination of the employee or an examination of the employee's medical history to determine whether there is a medical explanation for the positive test result. The employee also may be able to request a reanalysis of the same specimen.

Drug Testing

Although an employer's efforts at drug abuse prevention are necessarily broad based, highly focused programs can keep people from starting to use illegal drugs or help them to stop using them. One focused approach that has been found to be effective is drug testing. Drug testing is especially appropriate in safety-related work. It acts as a deterrent and as a mechanism for identifying drug use before addiction sets in. For working adults, drug testing is a powerful preventive tool because it carries the sanctions of peer worker disapproval and loss of job.

The circumstances that trigger drug testing could include preemployment screening, testing for reasonable cause, random testing, unannounced testing, postaccident testing, testing coincident with routine medical evaluations, return-to-duty testing, and testing during and following drug rehabilitation. A drug-testing program could contain an amnesty provision and be linked to procedures for referring drug users to treatment.

Drug testing can be a valuable deterrent. It can discourage nonusers from beginning to use drugs; it can deter experimental users from graduating to more serious abuse; it can motivate nonaddicted users to discontinue use for fear of getting caught; and it can challenge addicted users to seek medical help.

Management should not think of drug testing as a stand-alone substance abuse program or the primary component of a more comprehensive program. It is not a panacea or a substitute for sound management practices. It should be viewed as a complementary function of policy enforcement, education, training, and employee assistance.

Confidentiality

Principles of public safety, efficient performance, and optimal productivity must be balanced against worker expectations of privacy and confidentiality. In some cases, the safety of coworkers, customers, and the general public overrides an employee's right to privacy. But confidentiality is a must when dealing with drug testing. Because substance abuse is seen as a diagnosable and treatable illness, the results of drug testing should be treated with the same degree of confidentiality as are other medical or health-related conditions. Only certain employer representatives should have access to test results, and in some places, an employer might be required by law to ensure the confidentiality of drug test data, as well as information related to diagnosis, treatment, and rehabilitation.

The fear of being publicly identified as a drug user can turn employees against drug testing. Confidentiality makes sense, not just because it may be required by law, but also because it guarantees that employees be treated fairly and helps them overcome their apprehensions about drug testing.

A DRUG-TESTING PROGRAM

It helps to think of a drug-testing policy as a set of broad instructions from the company's management and a drug-testing program as the vehicle for carrying out those instructions. The policy and the program recommended in this book contain the following three components:

1. Educating employees generally to the dangers of drug abuse and specifically to the requirements of complying with the policy and its program
2. Training supervisors to recognize drug abuse and to intervene using particular techniques
3. Conducting urine drug tests so that drug-abusing employees can be identified and referred to treatment

Educating Employees

An antidrug program should inform employees about the dangers of illicit drug use, including its effects on health and job performance. An employer can generate goodwill by demonstrating a concern for the well-being of employees and for the provision of a safe and secure workplace. In addition, to the extent that health and safety are preserved, the employer obtains the benefits of improved productivity.

Employees deserve to know how the company plans to enforce the antidrug policy, to whom the policy will apply, the consequences of policy violations, and why the policy is needed. The educational component of an antidrug program will disseminate information about personal prevention at home and on the job, voluntary prevention activities (such as peer intervention), and the type of help that may be accessed through the organization's employee assistance program (EAP) (see the section on EAPs later in this chapter).

Training Supervisors

Supervisors must be given the skills and knowledge needed to recognize drug impairment and to take effective action that is consistent with the employer's policy and procedures. The employer must provide training in how to look for, respond to, and document illegal drug use, as well as how to encourage self-reporting by employees. Because supervisors are central to the success of an effective antidrug program, it is very important to identify their special roles and responsibilities. No one in the organization is better positioned to notice the telltale signs of drug abuse, to intervene when they appear, to document their appearance and the intervention action taken, and to make follow-up evaluations.

Training should consist of providing supervisors with a thorough understanding of the intent of the company's antidrug policy, its relevance to work performance and the problems associated with drug abuse, intervention tactics, and the legal and liability issues involved with intervention or the failure to intervene. The word *intervention* carries a connotation of no-nonsense action, which is appropriate in the context of workplace drug abuse. A quick, decisive, and determined response is necessary, but it should be tempered with sensitivity for the employee. Supervisors must balance the needs of the organization and the employee's personal need for privacy.

Confrontation is the supervisor's principal intervention tactic. It almost always occurs in a one-on-one meeting between the supervisor and the employee. The purposes of the meeting are to discuss the employee's unacceptable performance, agree on the improvement that must be made, set a timetable for improvement, and spell out the consequences of the employee's not making the necessary improvement.

If the topic of drug abuse is raised during the confrontation, it should be raised by the employee, not the supervisor. An admission of drug abuse is helpful because it is the abuser's first step in coming to grips with the problem and it allows the supervisor to meet his or her objective of leading the employee to professional assistance. Although identifying the source of the unacceptable performance is helpful, the supervisor's focus throughout the meeting and in all subsequent dealings with the employee should be job performance.

The supervisor may conclude from the meeting that the employee needs professional help. If so, he or she can inform the employee of this during the meeting and then send a follow-up memorandum. The memorandum should review the performance problem, the employee's actions to correct the problem, and the recommended assistance. It also should express concern for the employee and give notice that a failure to obtain the recommended assistance will be a factor in determining disciplinary action if such discipline becomes necessary.

Although supervisors are generally skilled at spotting performance problems, they are not usually skilled at diagnosing the sources of the problems. The immediate objective, then, is to bring the employee into contact with a professional diagnostician so that a treatment program can be formulated and therapy started. In most cases, therapy will consist of counseling that will help the employee to understand the dimensions of the problem, accept a course of action designed to solve it, and provide some skills that support the course of action.

Testing for Drugs

Drug testing is a deterrent and a response mechanism. It is a deterrent because people who know that they will be tested may be persuaded not to use drugs. It is a response mechanism because it identifies employees whose drug use may pose safety risks to themselves and their coworkers.

Testing Options

Preemployment Testing.   This form of testing is preventive because it denies employment to persons who are identified as drug users. Almost all companies that use drug testing include preemployment testing. It is the most frequently used form of situational testing. Part of the reason for widespread use of preemployment testing is that it poses less of a risk to an employer in terms of labor grievances and litigation because the employer has no obligation to a nonemployee.

Reasonable Cause Testing.   This form of testing is used when an employee's unsafe or unacceptable job conduct clearly points to drug use. The major obstacle to reasonable cause testing is the lack of training and encouragement given to supervisors to look for drug-abusing employees. A supervisor also might avoid reasonable cause testing because of a concern that (1) the team spirit or unity of employees will be hurt and thus productivity will decline, and (2) the supervisor's decision will be challenged by the employee or union and questioned by someone higher up in management.

In addition to these concerns, the company drug policy may be unclear or require the supervisor to file a large number of reports. The policy also may be legally unsound. Because the stakes can be high in a reasonable cause situation, the employer must provide supervisors with a well-structured testing process. For example, the company might require that the supervisor be sure that he or she can explain and substantiate the facts that led to the decision to test an employee; that the indicators are specific, contemporaneous, and tangible; and that they are associated with probable drug use.

The process also might require the supervisor to document behavioral changes and performance indicators over a period of time and to compare those observations with previous conduct. The unacceptable conduct might consist of repeated errors on the job, rule violations, and an unsatisfactory attendance record. The evidence of probable drug use might include any of the common physiological symptoms, such as a staggering gait, slurred speech, or unusual actions.

A common procedure in reasonable cause situations is to apply the "two supervisors rule," which requires that the testing decision be made jointly by two supervisors who have knowledge of the facts. Sometimes the rule is extended to require that one or both of the supervisors have received training in making reasonable cause determinations.

Another approach would be for the observing supervisor and one employee to confer and document the incident. The next best situation would be for the observing supervisor to confer with another supervisor who was not a witness. The last alternative would be for the observing supervisor to act on his or her judgment alone.

The decision-making process in reasonable cause determinations must be highly prescriptive and unambiguous. Ideally, every supervisor responsible for enforcing reasonable cause testing will have received training regarding the circumstances and evidence necessary to make these determinations.

The minimum length of training for reasonable cause testing in the federal programs is one hour, which is far too little training, especially since it must address several other major topics as well. At least four hours should be allocated for training, and the curriculum should include an examination of the employer's drug-testing policy and rules; identification of drug and drug paraphernalia; recognition of drug abuse indicators; a review of relevant legal concepts, intervention tactics, and referral and treatment procedures; and a layperson's view of drug-testing technology. At least one-third of the training time should be spent in hands-on activities such as making reasonable cause determinations in hypothetical situations.

The personnel files of supervisors who receive this training should be documented so that a defense can be made for the supervisor and the employer in case of charges of negligence, irresponsibility, or discrimination.

Random Testing. Random testing is the most controversial option because it pits the employer's desires, which often mirror broad societal interests, against individual workers' desires. Random testing is used to a greater extent in occupations where the public interest outweighs individual interests, such as in law enforcement and aviation. In some work situations, random testing may apply only to employees engaged in certain activities.

Random testing is also called *unannounced testing,* because the salient feature is the absence of advance notice, or *no-cause testing,* because selection of persons to be tested is not related to a specific reason for testing. These two factors—no notice and no cause—are the reasons why this type of testing is so unpopular.

The word *random* comes from the technique for selecting the persons to be tested. A random selection technique is one in which every person from a defined population has an equal chance of being chosen for testing. The number of persons chosen from the total population is often expressed as a percentage. The percentage is sometimes proportional to the employer's perception of the drug use problem—that is, a perception of widespread drug use requires that a high percentage of persons be randomly selected. The random technique also can be applied to the process of selecting from among many work sites one or a few sites where all employees are tested.

In the random testing programs of the Department of Transportation, an implementation procedure has been set up for an employer to phase in such testing during the first 12 months after starting a drug-testing program. The employer's obligation in the first year is to test at least 25 percent of all employees subject to random testing and to reach a random testing rate of 50 percent by at least the last test collection session in the first year. The phase-in procedure allows an employer to collect a smaller number of specimens at the beginning of the year and build up gradually.

Let's assume, for example, that 600 persons are subject to random testing and the employer has decided to conduct one collection session each month. To be in compliance with the 50 percent testing rate by the end of the year, the employer will need to test at least 25 persons in December—that is, 50 percent of 600 divided by 12. To be in compliance with the rule to have 25 percent of the affected employees tested by the end of the year, the employer will need to test 125 people in the first 11 collection sessions plus the 25 persons tested in the 12th and final session. During the second year, the employer would be required to maintain the 50 percent rate, which would mean that 300 persons would be tested, with collections spaced reasonably throughout the year.

The random testing rate is not to be confused with the percentage of employees who are selected for testing each time testing is conducted. Let us assume that the employer in the example above decides to conduct 10 testing sessions spread out through the year, with 30 employees tested each time. At the end of the year, 300 employees will have been randomly tested, which represents 50 percent of the total, but the percentage of employees tested each time will have been 5 percent (that is, 30 divided by 600).

Postaccident Testing. In this testing option, persons who are directly involved in an accident or a near miss are required to undergo testing. Postaccident testing is similar to reasonable cause testing because both are based on events that automatically call for testing. In postaccident testing, however, there need not be any indicators of impairment.

The employer establishes the types of accidents that call for testing. Two measures of severity—extent of injury and extent of monetary loss—are the usual determinants. The persons to be tested are identified as to their possible involvement in causing the accident.

Periodic Testing. This is a catchall category that includes drug tests conducted at designated intervals. The tests are usually conducted as an adjunct to things such as routine checkups or recertification of occupational licenses.

Periodic testing has limited efficacy in deterring or detecting drug use because users can simply abstain from use prior to the scheduled test. Also, the health professionals who collect specimens for drug testing as part of a medical evaluation are not always set up to guard against specimen substitution.

Rehabilitation Testing. The frequency and manner of testing employees in rehabilitation and before return to duty are determined by the professionals involved in the rehabilitation program. The key person could be a medical review officer (MRO) employed by the company. Although the principal function of an MRO is to evaluate positive test results, his or her role could be expanded to take on rehabilitation functions, such as setting an unannounced testing schedule for the employee and deciding when an employee is fit to return to work.

Making a determination that an employee is no longer drug dependent and therefore not a risk to the work environment always carries an element of controversy. The employee's nonabusing coworkers may view the decision, indeed the whole issue of rehabilitation, as being inconsistent with safety.

The use of unannounced testing after the employee returns to work is determined by management or senior supervisors close to the job and familiar with the employee's duties. When the job involves safety-sensitive duties, unannounced testing will occur more frequently and be more unpredictable, and the period of aftercare monitoring will be longer. This is done to gain maximum assurance that the employee will remain free from drugs. The frequency of unannounced testing following rehabilitation can vary from once every three months to once every three days, with the norm close to once a month. The length of after-treatment monitoring usually ranges from one to five years.

Drug testing can contribute to a rehabilitation program in the following three ways:

1. It can serve as a means for identifying employees who may be in need of treatment.
2. Because urinalysis reveals the types of drugs taken and provides some clues as to quantities taken, it can be used as a diagnostic aid in evaluating the nature of the involvement with drugs.
3. It can be used to monitor treatment progress and provide credible and timely information on an employee's continued use or abstinence from drugs.

With regard to the last point, drug testing can be used in a therapeutic sense as well. For example, a positive test during rehabilitation can be used to confront denial of continued drug use. Even occasional use can be spotted by drug testing so that steps can be taken by treatment professionals to keep the employee from reverting to a pattern of regular use. When handled skillfully, drug testing can help employees in rehabilitation to resist peer pressure and to attain a drug-free status.

Test results can be misleading if the test fails to look for all the drugs that an employee in treatment might be using. An initial diagnosis may reveal a cocaine dependence, so rehabilitation testing would focus on that drug. If the testing program does not include a full array of screens, however, the employee could shift to heroin or some other drug and escape detection.

Drug treatment professionals are generally supportive of urinalysis as a treatment aid, but they also have reservations about possible pitfalls. Their main concern is the possible use of testing for punitive instead of diagnostic and therapeutic purposes. They fret about employers wanting to take too narrow a stance on positive test results. They know from their experiences that relapse is common, and they expect employers to be forgiving when relapse occurs. This is certainly a matter for consideration by the employer, but it should not be a reason for withholding the established sanctions. The credibility and effectiveness of a rehabilitation program can be seriously undermined if positive tests are not always followed by the customary penalties. A rehabilitation program cannot become, in either fact or appearance, a safe haven for employees who continue to abuse drugs.

The Deterrent Effect of Testing

Some types of testing, such as postaccident, reasonable cause, and unannounced testing, have an important deterrent effect and can lead to the identification of employees who need help. Preemployment testing and periodic testing do not have much of a deterrent effect because the advance notice that customarily accompanies these forms of testing allows many drug users to abstain long enough to avoid detection. Employees who are so heavily dependent on drugs that they are unable to abstain for even a short period of time prior to a scheduled drug test will be identified, but deterrence is not an issue for them because of the overpowering nature of their dependence.

The extent of abuse perceived by management, the safety sensitivity of the work, and management's tolerance level are factors that will determine the types of testing to be applied and the frequency of testing. If management's desire is to establish a high deterrence level, a random testing schedule could be used and even adjusted to involve a larger percentage of the work force and to occur more frequently. For example, when the U.S. Navy was confronted with a serious drug problem, it set the random testing rate as high as 240 percent. The military generally maintains a random testing rate of 125 percent, while the federal drug-testing program operates at a 50 percent rate.

Advocates of drug testing believe that an optimum level of deterrence can be achieved by combining frequent, unannounced testing with a random selection method. For example, the employer might schedule testing at a frequency of not less than once a month, with the testing day not known until the day arrives. On that day, a percentage of the work force would be randomly selected. This technique has proven to be an effective deterrent, and when used consistently, it has resulted in a decline in accidents and the number of employees who test positive for drugs.

Collecting Specimens

An experienced drug-testing program coordinator will unhesitatingly say that the worst possible event is to experience a false-positive test result. The coordinator also will say that a false positive will most likely occur as a result of human error during the collection of specimens.

Specimen collection is an administrative process involving intense human labor. It is repetitive and demands constant attention to detail. When not downright boring, it can be downright confusing. The paperwork that accompanies each specimen can be overwhelming: consent, waiver, test order, log book, specimen labels, and chain of custody. These must be filled out, signed, collated, and arranged in a particular way. Collection of specimens is an operation in which mistakes are intolerable yet inevitable.

The employer must make sure that the specimens are collected and transported to the drug-testing laboratory in a manner that guards against switching, substitution, dilution, adulteration, and contamination. Chain of custody is the principal mechanism for ensuring the integrity of specimens. This refers to the procedures that govern collecting, handling, storing, and testing of specimens; disseminating results; and retaining specimens in a manner that ensures confidentiality and accuracy. The major purpose of

chain of custody is to incontrovertibly match three components: the specimen, the donor, and the results of the specimen.

The chain-of-custody process includes a signed consent by the specimen
donor in which he or she agrees to provide the specimen knowing that it
will be examined for the presence of drugs and knowing the consequences
of a positive test result. The consent form also may contain an acknowledgment that the employee understands the employer's policy and the consequences of refusing to provide a specimen or cooperating in the test.

As a part of the consent or on a separate form, the employee will acknowledge that the employer has access to the drug test results and can
disclose those results to specified persons or agencies. The employee's consent for the release and disclosure of the test results is indicated by his or
her signature on the form. An employer or an employer's agent who collects
the specimen also may want to obtain a signed waiver in which the specimen
donor agrees to release the employer or the agent from any damages or claims
arising from the drug test.

An important part of chain-of-custody documentation is the test report.
The report will typically include identifying numbers that link the report
with the corresponding specimen and donor. The report will reflect the drugs
looked for, the findings, the test methods, the date of testing, and the identity
of the person who conducted the test or who was responsible for laboratory
operations.

Analyzing Specimens

The standard procedure for urinalysis includes two steps. The first step is
to screen specimens for the presence of one or more drugs. The number or
combination of drugs is usually determined by the rules of the testing program (for example, the federal program specifies a particular combination
of five drug classes). Sometimes this number is selected by the employer,
often on the recommendation of the drug-testing laboratory or an outside
consultant. The recommendation is based on the types of drugs commonly
abused among the employee population to be tested.

Specimens that produce negative results in the screen are not tested
further. Specimens that produce positive results are referred to a second test
called a confirmation or verification. A confirmation test uses gas chroma-
tography/mass spectrometry (GC/MS) as the analytical methodology. A verification test uses any analytical methodology other than GC/MS. Confirmation
tests have wide acceptance in the scientific and legal communities.

Screens.   Almost all screens are done by immunoassay techniques. These
techniques depend on a chemical reaction between the specimen and an
antibody designed to react to a specific drug. The chemical reaction causes
a change in the specimen that is measured by a sensitive instrument, such
as a spectrophotometer. If the reading on the machine is higher than a given
standard, the specimen is presumed to be positive.

In enzyme immunoassays (EIA), an enzyme is used to create the chemical reaction. The change in enzyme activity indicates that a drug is present in the urine specimen. In radioimmunoassays (RIA), the specimen is exposed to a radioactive material. The presence of a drug is indicated by the amount of radioactivity produced by the reaction. In fluorescence polarization immunoassays (FPIA), a fluorescing material is added to the specimen. The degree of light polarization is the indicator of a drug's presence.

Thin-layer chromatography (TLC) is used both as a screening and a verifying technique. In TLC testing, a measured amount of urine is placed on a glass plate that has been coated with a thin layer of a material to which silicon or some other material will easily attach. The coated plate is put into a container that has a special chemical solution inside. The chemical solution moves up the plate. A reaction occurs in which the components of the urine separate according to their different abilities to move, or migrate. The separated components can then be identified by spraying the plate with a solution that causes the components to change color. The technician interprets the color and migration patterns to determine the presence of one or more drugs. TLC is not a favored form of drug testing because the test results are highly subjective—that is, they are based on the technician's ability to interpret the color and migration patterns.

Confirmation Tests.   As mentioned before, confirmation testing is by GC/MS. In this technique, a gas such as helium or nitrogen transports the urine specimen to a column where the components of the specimen are separated. The equipment used in this process is called a gas chromatograph (GC). The gas medium transports the separated components to a detector for precise identification and measurement. The detector is called a mass spectrometer (MS). The MS operates on a principle of identification called *mass-to-charge ratio*. The mass spectrum of a substance is specific for that particular substance. The task of the technician is to match the spectra of the urine specimen with the known spectra of drugs.

In-House versus Commercial Drug Testing

One of the questions that crops up in starting a drug-testing program is whether to conduct tests in-house or to contract with a commercial drug-testing laboratory. An in-house drug-testing program is one in which the employer performs all the functions related to specimen collection, analysis, and expert witness testimony. The major elements of the program are the staff, equipment, related supplies, and laboratory facility.

Typically, the staff consists of a combination of urinalysis technicians, office and supply clerks, and at least one manager or supervisor with a background in forensic toxicology. The companies that manufacture drug-testing equipment and reagents provide a modicum of entry-level training in how to operate the equipment. Advance training, which is more complex and expensive, will teach the various drug-testing techniques and test interpretation. Some equipment manufacturers provide technical assistance for problems that arise when the equipment is in operation.

The equipment for an in-house testing program is almost always less elaborate than that found in a commercial drug-testing laboratory. Generally speaking, in-house equipment will not match commercial equipment in terms of speed, automation, reliability, and accuracy. In many cases, in-house equipment is leased and comes with a service contract.

The testing reagents are sold by the equipment manufacturer and are very often the manufacturer's main source of income. Reagents are expensive when bought in small quantities, and they have a limited shelf life, which prevents users from buying them in large quantities. In addition, once a container of reagent is opened, it must be used immediately or discarded. In addition to reagents, an in-house testing program will stock specimen bottles, gloves, disinfectants, distilled water, and many other supplies.

The in-house test laboratory must be located in a hygienic environment, preferably isolated from the employer's other operations, and it must be equipped with particular electrical, air-conditioning/venting, and plumbing facilities.

Why would an employer want to have an in-house testing facility? The two reasons that stand out are control and cost. Control of the program on the premises provides rapid test results and reduces the administrative burdens of chain of custody and confidentiality. The lower cost results in more savings.

What are the disadvantages of in-house testing? Unless the employer is willing to pay the higher salaries for professional laboratory staff, the accuracy and reliability of test results will be subject to question. This extends to the equipment and facilities as well. The only way to overcome this limitation is to duplicate a full-scale commercial drug-testing laboratory, but this is not cost-effective.

One serious consequence of having less than a full testing capability is not being able to detect and measure all major drugs or their combinations. Another serious consequence is the lack of persons on staff who can serve as expert witnesses and answer technical questions in legal proceedings.

Perhaps the greatest drawback to an in-house testing program is the exposure to civil liability. The employer will be open to charges ranging from discrimination to negligence. Small mistakes in specimen collection, chain-of-custody documentation, and quality-assurance procedures can lead to major problems in litigation.

When one looks objectively at the pros and cons of in-house testing versus commercial testing, the latter appears to be a better choice. The in-house approach seems to make sense only when the volume of testing is high (at least 300 specimens per month) and the combination of staff, equipment, and facility guarantees a high degree of confidence in test results. Even in this scenario, the savings that can be realized through volume testing are offset by the greater investment required to attain high confidence.

If an employer decides to contract with a commercial drug-testing laboratory, what assurance is there that the selected laboratory has the requisite expertise and equipment and follows procedures for chain of custody, quality control, and confidentiality of test results? A simple answer is to select a laboratory that has been certified by the U.S. Department of Health and Human Services (DHHS). A better answer is to select a DHHS-certified laboratory and also to evaluate the analytical services through blind performance testing. Consulting firms such as those that provide specimen collection services can be of help in setting up blind performance tests and in ensuring that the laboratory meets its contractual obligations to provide strict chain of custody, case documentation, and frozen storage.

Not more than 20 years ago, when drug testing as we know it today was just beginning, the test procedures were much less sophisticated. False-positive results, while not common, occurred often enough to cause concern. Advances since then in the technology of collecting and analyzing specimens have made it possible to virtually eliminate false positives. For example, one major drug-testing laboratory conducted nearly 5 million distinct analyses of urine specimens involving nine different drugs and nearly 1.5 million analyses of urine for two different drugs, and not one analysis resulted in a false-positive finding.

Both the employer and the laboratory performing drug-testing services must be concerned about legal challenges of test results. A competent drug-testing laboratory will have staff capable of testifying, but an employer usually will not. Although an employer can expect the laboratory to provide most of the testimony, especially in the scientific area, the employer may be called to testify. Here are some actions an employer can take to prepare for this testimony:

- Become familiar with the various chain-of-custody forms.
- Know the procedures that are used to collect, package, and transport specimens.
- Know the testing techniques that are used for screening specimens and confirming positive results.
- Know the procedures for reporting test results and maintaining confidentiality.
- Become familiar with any federal or state laws relating to drug testing.
- Review the case being litigated, and be familiar with the details of what happened and what the plaintiff has alleged.

The employer can expect to be severely challenged by the plaintiff's attorney. The major lines of attack will be the employer's credibility, fairness, and good faith in conducting drug tests. The best defense is to be prepared.

A Consortium Approach to Testing

Small to medium-size companies that wish to start drug-testing programs might find it easier and more economical to form a consortium. The federal government encourages consortia for companies that are required to comply with federal drug-testing rules.

An example of a consortium would be the hiring of a contractor to administer the drug-testing programs of many employers. The contractor would help the consortium members write their drug-testing policies, educate their employees, and train their supervisors. The contractor also would collect specimens, transport specimens to the testing laboratory, perform or arrange for the testing of the specimens, maintain chain-of-custody documentation, report or arrange for the reporting of test results, provide MRO evaluation of positive test results, maintain test records, and provide an annual summary of information.

The consortium approach offers small companies the advantage of not having to perform the above functions with limited internal resources. In addition, the consortium can buy supplies in larger quantities, thus offering employers the advantage of lower costs.

Record Keeping

One reason often cited for management's weakened support of a drug-testing program is the failure of program administrators to produce good cost-benefit analyses and solid numbers pointing to cost savings in areas such as employee attendance, product waste and loss, productivity, accidents, injuries, and medical benefits. The failure lies not with the unavailability of numbers but with efforts to gather and massage them to create reports for management's attention.

Data collection and record keeping are essential in making objective assessments of the effectiveness of an antidrug program. The kind of data referred to here are not associated with employees by name but with the incidence, prevalence, and extent of drug use in the workplace. The numbers can be examined in relation to points in time—for example, before the antidrug program began and one year later. Without reliable numbers, an employer will be unable to know whether the investment in an antidrug program is producing the intended benefits.

FACILITATING DRUG TESTING AND TREATMENT

An employee assistance program (EAP) is a formal system for identifying unacceptable job performance and for referring the employee to a professional who is capable of dealing with the personal problem that underlies the poor performance. An EAP deals with all types of problems, including financial, legal, and family problems as well as drug abuse. It offers a humanitarian, job-based strategy for conserving human resources through a balancing of economics and empathy. It is designed to be cost-effective for the employer and to produce positive results for the employee. Because of this, it is sometimes described as a win-win proposition for both management and workers. An EAP is always confidential and nonpunitive, and it affirms three important propositions:

1. Employees are valuable members of the organization.
2. It is better to help troubled employees than to discipline or discharge them.
3. Recovered employees are better employees.

Unions in many industries and trades also have adopted EAPs.

An EAP can be operated internally, from within the sponsoring organization, or externally on a contract basis. Larger organizations usually lean toward the internal EAP, whereas smaller or widely dispersed organizations usually opt for external programs. External providers of EAPs range in scope from large national and regional operations to providers that operate locally or as components of hospitals or treatment centers.

The nature of EAP services can vary considerably from one employer to another. Each workplace has unique characteristics and dynamics, which in turn dictate its EAP needs. In some cases, supervisors feel more comfortable dealing with an internal EAP specialist, while in others the anonymity of an external specialist may be more appealing.

An EAP can be a valuable organizational mechanism for dealing with drug-abusing employees because it offers an opportunity for salvaging valuable employees within a structured process that includes cost control. The process places the major responsibility for success where it belongs—on the shoulders of the employee receiving the benefits—and for all practical purposes, it is free from the legal problems that usually accompany efforts by an employer to change employee behavior. The most positive feature may be that labor and management often agree on matters of employee assistance.

The union's interest in supporting an employer's EAP is usually predicated on obtaining specific assurances that the employee's job security and promotional opportunities will not be jeopardized by a request for diagnosis or treatment and that interviews of the employee will be restricted to issues of job performance. When an employee's job performance deteriorates to a clearly unacceptable level and the employee has not asked for help from the EAP, the union can be expected to work in cooperation with management to advise the worker in a confidential, nonthreatening manner of the availability of EAP services, encourage acceptance of the services, and make it clear to the worker that failure to correct unacceptable job performance can lead to disciplinary action, including termination.

A well-rounded EAP will include diagnostic counseling, referral for treatment and rehabilitation, and supportive long-term follow-up care to reinforce rehabilitation. It also will be conducted with confidentiality. The argument for providing medical treatment benefits can be supported by the belief that valued employees are not easily replaced and that investments in rehabilitation are preferable to investments in recruiting, training, and developing replacement employees. An extension of this argument is that a rehabilitated employee serves as a model for others and can be a valuable asset in promoting prevention.

The extent of rehabilitation offered by a company tends to vary with management's view concerning whether drug users are violators or victims, the cost-effectiveness of rehabilitation, the financial ability of the company to provide significant benefits, and the availability of rehabilitation resources.

While it may be true that many companies will not or cannot fund a full rehabilitation program, nearly every company can afford an EAP. A modestly funded EAP can at least provide employees with information on where to obtain assistance.

CHALLENGES TO DRUG-TESTING PROGRAMS

It is important to use testing systems that are based on state-of-the-art methods and rigorously controlled procedures, especially if the consequences of a positive result are great. Where reputation, livelihood, or continued employment is an issue, maximum accuracy and reliability of the detection and deterrence process are essential.

The following subsections deal with some challenges that employees may present in response to positive test results.

Passive Inhalation

Passive inhalation of marijuana smoke is not a viable challenge for at least two reasons. First, the cutoff levels of drug tests are set sufficiently high so as to preclude the possibility that a positive finding will result from passive inhalation of marijuana smoke. Also, studies to determine whether false positives could result from passive inhalation were conducted in small, poorly ventilated areas that did not correspond with real-life conditions. To obtain a positive result from passive inhalation, the researchers had to conduct the tests almost immediately following prolonged and intense exposure to marijuana smoke.

Use of Prescription Medication

A problem arises when an employee is reluctant to tell an employer about the use of a prescribed drug. The employee's reluctance might stem from a sense of privacy or fear about revealing the medical condition being treated.

This reluctance could cause an employee to withhold information that might affect a drug test even when the information is specifically requested. Thus, the employee would test positive for the improper use of a controlled substance. Clarification of this result should come from the employee in the form of clear and convincing proof documenting the lawful use of a prescribed medication.

This problem can be avoided if employees understand that a positive test result for a prescription drug taken as prescribed will carry no adverse action. Persons in safety-sensitive positions may be required to change duties until they have stopped using a potentially impairing drug, but such a change is not required for most employees. The usual practice is to keep intact the prohibition against the use of any drug that is likely to cause impairment in safety-sensitive work but to reserve the right of management to make case-by-case determinations for employees who use legally prescribed drugs.

Ingestion of Certain Food Substances

Research has shown that some food substances will trigger a positive test result. This can be prevented by instituting three safeguards:

1. The person giving the urine specimen is specifically requested to identify any foods, such as poppy seeds, that he or she recently ingested. This information accompanies the specimen to the laboratory and is considered by laboratory personnel when analyzing the specimen.
2. The testing methodology includes confirmation by GC/MS.
3. A medical review of each positive test result is required, along with an interview and/or physical examination of the tested person by a professional who is trained in drug test interpretation and substance abuse disorders.

STATE AND LOCAL LEGISLATION

A number of states and cities have enacted or are considering laws to restrict workplace drug testing. These laws generally restrict the scope of testing by both public and private employers and set down procedural safeguards and privacy protections. The laws generally do not forbid drug testing entirely but require only that testing be done situationally (for instance, for reasonable cause) or that particular procedures be followed to ensure accurate test results and to protect employees' rights.

Six states—Vermont, Iowa, Minnesota, Montana, Connecticut, and Rhode Island—have already enacted drug-testing laws. These laws restrict drug testing to reasonable suspicion and limit the disciplinary actions that employers may take. Many more states are considering such legislation. A broad consensus appears to be emerging that drug testing is too valuable a tool to ban entirely, but in light of its potential for misuse, it could stand some government regulation.

In some jurisdictions, the courts have prohibited private-sector employers from terminating employees who do not have "at will" employment contracts. In such cases, termination would be in conflict with an implied contractual obligation (such as might be found in an employee handbook, a personnel manual, or a public policy as expressed in federal or state laws). In such a jurisdiction, an employee could have a claim against an employer for being discharged as the result of a positive test or for a refusal to take a test.

FEDERAL LEGISLATION

Federal Rehabilitation Act of 1973

This act prohibits federal contractors, federal agencies, and recipients of federal financial assistance from discriminating against qualified handicapped persons. Under the act, alcoholics and drug addicts may be considered handicapped persons unless their use of alcohol or drugs would prevent successful job performance or threaten the safety or property of others. Employers must attempt to accommodate substance abusers in the workplace unless, based on consideration relating to business necessity and cost, accommodation would impose an undue hardship.

The act permits employers to require applicants and employees to undergo comprehensive physical examinations, including drug and alcohol testing. The question of whether employers may discharge or refuse to hire an individual solely on the basis of a positive test result—that is, without evidence that the individual's use of alcohol or drugs would significantly affect job performance or safety—is unresolved. In this circumstance, the prudent employer will limit decisions to discharge or not hire to situations in which there is clear and convincing evidence that job performance or safety would be negatively affected.

Under this act, employers must implement affirmative-action plans that include "a description of the extent to which and the methods whereby the special needs of handicapped employees are being met." As mentioned earlier, employers in the federal government have recognized that alcohol and drug abuse are handicapping conditions as contemplated by this act.

Drug-Free Workplace Act of 1988

When Congress passed Title V of the Omnibus Drug Initiative Act of 1988, it included a provision with the short title of the Drug-Free Workplace Act of 1988 (Pub. L. 100-690, Title V, Subtitle D). This act (see Appendix C) provides that all businesses contracting with the federal government and all grantees receiving federal financial assistance must certify that they have in place policies directed toward the creation and maintenance of a drug-free workplace.

The act applies to any contract over $25,000 and to any grant from any federal agency regardless of the amount. It became effective on March 18, 1989. The rules specify that the act applies only to the direct recipient of the federal funds. Therefore, if a federal agency provides financial assistance to a state agency, which then distributes the funds to several local agencies, only the stage agency that received the funds would have to meet the drug-free workplace requirements. Significantly, neither the act nor the regulations require contractors or grantees to conduct drug tests of employees.

The certification requirements are spelled out in detail in the act. A contractor or grantee is required to certify that it will provide a drug-free workplace by doing the following:

- Publishing a statement notifying employees that the distribution, possession, or use of a controlled substance is prohibited in the workplace and specifying the actions that will be taken against employees for violation of probation
- Establishing a drug-free awareness program to inform employees about the dangers of drug abuse; the grantee's policy of maintaining a drug-free workplace; any available drug counseling, rehabilitation, and EAPs; and the penalties that may be imposed on employees for workplace drug abuse violations
- Providing employees who work on the grant with a copy of the statement required by the first item in this list
- Notifying employees who work on the grant that as a condition of employment under such grant, the employee is to abide by the terms of the statement described in the item in this list and notify the employer of any criminal drug conviction for a workplace violation within five days after such conviction
- Notifying the granting agency within ten days after receiving notice of a conviction from an employee
- Imposing a sanction on, or requiring participation in a drug abuse assistance or rehabilitation program by, a convicted employee
- Making a good-faith effort to continue to maintain a drug-free workplace

If a grantee fails to comply with the certification requirements, the result could be suspension of payments, termination of the grant, or debarment (a declaration of ineligibility for any federal grant or contract for up to five years). Appendix 1–A offers two forms for making certification of compliance with the act.

The Drug-Free Workplace Act does not require the employer to provide any guarantees of success in attaining a drug-free workplace, only to show a good-faith effort to do so. This effort is demonstrated in four ways:

1. By having and distributing to employees a policy that states the employer's intention to maintain a drug-free workplace
2. By informing employees of the dangers of drug use on the job and the availability of counseling and rehabilitation
3. By requiring employees convicted of an on-the-job drug-related offense to report the conviction within five days
4. By imposing sanctions on employees who are convicted of such offenses

An employee who is convicted for a drug violation that is not connected with work is not covered by the act, although this could be covered by the employer's policy and rules.

The act does not specify the sanctions that should be imposed on employees who are convicted of on-the-job drug-related offenses, nor does it mention disciplinary actions to be imposed for violations of the employer's drug-free workplace policy. The penalties can range from termination to rehabilitation or any combination thereof. Although counseling and rehabilitation are mentioned, the act does not require the employer to pay those costs, only that the employer provide information about where diagnosis and treatment can be obtained.

Alcohol is not covered. The reasoning appears to be that alcohol is not a controlled substance and that an employer will already have an alcohol abuse policy.

The intent of the act is commendable, but it falls far short of the serious effort that will be required to bring about a drug-free workplace. Does anybody really think that employees will march into their bosses' offices to announce their drug convictions so that they can be punished? The only lasting value of the act may turn out to be the promotion of EAPs. Every employer that wishes to continue receiving federal funds will be compelled to at least consider setting up an EAP, even if it is only on paper.

CONCLUSION

Drug abuse prevalence in a work force is related to many variables, including the nature of the work, the culture and traditions of the industry, the operating philosophies of management, the orientation of supervisors, and the social mores of the employee population. A direct variable is the influence of countermeasures effected by the employer. Countermeasures are effective to the extent that they are weighed against actual (not imagined) prevalence. The use of drug testing as a countermeasure should be based on an objective analysis of need. For example, it would not be effective to conduct random tests of office workers when the drug problem exists in the plant.

A business that demonstrates zero tolerance for illegal drugs in the workplace can be a model for spreading the antidrug message to the community. At only marginal cost, an employer can link the company's drug education and training programs to similar programs conducted in schools, churches, private organizations, and other community agencies.

The success that an employer will have in ridding the workplace of drug abuse depends to a large extent on employee perceptions. Enforcing an antidrug policy, testing for drugs, educating employees, and training supervisors are activities that strongly shape employee perceptions. Another activity that influences these perceptions is respect for employees' privacy expectations.

Many companies that have initiated drug-testing programs report dramatic reductions in medical costs, accident rates, and absenteeism, as well as increased productivity and morale. Successful programs integrate employee education, supervisory training, and employee assistance. The companies that have achieved good results have managed to satisfy both the needs of employees to feel safe and secure at work and the needs of management to maintain a safe, secure, and productive environment.

Appendix 1–A

Sample Certifications Regarding Drug-Free Workplace Requirements

ALTERNATE I

I. The grantee certifies that it will provide a drug-free workplace by:
   A. Publishing a statement notifying employees that the unlawful manufacture, distribution, dispensing, possession, or use of a controlled substance is prohibited in the grantee's workplace and specifying the actions that will be taken against employees for violation of such prohibition
   B. Establishing a drug-free awareness program to inform employees about the following:
      1. The dangers of drug abuse in the workplace
      2. The grantee's policy of maintaining a drug-free workplace
      3. Any available drug counseling, rehabilitation, and employee assistance program
      4. The penalties that may be imposed on employees for drug abuse violations occurring in the workplace
   C. Making it a requirement that each employee to be engaged in the performance of the grant be given a copy of the statement required by paragraph A
   D. Notifying the employee in the statement required by paragraph A that as a condition of employment under the grant, the employee will do the following:
      1. Abide by the terms of the statement
      2. Notify the employer of any criminal drug statute conviction for a violation occurring in the workplace no later than five days after such conviction
   E. Notifying the agency within ten days after receiving notice under subparagraph D2 from an employee or otherwise receiving actual notice of such conviction
   F. Taking one of the following actions within 30 days of receiving notice under subparagraph D2 with respect to any employee who is so convicted:
      1. Taking appropriate personnel action against such an employee up to and including termination
      2. Requiring such employee to participate satisfactorily in a drug-abuse assistance or rehabilitation program approved for such purposes by a federal, state, or local health, law enforcement, or other appropriate agency

    G.   Making a good-faith effort to continue to maintain a drug-free workplace through implementation of paragraphs A–F

II.   The grantee shall insert in the space provided below the site(s) for the performance of work done in connection with the specific grant.

Place of performance (street address, city, county, state, zip code)

_____

_____

ALTERNATE II

The grantee certifies that as a condition of the grant, he or she will not engage in the unlawful manufacture, distribution, dispensing, possession, or use of a controlled substance in conducting any activity with the grant.

_____

Signature

_____

Date

Chapter 2

Defining the Problem

THE DIMENSIONS OF ABUSE

This book contains a variety of descriptors for the phenomenon we generally call drug abuse. Among these are *substance abuse, chemical abuse,* and simply *use,* which in fact may not necessarily indicate abuse at all. No special meaning should be attached to the different terms, except where differentiation is specifically indicated.

Abuse Defined

Abuse cannot be precisely defined in reference to an actual phenomenon. What one person or group may deem harmful to the individual personally or to society as a whole may not be so perceived by others or by the drug user. Implicitly, the term *abuse* has come to mean badness or any use of which one does not approve, and this notion has become the most common component of all definitions. As such, the use of the term often depends as much, if not more, on political and moral judgments than on considerations of the actual pharmacological action of a drug on an individual's health and the impact of drug-using actions on social welfare.

The abuse concept carries connotations about what is bad, deviant, or excessive. It is an apt concept to use in reference to an attitudinal response to drug use that incorporates these judgments. Many authorities suggest that the term should be avoided entirely as too polemical and too inclusive to be scientifically useful in trying to understand various degrees of drug use. Some emphasize that the term *drug use* should be used instead, a change that may draw attention to the need to know more about the pharmacology of drugs. Others suggest that the terms *nonmedical use* and *illicit drug use* (that is, use that is illegal according to federal or state laws) are more descriptive of certain kinds of drug use. Also, since *abuse* is more appropriately applied to people than to drugs, the term *drug misuse* is often used as a substitute.

The lack of a standard frame of reference is one problem that stands in the way of identifying abusers and bringing them into contact with appropriate treatment modalities. Perhaps more than anything else, drug abuse evades accurate definition because of the large number of drugs that can be used, their various physiological and psychological effects, and the varying lag times between onset of initial use and the appearance of medical and behavioral problems. In the absence of well-defined guidelines, little opportunity is present for early diagnosis, and the odds for preventing dependence and attaining recovery decline significantly as time passes.

The most frequently accepted definition of *substance abuse* is the clinical definition given in the *Statistical Manual of Disorders* published by the American Psychiatric Association. A substance abuser is a person who (1) is usually intoxicated throughout the better part of the day; (2) has behavioral problems in which the person cannot moderate or stop usage, continues in spite of medical contributions, and must use the substance to remain functional in social and work situations; and (3) has used the substance for at least one month.

This definition of a substance abuser differs from the definition of a chemically dependent person. To be dependent, the individual must display either tolerance for the drug (that is, larger and larger doses are required to attain the same effect) or withdrawal symptoms when use is discontinued.

Definitionally, let us say that a substance abuser who is not diagnosed and brought into treatment in an early stage of use stands a fair chance of progressing to the chemically dependent state. Let us add the observation that the odds for rehabilitation are much lower for chemically dependent persons and that the range and severity of social and work problems that accompany chemical dependence are enormous in comparison to those that accompany substance abuse.

Abuse Factors

Despite the many untruths and myths associated with drugs, several factors have been found consistently to play a part in abuse and dependence. One important factor is the nature of the drug. Some drugs, such as cocaine, produce powerful main effects, few negative side effects during initial use, and a potential for rapid dependence. Other factors are drug availability and affordability. Crack, a derivative of cocaine, is a common commodity even in the best neighborhoods and is affordable to pre-high-schoolers. The combined factors of drug effects, availability, and affordability may help explain why the use of crack has grown so rapidly and is so difficult to deal with.

Other factors are the influences of family and personality. Children from homes where a parent or sibling was or is chemically dependent are five times more likely to become substance abusers. Persons who are markedly rebellious, have low self-esteem and low self-confidence, and display exaggerated independence tend to be associated with abuse and dependence. These factors can serve as warning signs.

Recent drug use research has turned up some interesting findings:

- Alcohol use in this country has been stable during the past decade.
- Whites are slightly more likely to be drug dependent than blacks.
- Males are more at risk than females.
- A substance abuser who is married and still working has a 60 to 80 percent chance of recovery, while an unattached abuser who has no dependable source of income has only a 20 to 30 percent chance of recovery.

What can be applied to the workplace from these findings? For one thing, employers should not be fooled by a substance-abusing employee who points to his or her elevated status as proof of immunity from dependence. For another, having a job is important in preventing abuse and in promoting a successful recovery.

DEFINING THE PROBLEM AND THE EMPLOYER'S NEEDS

What is the extent and nature of drug abuse in the workplace? What can be done to deal with it, and what resources will be needed? These preliminary questions need to be asked before going any further, and there are several possible approaches to obtaining the answers:

- Refer to the findings of studies of occupational drug abuse. National, regional, and state studies may serve as rough guidelines in defining a probable range of abuse affecting either the industry or geographical area.
- Contact the professional association for the industry. Other companies in the industry may have asked the association for guidance in solving a similar problem. Chances are that the staff has already conducted research and developed usable materials. In many instances, a professional association can provide consultations, program recommendations, implementation assistance, and follow-up evaluations.
- Talk to competitors or companies in the same general line of business. Another company whose employees have similar demographic characteristics may be able to provide relevant information based on its own experiences.
- Consult with government agencies that have addressed drug abuse issues. Of particular interest are state agencies that deal with unemployment, workmen's compensation, and labor grievances.
- Assess the character of drug abuse in the communities from which labor is drawn. Ask questions of health offices, social service agencies, drug treatment facilities, and law enforcement agencies. The answers may provide insights into the extent of drug use in the communities, the age-groups of users, the preferred drugs of abuse, and the methods of drug administration.

- Arrange for drug awareness speakers and seminars. Tap the speaking resources of local drug councils, treatment facilities, and self-help groups.
- Analyze internal company operations. Focus on indicators of substandard performance, such as absenteeism, tardiness, unexplained absences from workstations, sick leave, medical claims, workmen's compensation claims, accidents, security breaches, theft and property losses, training costs, productivity, and problems in handling troubled employees.
- Consult with representatives of key departments such as occupational health, safety, security, and human resources to get an organization-wide sense of the problem.
- Conduct a voluntary, anonymous urine drug screen. Assure the employees tested that the specimens they contribute will not be traced to them. A survey of this type has few legal ramifications and can be a strong deterrent by conveying to employees the seriousness of the problem. This approach can be especially helpful in identifying the types of drugs being abused.
- Ask the employees, either one-on-one or in small groups, about the presence of drug abuse and whether it is undermining health, safety, security, or other aspects of work.
- Conduct a survey of employees. If handled sensitively, the survey can guarantee the anonymity of respondents and provide high-quality answers at a modest cost. The survey results can provide a foundation for decisions relating to policy sanctions and penalties, managerial training, and education of the work force.

USING A DRUG ABUSE SURVEY

Appendix 2–A is a sample survey that uses a questionnaire format to gather information concerning drug abuse within the work environment. The survey seeks to determine whether drug abuse is present and, if so, to assess the approximate extent and nature of the problem and discover employee attitudes that may assist or obstruct management's efforts to attack it.

The survey process has three distinguishing features:

1. Employees complete the questionnaire on a voluntary basis only.
2. The process guarantees employee anonymity.
3. Survey results are not used for security investigation purposes.

This particular survey would be administered by an outside contractor in conjunction with the employer. After the employer reviewed the questionnaire and made suggestions to tailor the content to its needs, the employer would mail the questionnaire to employees or provide the contractor with a mailing list for that purpose. A stamped envelope addressed to the contractor would be attached to each questionnaire. The completed questionnaires would be mailed directly to the contractor, which would tabulate the results and report them to the employer.

Survey findings help management to define any possible drug problems and to develop a response strategy that addresses these problems. Survey findings can be used to define and redefine drug abuse policy; select enforcement tactics, sanctions, and penalties; and determine the appropriateness of company-paid rehabilitation.

IDENTIFYING AND EVALUATING RESOURCES

The assessment of drug abuse in a particular workplace is logically accompanied by an identification of the resources available inside and outside the company. Resources within the company might include the following:

- Expertise of key staff in the company's medical, industrial health, safety, human resources, and security departments
- Office space, equipment, and clerical support staff
- An existing EAP, which might provide the foundation for drug abuse treatment
- The company's group health insurance plan, which might provide coverage of drug abuse treatment costs or provide that option at an affordable cost

Resources to be explored outside the company include the following:

- Community health agencies, hospital drug clinics, detoxification centers, psychiatric care facilities, methadone maintenance programs, therapeutic communities, and halfway houses
- Local drug abuse councils, safety associations, and self-help groups
- Consultants who specialize in helping companies develop and implement drug abuse policies and programs

Once the available resources are identified, the employer must evaluate them in relation to its particular work force. The following questions can guide the evaluation process:

- Does management want to exercise a high degree of program control by providing in-house treatment? Keep in mind that some forms of counseling and treatment are well beyond the expertise and facilities of even the best staffed and equipped companies.
- Is management prepared to commit the financial and staff resources required? If a company is too small or too fragile economically to permit such expenditures, it should at least encourage needy employees to obtain

treatment even though the company is not in a position to assist them financially.
- Does the local community have good treatment resources? Are the resources affordable and accessible?
- Is it possible to set up a pooling arrangement in which two or more companies share the financial and staff burdens of a fully developed program? Arrangements of this type tend to work best when the consortium, though jointly funded, operates with some degree of independence.

TREATMENT MODALITIES

Drug abuse programs that include treatment are generally based on the community model or the in-house model.

The Community Model

Companies that have limited resources or operate in areas with existing quality treatment services are logically attracted to the use of community resources. The company's treatment staff is likely to consist of a single coordinator and clerical support. The coordinator typically possesses a combination of interactive and administrative skills and has a good knowledge of available treatment resources. While not necessarily a trained counselor, the coordinator is sufficiently skillful in evaluating the gross dimensions of an employee's problems so that a correct referral can be made.

Contact with a program coordinator can be made through one of four channels:

1. Identification by supervisors and managers who have been trained to observe and document unsatisfactory job performance
2. Self-identification by employees seeking assistance
3. Peer referral
4. Identification through drug testing

After consultation with an employee, the coordinator proposes a rehabilitation strategy, obtains the employee's agreement, and then makes arrangements for him or her to receive the proposed treatment through a facility located in the community. The coordinator monitors the employee's progress during and after treatment. The criterion for successful therapy might be the correction of unsatisfactory performance indicators. A return to unsatisfactory performance after treatment would indicate a relapse requiring additional therapy.

The major advantage of the community model is the minimal commitment of company staff. A disadvantage is that community resources are not usually designed for resolving drug abuse problems as they relate to work environments generally or to a company's specific characteristics.

The In-House Model

This approach is almost always reserved for companies that are willing and able to commit substantial in-house resources. Counseling services are provided by staff members, with some forms of treatment provided in the community.

The program staff typically consists of a coordinator and clerical support staff. The coordinator is a trained counselor who works with a medical director or medical complement (doctors, nurses, and technicians), which also may provide relevant services or guidance.

The major advantage of the in-house model is that it allows counseling to be tailored to the employee's unique work situation. The counselor is better positioned to monitor improvement or deterioration of the employee's job performance and to intercede where necessary to keep the employee on track with the prescribed rehabilitation strategy. The chief disadvantage of this model is cost.

The Troubled Employee Concept

A program that includes treatment services may be designed to deal specifically with drug and/or alcohol abuse. Another approach would be to include drug abuse treatment in an EAP, a program based on the troubled employee concept. There has been a general trend away from specific programs and toward more general EAPs primarily because the broader troubled employee concept implies assistance for an employee, no matter what the problem may be.

The troubled employee approach offers two distinct advantages when an employee's problems stem from drug abuse. The first is that employees are more likely to seek help when the assistance program is not identified specifically as a drug abuse program. The second advantage is that drug-abusing employees may seek help in dealing with secondary problems that result from drug abuse, such as child neglect and financial difficulties. It may become evident during counseling that the presenting problem is really a symptom of the larger problem of drug abuse.

CONCLUSION

Determining a company's needs in respect to the problem of drug abuse follows a process in which the nature of the problem is objectively assessed and the company's and community's resources are evaluated. From this assessment, the broad outlines of a policy are determined and choices are made with respect to a specific antidrug program.

Appendix 2–A

A Sample Drug Abuse Survey

Here are a few important points about this survey:

- It is strictly voluntary. Please do not complete it unless you wish to do so.
- The survey is designed and planned to be carried out with absolute anonymity. Please do not identify yourself anywhere in the survey.
- The results of the survey will be used by your employer to make planning and policy decisions. The results will not be used to conduct investigations.

Note that the survey is to be returned by mail to an outside contractor. Your answers will be tabulated by the contractor, not your employer.

The survey contains no questions that will reveal your identity. If you write something that could reveal your identity or the identity of some other person, the contractor will exclude it from any information reported to your employer.

INSTRUCTIONS

1. Do not write your name, address, or any other identifying information on this survey or the return envelope. Also, do not identify other persons, work processes, or job positions that might point to particular persons.
2. Fill out the survey only if you want to. Obviously, your employer wants to have your insights concerning an important and sensitive matter, but at the same time your employer does not want you to feel compelled to participate.
3. You do not have to answer every question. If you don't want to give a response to a particular question, pass over it.
4. Please complete the survey in privacy and avoid discussing your answers with other employees.
5. Mark your answers with dark pencil or ink.
6. Within five days after receiving this survey, please fill it out and mail it in the return envelope.

SECTION I

For the purpose of this survey, the term *legal drugs* means prescribed medicines that have been legally obtained and are being used in accordance with a physician's instructions. The term also includes nonprescription medicines that have been legally obtained and are being used for their intended purpose.

1.   Are you currently using a legal drug?

Yes [ ]   No [ ]

If No, go to Section II.

If Yes, please continue.

a.   Is the legal drug that you are using

[ ]   a prescription drug?
[ ]   a nonprescription drug?

b.   Are you using the legal drug on a

[ ]   short-term basis?
[ ]   long-term basis?

c.   Is the legal drug you are using a type that may cause drowsiness or dizziness?

Yes [ ]   No [ ]

d.   Do you operate machinery or perform duties that can cause harm to yourself or others?

Yes [ ]   No [ ]

e.   Does your supervisor know that you are using the legal drug?

Yes [ ]   No [ ]

SECTION II

For the purpose of this survey, the term *illegal* drug means any drug (1) that is not legally obtainable or (2) that is legally obtainable but has not been legally obtained. The term includes prescribed drugs not legally obtained and prescribed drugs not being used for prescribed purposes.

For example, marijuana and cocaine are illegal drugs because they are not legally obtainable; a drug prescribed for weight loss is illegal if the user takes it mainly to stay awake or takes it in excess of the prescribed dosage.

The terms *on the job* and *while at work* include lunch periods, break periods, and time spent traveling on company business.

1. Do you currently use any illegal drugs such as marijuana, cocaine, or prescription drugs that are not being used for prescribed purposes?

    Yes [ ]   No [ ]

    If No, go to Section III.

    If Yes, please continue.

2. What type of drug or drugs do you take?

    [ ]   Narcotics

    This class includes opium, morphine, codeine, heroin, hydromorphone, meperidine, pethidine, and methadone.

    The trade names include Dover's Powder, Paregoric, Parapectolin, Pectoral Syrup, Empirin Compound with Codeine, Robitussin A-C, Dilaudid, Demerol, Pethadol, Dolophine, Methadone, LAAM, Leritine, Percodan, Tussionex, Fentanyl, Darvon, Talwin, and Lomotil.

    The street names include M, morpho, tab, white, stuff, Miss Emma, monkey, schoolboy, horse, smack, H, junk, little D, lords, dollies, dolls, T and Blues, and China White.

    [ ]   Depressants

    This class includes barbiturates, methaqualone, and benzodiazepines.

    The trade names include Amobarbital, Phenobarbital, Butisol, Phenoxbarbital, Secobarbital, Tuinal, Ativan, Azene, Clonopin, Dalmane, Diazepam, Librium, Serax, Tranxene, Valium, Verstran, Equanil, Miltown, Noludar, Placidyl, and Valmid.

    The street names include yellows, yellow jackets, barbs, reds, redbirds, tooies, phennies, ludes, quays, quads, mandrex, downers, goofballs, sleeping pills, and candy.

    [ ]   Stimulants

    This class includes cocaine, amphetamines, phenmetrazine, and methamphetamine.

    The trade names include Biphetamine, Desoxyn, Dexedrine, Mediatric, and Preludin.

    The street names include bump, toot, C, coke, flake, candy, snow, pep pills, uppers, truck drivers, dexies, black beauties, speed, peaches, hearts, meth, crystal, crank, go fast, and crack.

[ ] Hallucinogens

This class includes LSD, mescaline, peyote, amphetamine variants, and phencyclidine (PCP).

Other names include lysergic acid diethylamide, PMA, STP, MDA, MMDA, TMA, DOM, DOB, DMT, DET, psylocybin, and psylocin.

The street names include acid, microdot, cubes, mesc, buttons, cactus, ecstasy, designer drugs, angel dust, hog, peace pill, sacred mushrooms, magic mushrooms, and mushrooms.

[ ] Cannabis

This class includes marijuana, tetrahydrocannabinol, hashish, and hashish oil.

Other names include Acapulco gold, Sinsemilla, Thai sticks, THC, hash, and hash oil.

The street names include pot, grass, reefer, roach, Maui wowie, joint, weed, loco weed, and Mary Jane.

[ ] Organic solvents

This class includes inhalants such as gasoline, airplane glue, hair spray, deodorants, spray paint, Liquid Paper, paint thinner, and rubber cement.

3. Do you currently take illegal drugs while on the job?

Yes [ ]   No [ ]

4. Have you ever reported to work while under the influence of an illegal drug?

Yes [ ]   No [ ]

5. Do you use illegal drugs when off the job?

Yes [ ]   No [ ]

6. How often do you take illegal drugs?

[ ] More than once a day
[ ] Once a day
[ ] Two or three times a week
[ ] Once a week
[ ] Two or three times a month
[ ] Once a month
[ ] Less than once a month

7. Where do you obtain your illegal drugs?

    [ ] Off the job
    [ ] On the job

    a. If you obtain your illegal drugs on the job, do you get them from

        [ ] a fellow employee?
        [ ] someone connected to the company but not an employee?
        [ ] someone not connected to the company?

    b. If you obtain your illegal drugs on the job, do you

        [ ] buy them?
        [ ] trade for them?
        [ ] get them as a gift?
        [ ] get them as a loan?
        [ ] steal them?
        [ ] Other _____

SECTION III

1. Have you used illegal drugs at any time in the past while employed by your present employer?

    Yes [ ]   No [ ]

    a. *If Yes,* did you use the drugs

        [ ] while on the job?
        [ ] while off the job?
        [ ] just before going on the job?

    b. Where did you obtain the drugs?

        [ ] On the job
        [ ] Off the job

    c. If you obtained the drugs while on the job, did you get them from

        [ ] a fellow employee?
        [ ] someone connected to the company but not a fellow employee?
        [ ] someone not connected with the company?

2. While employed by your present employer, have you received medical treatment related to drug abuse?

    Yes [ ]   No [ ]

a. *If Yes,* did your present employer pay all or part of the medical treatment costs?

Yes [ ]   No [ ]

3. Have you ever been taken into custody by the police or arrested for a drug violation?

Yes [ ]   No [ ]

a. *If Yes,* how many times?

[ ] Once
[ ] Two or three times
[ ] More than two or three times

b. What was the drug violation related to?

[ ] Use
[ ] Possession
[ ] Purchase
[ ] Sale
[ ] Swap or trade
[ ] Distribution
[ ] Growing or making
[ ] Other _____

c. Did any drug violation occur while you were employed by your present employer?

Yes [ ]   No [ ]

SECTION IV

1. Has anyone at your present place of employment ever offered to provide you with illegal drugs?

Yes [ ]   No [ ]

2. Have you ever observed anyone at your present place of employment selling, trading, loaning, or in some way transferring illegal drugs to another person?

Yes [ ]   No [ ]

a. *If Yes*, about how many different employees are involved in the selling, loaning, or transferring of illegal drugs?

[ ] One
[ ] Two or three
[ ] More than two or three
[ ] Ten or more

3. Has anyone at your present place of employment offered to put you in contact with someone who can provide you with illegal drugs?

Yes [ ]   No [ ]

4. Have you ever observed a fellow employee using illegal drugs while at work?

Yes [ ]   No [ ]

a. *If Yes*, about how many times?

[ ] Once
[ ] Two or three times
[ ] More than two or three times
[ ] Ten or more

b. What were the methods of abuse?

[ ] Smoking
[ ] Taking pills, tablets, capsules, etc.
[ ] Injecting
[ ] Snorting
[ ] Inhaling

c. About how many persons have you observed using illegal drugs at your present place of employment?

[ ] One
[ ] Two or three
[ ] More than two or three
[ ] Ten or more

5. Do you believe that any of your fellow employees are currently using drugs on the job or reporting to work while under the influence of drugs?

Yes [ ]   No [ ]

a. *If Yes*, what is your belief based on?

[ ] Erratic behavior by the employees involved
[ ] Overheard the involved employees talk about it

[ ] Remarks made directly to me by the employees involved
[ ] Unexplained absences from the job, followed by a change in behavior
[ ] Other _____

6. Do you believe that some on-the-job accidents at your present place of employment have been caused by drug abuse?

Yes [ ]   No [ ]

a. *If Yes*, what is your belief based on?

[ ] I observed that an involved employee was acting erratically just before or at the time the accident occurred.
[ ] An involved employee made specific remarks to me.
[ ] I overheard an involved employee talking about it.
[ ] Other _____

SECTION V

1. An employee who is caught using illegal drugs on the job should be

[ ] reprimanded.
[ ] given a second chance.
[ ] discharged.
[ ] discharged and reported to the police.

2. An employee who takes an illegal drug off the job and reports to work while the drug is still in his or her system should

[ ] not be subject to action by the company.
[ ] be reprimanded.
[ ] be given a second chance.
[ ] be discharged.

3. An employee who is caught selling illegal drugs on the job should be

[ ] reprimanded.
[ ] given a second chance.
[ ] discharged.
[ ] discharged and reported to the police.

4. An employee who buys, possesses, loans, or trades illegal drugs on the job should be

[ ] reprimanded.
[ ] given a second chance.
[ ] discharged.
[ ] discharged and reported to the police.

5. With regard to controlling the use of illegal drugs by employees, it is my opinion that the company should

    [ ]   do nothing more than it is currently doing.
    [ ]   do a little more to control the problem.
    [ ]   do a lot more.

6. In my opinion, the company's supervisors are

    [ ]   very knowledgeable about the use of illegal drugs by employees and are very attentive in looking for it.
    [ ]   somewhat knowledgeable about the problem and generally alert to it.
    [ ]   not very knowledgeable and not very attentive in looking for it.

7. In my opinion, the company's effort to educate employees about the dangers of using illegal drugs has

    [ ]   been very effective.
    [ ]   been somewhat effective.
    [ ]   not been effective.
    [ ]   been almost nonexistent.

8. In my opinion, the company's overall effort to deal with the use of illegal drugs by employees has

    [ ]   been very effective.
    [ ]   been somewhat effective.
    [ ]   not been effective.
    [ ]   been almost nonexistent.

9. Of the following methods for dealing with the use of illegal drugs by employees, I would like to see the company use

    [ ]   undercover operatives from an outside investigative agency.
    [ ]   informants recruited from the company's work force.
    [ ]   searches of the workplace and of employees and their belongings, including personal vehicles on the company's premises.
    [ ]   periodic urine testing of employees.

10. If the company decided to conduct urine tests of current employees, I would

    [ ]   be against the idea.
    [ ]   not like it but would cooperate.
    [ ]   gladly cooperate.

11. If the company decided to conduct urine tests of job applicants, I would

    [ ]   be against the idea.
    [ ]   not care one way or the other.
    [ ]   like the idea.

12. My attitude about giving a urine specimen for drug testing is that the procedure

       (Choose one)
[ ] is personally degrading.
[ ] is routine and not much different from any other health test.

       (Choose one)
[ ] is a violation of my privacy.
[ ] is not a violation of my privacy.

       (Choose one)
[ ] should not be used by the company.
[ ] should be used by the company.

Chapter 3

Developing a Drug-Testing Policy

OBTAINING INPUT

Soliciting input from a lawyer, a drug abuse consultant, managers in operating groups, union representatives, and senior staff from personnel, safety,
security, and occupational health is an important part of developing a policy.
Input from legal counsel may be disappointing because few lawyers have
extensive practical experience in drug testing and there is no foundation of
case law in this area. The best resource for policy development could turn
out to be an experienced drug abuse program consultant.

Legal Input

Some fairly general legal issues have been raised with respect to drug testing,
and these deserve consideration before the policy writer gets down to the
serious task of putting pen to paper. Express prohibitions against drug testing
do not appear in the Constitution or in federal or state law. The right to
privacy has not been clearly established in this area. Privacy can be an issue,
however, primarily in relation to confidentiality. For example, an employer
who discloses an employee's drug test results to a third party without permission may be open to a charge of invasion of privacy. Application of the
Fourth Amendment to drug testing can be used only by federal employees
because the Fourth Amendment is directed against unreasonable searches
by the government, not by private employers.

An employer has both a right and an obligation to maintain a safe and
sound workplace. The employer's right is to ensure that employees perform
their jobs competently; the employer's obligation is to ensure that employees
do not injure themselves or others. An employer is on firm legal ground in
exercising both the right and the obligation. The potential for liability occurs
in the methods used to control the working environment. Generally, the
employer's goal of orderliness in the workplace is not subject to litigation,
but the tactics for achieving that goal are.

The following guidelines may help avoid legal entanglements:

- A positive test result is not evidence of a crime. It is not illegal to have a drug in the body system. Make a distinction between employees who test positive and those who are caught using, possessing, distributing, or selling illicit drugs.
- Treat drug test results as confidential information. Collect and keep only essential information and keep confidential information under lock and key.
- Do not force employees to consent to a drug test, but do inform them that employees who refuse may be subject to disciplinary action, including discharge. Spell this out in the policy.
- If employees are selected for testing on a random basis, care must be taken to avoid the appearance of discrimination. A selection technique that appears to focus on race, sex, or lifestyle can lead to employee grievances.
- If certain positions are selected for testing, document a relationship between the performance of the jobs and the effects of drug abuse.
- If the work force is unionized, develop the policy with union input and modify the union contract as needed.
- Use a qualified laboratory to process tests and make sure that test methods are state-of-the-art. For example, select an enzyme or radioimmunoassay method for preliminary screening and confirm positives by the GC/MS method.
- Obtain each tested employee's consent at the point of collection. Do not rely on a timeless consent obtained from the employee when the policy was first announced.
- Take safeguards in the collection of specimens to prevent contamination, switching, and mislabeling. Initiate chain-of-custody documentation at the time of collection.
- Avoid any appearance that the drug-testing program is being used for anything other than its intended purpose. When specimens are collected and/or tested by in-house resources, the door is open to claims that management is falsifying test results in order to discharge certain employees, such as members of the union or minority groups. Using an outside vendor to collect and analyze specimens will prevent this from becoming an issue.
- Refer all positive test results to a physician or trained professional for the purpose of ruling out any alternative explanations for the positive results.
- Notify employees who test positive and allow them to confer with a supervisor or manager. Recognize that a positive test result does not automatically mean illicit drug use. For example, an employee may have failed to declare the use of prescribed medication just prior to the test. Giving the employee an opportunity to explain, followed by a reevaluation of the test results, might reverse the finding.
- Set up an appeal process for employees.
- Enforce the policy consistently and uniformly. Be fair when administering discipline.

Union Input

Collective bargaining will be a major issue in policy development. An employer who is party to a collective bargaining agreement is required under the National Labor Relations Act to bargain in good faith with a labor union on issues involving conditions of employment. A debatable matter between management and the union could be whether or not drug testing constitutes a condition of employment. Arguments can be made either way, but the greatest determinants are likely to be the language of the collective bargaining agreement and existing practices. If drug testing is an extension of an established working condition, such as evaluations to determine fitness for duty, there may be no requirement to bargain. If this is not the case, the move to institute drug testing might represent a substantial change in working conditions and would require negotiation with the union.

When bargaining is required, an employer can expect to negotiate on the positions that would be affected by drug testing, the drugs to be tested for, the testing methodologies, selection of the testing laboratory, chain-of-custody procedures, safeguards against false positives, the circumstances under which drug testing can be conducted, privacy in the collection process, the discipline to be meted out for violations, the methods for reviewing and appealing positive tests, employee assistance benefits, rehabilitation, and grievance and arbitration procedures.

In general, unions oppose drug testing and support EAPs and broad rehabilitation rights for drug-affected employees. They particularly dislike random testing but, with qualifications, show some acceptance of preemployment testing, postaccident testing, reasonable cause testing, and testing related to rehabilitation. Unions want limitations on an employer's right to fire an employee for a drug violation or to exclude an employee from drug rehabilitation assistance. Most unions and employee organizations want regulations or bargaining agreements that require an employer to establish comprehensive, nonpunitive EAPs that cover drug abuse and other problems confronting employees.

Other Input

A great deal of valuable information can be obtained from people in other departments of the organization. The health or medical department can provide guidance concerning the technical aspects of drug testing; the human resources department can clarify the disciplinary and employee assistance aspects; the safety department can help identify the safety-sensitive job positions that might be specifically targeted for drug testing; and the security department can help define the organization's responsibilities for cooperation with law enforcement agencies and the disposal of confiscated drugs and drug paraphernalia.

A useful by-product of the interplay with and among these various representatives can be a collective proprietary desire to create a quality policy, in terms of both the document itself and the implementation of its provisions. In the give-and-take of discussion, the policy writer has the chance to obtain from the participants some commitments to accept responsibilities and carry out functions that could be critical to policy execution. The policy writer should cultivate cooperative relationships with key persons in the organization for the immediate purpose of obtaining conceptual input and for the long-term purpose of ensuring support for the drug-testing program.

One other good source of ideas about policy development are companies that have already gone through the process. Much can be learned from someone who has been down the same road. Appendix 3–A contains a number of sample policies adapted from those developed by major corporations in a variety of industries. They present ideas that may be useful in choosing a format or general structure and in deciding an appropriate level of detail.

DRAFTING THE POLICY

A policy can range from very general to very specific. Many of the better policies lie somewhere in between. The degree of detail is a function of the need to cover all the bases and the preferences of management. Apart from length and style, it is important to express the policy in terms that employees can readily understand. Legalese and bureaucratic mumbo jumbo are the natural enemies of a workable policy.

Resist the temptation to adopt some other company's policy in toto. There is no such thing as a generic drug abuse policy. Do not hesitate to use another policy as a model, but make sure it is restructured to incorporate your organization's unique characteristics and conditions.

The policy-writing process can be facilitated by starting with a checklist of the elements or issues that will be addressed in the policy. Appendix 3–B is a sample checklist to help you get started.

FINAL POLICY CONTENT

At this point, the employer should have obtained some understanding of the dimensions of the drug use problem in the workplace, input from key departments and persons, and a rough draft of the policy. The content of the final document will include the elements described in the following sections.

Management's Philosophy

The policy needs to spell out why drug abuse is unacceptable and why testing is necessary. There should be some explanation of the "reasonable business necessity" that serves as the foundation of the policy. A drug-testing policy should not be implemented just because other employers are doing so. Rather, it should explain why this particular organization needs such a policy.

The usual reasons are related to job safety, public safety, loss prevention, productivity, and protection of reputation. One reason will probably stand out above the others. Focus on it and emphasize how it is adversely affected by drug use.

The philosophy or rationale of a policy is usually the first section of the policy document. It sets the tone and intent of following sections.

Prohibited Activities

The policy should describe the forbidden behaviors. Sometimes a policy will mention the undesirable consequences of drug abuse in the workplace but not specifically prohibit the activities that lead to the undesirable consequences. The prohibited activities would include using and possessing drugs at work.

The activities most often prohibited in a drug policy include the use or the possession, sale, or transfer of illicit drugs, as well as being on the job with a detectable amount of an illicit drug in the body system. The detectable amount violation can be described as a form of possession—that is, an individual possesses the drug when a scientific test reveals its presence in his or her system.

It could be a mistake to name the drugs that are prohibited or subject to testing. When the policy is written, eight major drug classes might be commonly abused, but that number may increase in the next year or two. The drug abuse patterns of employees and applicants also might change relative to the drugs that are included in the employer's drug-testing program. When a program consistently tests for some but not all of the major drug classes, the users subject to testing have an incentive for switching to drugs that are not included in the testing scheme. The federal program, for example, tests only for five drug classes. Barbiturates and benzodiazepines, which are commonly abused substances, are not included in this program, even though these drugs have strong impairing and addictive effects.

Prohibited drugs should be described according to their sources, uses, or effects rather than their chemical properties, and it might be helpful to provide examples, for instance:

> The term illegal drug as used in this policy means any drug that is not legally obtainable; any drug that is legally obtainable but has not been legally obtained; any prescribed drug not legally obtained; any prescribed drug not being used for the prescribed purpose; any over-the-counter drug being used at a dosage level different than recommended by the manufacturer or being used for a purpose other than intended by the manufacturer; and any drug being used for a purpose not in accordance with bona fide medical therapy. Examples of illegal drugs are Cannabis substances, such as marijuana and

hashish, cocaine, heroin, phencyclidine (PCP), and so-called designer drugs and look-alike drugs.

A policy also might mention other prohibited activities that are not necessarily related to drugs. For example, there may be provisions that prohibit the possession of contraband. The issue of contraband often arises when the policy provides for the seizure of unauthorized items while conducting searches for drugs on the premises. The unauthorized items, such as lethal weapons, explosives, and stolen property, will in most cases not relate to drug use, but the possession of them in the workplace could be cited in the drug policy as a violation. Mention of contraband is done for the sake of administrative convenience and can be avoided by identifying contraband violations in other policies or procedures.

Affected Employees

In some companies, drug testing applies to all employees, but in others it applies only to certain positions or groups of employees. If the rationale for drug testing is job safety, only those persons who hold hazardous jobs should be tested. An employer invites legal challenge when a policy is founded on certain reasons and tests are conducted for unrelated reasons.

Enforcement Actions

The actions that the company will take to detect violations of the policy should be described. For example, enforcement actions might be intervention by supervisors in reasonable cause situations; preemployment, random, and postaccident testing; inspections at entry points; unannounced general searches; security audits; and law enforcement investigations.

Penalties for Violations

The policy should state the action that will or may be taken by the company when offenses are detected. It should discuss the consequences of a positive drug test and an employee's opportunities to explain why a test showed positive. Also mention any appeal or grievance procedures that may apply. When the policy is implemented, it is important that similar punishments be routinely administered for similar violations.

Appeal Process

One of the best protections an employer has against charges of unfairness in the administration of the drug policy is to include an appeal provision. The provision can be as simple as saying that every employee will have an opportunity to confer privately with the person charged with taking disciplinary action before any disciplinary action is taken in connection with a violation of this policy. The appeal process can include more elaborate safe-guards, such as the opportunity to appear before a grievance committee or an administrative hearing officer, to be represented by legal counsel, or to present evidence, question witnesses, and challenge the employer's case.

One type of appeal might be the employee's right to have his or her original urine specimen retested for the purpose of challenging a positive test finding. This right should be conditional on requirements that the request be made in writing within a certain number of days following notice of the positive test to the employee; that the employee pay in advance the cost for reanalysis, subject to reimbursement if the retest is negative; and that the original specimen be retested at the same laboratory or transferred to another competent laboratory of the employee's choice in a manner that ensures the integrity of the specimen. A competent laboratory will routinely maintain positive specimens in controlled and refrigerated storage for at least one year.

Voluntary Alternatives

A company may offer treatment and rehabilitation benefits to employees seeking to resolve personal drug abuse problems. The investment already made in developing a productive employee may be reason enough for a company to provide assistance in lieu of automatic termination. If a com-pany's economic situation does not allow the provision of such benefits, the policy might provide for continued employment or return to employment for employees who undergo successful therapy at personal or public expense.

Even when an employer chooses not to provide financial assistance for treatment of drug problems, there is good reason to recognize the concept that drug problems are treatable and to encourage early referral to diagnosis and treatment. It does not hurt an employer to express concern for workers and their families who are adversely affected by drug use.

If the company has an EAP, it can be used for referring drug abusers to diagnosis and treatment. If an EAP does not exist, very serious consideration should be given to creating one. An EAP can be internal or external—that is, it can be conducted within the organization's resources or through an outside contractor.

The services of an EAP can be modest, such as simply referring em-ployees to nonreimbursed treatment, or generous, such as providing inpa-tient detoxification or long-term therapy at the employer's expense. A practical provision of the policy would be not to penalize an employee who seeks drug abuse assistance through the EAP but at the same time to make clear that the EAP will not protect an employee from disciplinary action for a policy infraction or substandard work performance.

The policy writer should outline the procedures for referring employees to drug treatment. Referrals can be self-initiated or made by supervisors, peers, or union representatives. The policy also must spell out the provisions for return to work of employees who have been suspended pending completion of treatment.

Confidentiality

The policy should reflect a concern for the privacy of employees and stress the special responsibilities assigned to supervisors and drug abuse program coordinators for the protection of information relating to drug test results, referrals to the EAP, diagnosis, and treatment.

Definitions

An employer can anticipate close scrutiny of a drug-testing policy. Where interpretations are possible, attempts will be made to sustain self-serving and narrow points of view that may have little relevance to what is intended. Small ambiguities in important language can create large loopholes. What may seem to the policy's author straightforward, nonarguable language will not necessarily come across that way to employees. Terms such as *detectable amount* and *reasonable cause* require explicit definition because they can be interpreted in different ways.

A definitions section will help eliminate the problem of conflicting interpretations. It also will facilitate understanding. For example, it may be necessary to let the reader know repeatedly that the policy is applicable "in the plant facility, surrounding areas on owned or leased property, parking lots, storage areas, and owned or leased vehicles wherever located." This cumbersome description can be replaced with a shorter term—for example, "company premises"—that is defined on its first appearance or in a separate definitions section.

Sometimes different terms are used to describe the same concept. The terms *illegal drugs, illicit drugs,* and *controlled substances* tend to be used interchangeably and thereby imprecisely. A single term should be selected for each concept, the concept should be clearly defined, and the term should be used in the policy without variation.

PROBLEMATIC ISSUES

Privacy

Test results that reveal medical use of a legal drug are subject to the employee's personal privacy interest. The same would apply to drug use information provided by the employee to permit informed interpretation of test results. Test results that indicate nonmedical use of a controlled substance are not subject to any recognized privacy interest, but the employer should still handle such results confidentially. Much can be gained by showing a sensitivity for employee privacy and by reducing any anxiety about the testing process.

In at least two circumstances, however, an employer will want to be able to divulge test results: pursuant to an official inquiry or discovery request and to defend in legal proceedings. The release of drug test results for the purpose of determining a former employee's suitability for employment elsewhere could be a third circumstance, but the former employer would require a written consent before releasing the information.

In all other cases, a specific, written release signed by the employee is always necessary before permitting the release of drug test results or information about an employee's rehabilitation program.

Rehabilitation

Three options for rehabilitation are the most appealing. The sympathetic approach for handling an employee who needs assistance to overcome a drug problem offers the employee the option of entering a rehabilitation program in lieu of discharge. The opportunity for rehabilitation can be enhanced or conditioned. Enhanced options, for example, would be to allow the employee to remain on the job while enrolled in rehabilitation and to reinstate the employee in the same or a similar job following rehabilitation.

The conditional option requires the employee to qualify for rehabilitation. The qualifications might include voluntary self-referral and not having been identified as a drug user through a drug test or other means. Eligibility to remain in employer-supported rehabilitation might require that the employee abstain from drug use completely and undergo frequent unannounced drug tests.

An employer may take an unsympathetic approach: not to provide rehabilitation under any circumstances. After all, drug abuse is a self-induced illness and the principal beneficiary of rehabilitation assistance is a violator of work rules. While some benefit of rehabilitation may accrue to the employer, a multitude of financial, managerial, and labor relations problems are associated with the implementation of a rehabilitation program. Included among these is the questionable practice of returning formerly dependent drug users to potentially hazardous positions and requiring drug-free employees to work alongside employees who have demonstrated a disregard for workplace rules and state or federal laws.

Whether, and under what circumstances, to offer rehabilitation are hotly debated issues. Many employers understand and sympathize with the arguments raised in support of broad rehabilitation opportunities, but most cannot afford to carry them out.

Economic considerations aside, what is the employer's first duty in the overall scheme of things? Is it to provide assistance to employees in need of help, or is it to provide a safe and productive workplace for everyone?

Should the employer, for instance, provide rehabilitation to an employee who fails to discontinue drug use and waits to be detected through drug testing, or should the employee be discharged without benefit of rehabilitation, thereby sending a strong signal that drug use will not be tolerated?

Off-Duty Use

An employer's evaluation of drug abuse in the organization may present compelling reasons for prohibiting off-duty use of drugs. Recent studies indicate that many of the commonly abused drugs can cause lingering impairment. In addition, dependent users are likely to use drugs at work as well and to be distracted by anxiety about the next fix. A policy provision against off-duty drug use is an employer's way of stating that the risk of on-duty impairment resulting from off-duty use is not acceptable and that the only responsible recourse is to make it a punishable violation.

CONCLUSION

In this chapter, a framework has been presented for crafting a drug-testing policy. The framework can be adapted to integrate rules pertaining to alcohol abuse and to link medical treatment of abuse to a company's EAP.

Appendix 3–A

Sample Drug-Testing Policies

DRUG-TESTING POLICY
FOR A CHEMICAL PRODUCTS MANUFACTURER

I. Policy Statement

It is the policy of the Company to maintain a safe work environment conducive to effective business operations. The Company requires that personnel, equipment, and operating practices be consistent with the highest standards of health and safety.

The presence of drugs and alcohol in the workplace and the influence of these substances on employees during working hours, while often violative of law, is also inconsistent with effective business operations and is grounds for disciplinary action.

While the Company has no intention of intruding into the personal lives of its employees, the Company recognizes that alcohol and drug abuse, as well as other problems in living, can be successfully treated and provides a program designed to assist affected employees and their dependents. The Company's policy is to make help available and to support employees in solving these problems, providing job performance remains satisfactory.

A corporate-wide Substance Abuse Screening Program will be adopted and maintained for the screening of all prospective employees and current employees in sensitive positions at all domestic facilities and, where feasible, abroad.

II. Screening Programs

Pursuant to and consistent with Corporate Policy, substance abuse screening programs will be adopted and maintained at all domestic facilities and, where feasible, abroad. The programs shall be applicable to all prospective employees offered a position and to current employees in sensitive positions, as defined hereafter. All substance abuse screening programs will meet with the following conditions:

- Location/plant management must adopt the Substance Abuse Screening Program as set forth herein.
- Prior to adoption of the Substance Abuse Screening Program, a comprehensive Preemployment Physical Examination Program approved by the Sector Medical Director and consistent with corporate guidelines must be operational at all locations.
- Prior to implementation of the Substance Abuse Screening Program, an Employee Assistance Program (EAP) must be available through each location for current employees and, for prospective employees, by referral to a community or private program.

III. Preemployment Screening

A. Prior Notice

All applicants shall be informed in writing of the Company's substance abuse policy and drug screening procedure. This information will include the following:

- A request to sign the informed consent form for substance abuse testing, which includes notice that a confirmed positive result will be reported to Employee Relations and may result in rejection of employment
- Notice that failure to consent to the test will result in the remainder of the preemployment examination not being completed

B. Screening Tests

Screening tests will be performed on urine specimens, except for blood alcohol determination. The location must establish procedures to ensure that specimens are obtained from the prospective employee (e.g., examine for color, specific gravity, and temperature).

Specimens should be labeled to ensure correct identification, and an appropriate chain of custody of all collected specimens must be implemented. Only laboratories and protocols approved by Corporate Medical Services shall be used. Such protocols will detect levels high enough to minimize false positives. The corporation has contracts with approved laboratories to maximize accuracy and minimize cost.

C. Positive Test Confirmation

All positive test results will be confirmed by a different test with greater specificity than the initial laboratory procedure. For example, an initial test by EMIT, an enzyme immunoassay (EIA), can be confirmed by gas chromatography/mass spectroscopy (GC/MS). Thin-layer chromatography (TLC) is not an acceptable screening test. The laboratory will confirm a positive test result on either the initial sample or on a second sample. The first option is preferred. If the latter option is chosen, the second sample must be obtained within five days of notification to the applicant if originally positive for marijuana or within one day of notification if positive for any other substance.

D. Failure to Provide a Specimen

Prospective employees who cannot or refuse to provide a urine sample on the day of their preemployment physical examination will be reported to Employee Relations as having an incomplete physical examination.

E. Inquiries Regarding Test Results and Employment

Any inquiries regarding employment decisions will be referred to Employee Relations. Inquiries by applicants regarding preemployment physical examination results will be referred to the Medical Department.

F. Case-by-Case Determination

A prospective employee with a confirmed positive test shall not, for that reason alone, be rejected for employment. In light of the corporate obligations under various federal and state laws protecting the handicapped, the Medical Department staff and Human Resources will determine whether an applicant with a confirmed positive test is nevertheless qualified to perform the job in question. The Medical Department staff and Human Resources personnel will treat the specific test results as confidential. The law does not require the employment of those whose current alcohol or drug use constitutes a threat to the property or safety of others. Given the nature of our products and operations, employment of an individual who tests positive would usually pose an unacceptable safety risk to fellow employees and product integrity.

G. Substance Abuse Rehabilitation

A prospective employee who is found to have a confirmed positive test will be given the opportunity to voluntarily accept a referral to a Substance Abuse Rehabilitation Program. Any consultation, treatment, or other costs will be the sole responsibility of the applicant. Following successful rehabilitation and if a position is available, the applicant may be reconsidered for employment after undergoing a required drug screen at the time of reapplication and upon agreement to future random testing.

IV. Employee Screening

A. Prior Notice

Employees will be advised of the adoption of the Substance Abuse Screening Program. The program will be implemented by plant or location management in consultation with Human Resources, Medical Department personnel, Security, and the Law Department. In unionized situations, upon agreement with the union so as to ensure compliance with the labor agreement and any duty to bargain, the program will be applied to current employees.

B. Content of Notice

Employee notification will include reference to Corporate Policy and briefly describe the procedures to be followed. Employees should be advised that disciplinary action, including discharge, may be taken as a result of confirmed substance abuse on the job; working while under the influence of drugs or alcohol; sale, use, or possession of illegal substances on company premises; or declining to submit to a substance abuse test.

C. Informed Consent

All employees to be tested will be required to sign the approved informed consent form for substance abuse testing. The range of disciplinary actions that may be taken for failure to submit to the test should be based on both the refusal to take the test and the circumstances indicating the need for such testing.

D. Screening of Employees Under the Influence

Screening of current employees, without corporate approval, may be appropriate under circumstances where there is reason to believe that the employee is under the influence of alcohol or drugs and cannot safely perform his or her duties, for example:

- When an employee appears intoxicated, confused, or uncoordinated, or when he or she exhibits marked personality changes or obviously irrational behavior
- Following accidents or serious incidents where there is reason to believe the employee was similarly under the influence of alcohol or drugs

E.   Screening for Sensitive Job Classifications

Employees in sensitive positions will be subject to periodic or random screening. Such classifications would include positions where substance abuse is particularly dangerous to the life, safety, or health of the employee, coworkers, or the public. This would generally include Company pilots; those who work with highly toxic materials, explosives, or other ultrahazardous materials; armed guards; and Department of Transportation certified truck drivers. To ensure consistency and compliance with local laws, locations with employees in sensitive job classifications should obtain prior approval through their sector from the Corporate Task Force, which includes representatives from Human Resources and the Medical and Law departments.

F.   Recall

Employees who are being recalled from layoff or approved leaves of absence for reasons other than substance abuse will not be required to undergo screening at the time of their return to work.

G.   Help Yourself Program

Employees whose tests are positive under the Substance Abuse Screening Program or who have a medical problem will be referred to the Help Yourself EAP to aid the employee with respect to his or her medical problem. At the same time, it should be recognized that disciplinary measures such as suspension or discharge may be necessary to protect the health and safety of the employee, coworkers, or the local community.

H.   Reporting Results

Results of urine drug tests (or blood alcohol determinations) will be reported by the Medical Department staff to the appropriate Employee Relations office. The confidentiality of the information will be respected.

V.   Administrative Guidelines

A.   Employment Applications

All employment applications should include the following advice: "The preemployment physical examination includes a screening for drug abuse."

B.   Employment Offers

Employment offers should expand the reference to the preemployment physical to advise of the substance abuse screening—for example, "This offer is subject to your passing a preemployment physical examination, which includes a substance abuse screening test."

C. When Applicants Test Positive

A positive test will be reported by the Medical Department staff to Employee Relations. Employee Relations, in consultation with the Medical Department staff, will determine employability. An applicant who tests positive is not, for that reason alone, to be rejected. But given the critical nature of so many of our products and the hazardous characteristics of so many of our raw materials, it would be unusual for us to employ someone who tested positive. An applicant who has tested positive is free to reapply for a position if and when one becomes available and following successful rehabilitation. Applicants who are rejected because of a positive test should be so advised by Employee Relations: "You have failed the substance abuse screening portion of the physical, and, as a result, the offer of employment has been withdrawn. Please call the plant Medical Department if you have any questions. The doctor or nurse will also be able to recommend an assistance program [not Company paid] in which you might enroll."

D. Designating Sensitive Positions

Under the Substance Abuse Screening Program, employees in sensitive positions will be subject to screening. Such classifications include positions where substance abuse is particularly dangerous to the life, safety, or health of the employee, co-workers, or the public. This would generally include Company pilots; those who work with highly toxic materials, explosives, or other ultrahazardous materials; armed guards; and Department of Transportation certified truck drivers.

E. Use, Sale, or Possession

The use, sale, or possession of illegal drugs or the unauthorized use of alcoholic beverages on Company premises continues to constitute grounds for dismissal or such other lesser discipline as the Company determines. But violators may be referred to the EAP based on the facts and circumstances of each individual situation.

F. Prior Notice of Employee Tests

An employee should receive prior notice within three to four weeks of his or her substance abuse screening test. This should encourage early access to the location's EAP and minimize any adverse impact on employee relations.

G. Refusal to Submit to Screening

Employee Relations will be notified whenever a prospective employee refuses to consent to screening. Such individuals will be advised that the job offer has been withdrawn in light of their refusal to complete the preemployment process. A current employee who refuses the substance abuse screening test will ordinarily be terminated. Termination will generally be the response when a current employee refuses a test, since the employee would usually be in a sensitive position involving ultrahazardous activities. The screening test also might have been requested because the employee's behavior indicated that he or she was under the influence of drugs or alcohol. In the latter circumstance, discharge or, at Company discretion, some lesser discipline would be appropriate because of the conduct in question and only incidentally for refusal to take the screening test.

H. When Current Employees Test Positive

Employee Relations will coordinate the response to a positive test. Bear in mind that we reserve the right to discharge or otherwise discipline employees who test positive. But usually we will try to assist the employee through a rehabilitation program, using the EAP. An employee may be allowed to return from a leave of absence in conjunction with the EAP or, when considered appropriate by the Company, to remain on the job. However, any return to work or continuation on the job will be subject to reports from the EAP to Employee Relations of satisfactory participation in a rehabilitation program, consent to periodic testing thereafter, and passing of such tests. Employees who test positive a second time will ordinarily be terminated.

I. Collective Bargaining Obligations

Drug screening for employees represented by a union is ordinarily a mandatory subject for bargaining. As a result, current employees covered by labor agreements will normally be tested only after successful negotiations with their union. Some unions, such as the Teamsters, have indicated a willingness to agree to drug-screening programs.

J. Contract Employees

Locations using contract employees on a regular basis for other than casual employment should implement programs whereby contractors will adopt and maintain screening programs for their prospective employees comparable to the Company's program.

DRUG-TESTING POLICY FOR A TRUCKING COMPANY

This trucking company was subject to the drug-testing rules of the Federal Highway Administration, U.S. Department of Transportation.

I. Purpose

A. A major purpose of this policy is to reduce highway accidents, fatalities, injuries, and property damage that result from driver use of controlled substances and alcohol.
B. This policy is also intended to promote a safe, healthful, and efficient working environment for all employees. Being under the influence of a controlled substance or alcohol on the job poses serious safety and health risks to the user and to all those who work with the user. The use, sale, purchase, transfer, or possession of an illegal drug in the workplace and the use, possession, or being under the influence of alcohol also pose unacceptable risks for safe, healthful, and efficient operations.
C. The Company recognizes its contractual obligations to its clients for the provision of services that are free of the influence of controlled substances and alcohol and will endeavor through this policy to provide such drug-free services.
D. Furthermore, the Company takes note of requirements to comply with Federal Highway Administration (FHWA) and Department of Transportation (DOT) regulations relating to controlled substance use and will endeavor through this policy to maintain compliance.

II. Definitions

alcohol   Any beverage that contains ethyl alcohol (ethanol), including but not limited to beer, wine, and distilled spirits.
biological testing   The scientific analysis of urine, blood, breath, saliva, hair, tissue, and other specimens of the human body for the purpose of detecting a drug or alcohol.
chemical testing   See *biological testing.*
collection site   A place where individuals present themselves for the purpose of providing body fluid or tissue samples to be analyzed for specified controlled substances. A collection site will have all necessary personnel, materials, equipment, facilities, and supervision to provide for the collection, security, temporary storage, and transportation or shipment of the samples to a laboratory.
commercial motor vehicle   Any self-propelled or towed vehicle used on public highways in interstate commerce to transport passengers or property when the vehicle (1) has a gross vehicle weight rating or gross combination weight rating of 26,001 or more pounds; (2) is designed to transport more than 15 passengers, including the driver; or (3) is used in the transportation of hazardous materials in a quantity requiring placarding under regulations issued by DOT under the Hazardous Materials Transportation Act (49 USC App 1801–1813).
Company facilities   See *Company premises.*
Company premises   All property of the Company, including but not limited to buildings and surrounding areas on Company-owned or leased property, parking lots, and storage areas. The term also includes Company-owned or leased vehicles

and equipment wherever located. It also includes premises where the Company performs contract services.

contraband   Any article, the possession of which on Company premises or while on Company business, causes an employee to be in violation of a Company work rule. Contraband includes illegal drugs, alcoholic beverages, and drug paraphernalia.

controlled substances   Defined by 21 USC 802; includes all substances listed in Schedules I through V as they may be revised from time to time.

driver subject to DOT testing   An employee driver or contract driver under contract for 90 days or more in any period of 365 days. A driver subject to DOT testing is a person who operates a commercial motor vehicle in interstate commerce and is subject to the driver qualification requirements of DOT.

drug   Any substance (other than alcohol) that is a controlled substance as defined in this policy.

drug testing   See *biological testing.*

employee   An employee, contractor, subcontractor, agent, officer, or representative of the Company.

illegal drug   Any drug that is not legally obtainable; any drug that is legally obtainable but has not been legally obtained; any prescribed drug not legally obtained; any prescribed drug not being used for the prescribed purpose; any over-the-counter drug being used at a dosage level different from that recommended by the manufacturer or being used for a purpose other than that intended by the manufacturer; any drug being used for a purpose not in accordance with bona fide medical therapy. Examples of illegal drugs are Cannabis substances, such as marijuana and hashish, cocaine, heroin, phencyclidine (PCP), and so-called designer drugs and look-alike drugs.

interstate commerce   Trade, traffic, or transportation in the United States that is between a place in a state and a place outside of such state (including a place outside of the United States) or is between two places in a state through another state or a place outside of the United States.

legal drug   Any prescribed drug or over-the-counter drug that has been legally obtained and is being used for the purpose for which it was prescribed or manufactured.

medical practitioner   A licensed doctor of medicine (MD) or osteopathy (DO) or a doctor of dental surgery (DDS) authorized to practice by the state in which the person practices.

medical review officer (MRO)   A licensed doctor of medicine or osteopathy with knowledge of drug abuse disorders. The MRO has the knowledge and medical training to interpret and evaluate an individual's positive test result together with his or her medical history and any other relevant biomedical information.

possession   Meant to also include the presence of any detectable amount of an illicit drug in the body system.

random testing   A testing process in which selection for testing is made by a method using objective, neutral criteria ensuring that every person subject to testing has a substantially equal statistical chance of being selected. The method does not permit subjective factors to play a role in selection—that is, no person may be selected as a result of discretion.

reasonable cause   A belief that the actions, appearance, or conduct of a person are indicative of the use of a controlled substance or alcohol. Such a belief is based on objective, articulable facts. A reasonable cause or for-cause situation is any situation in which an employee's job performance is in conflict with established job standards relating to safety and efficiency. The term includes accidents, near accidents, erratic conduct suggestive of drug or alcohol use, any unsafe performance behaviors, and unexplained deviations from productivity.

under the influence   A condition in which a person is affected by a drug or alcohol in any detectable manner. The symptoms of influence are not confined to those consistent with misbehavior or to obvious impairment of physical or mental ability, such as slurred speech or difficulty in maintaining balance. A determination of being under the influence can be established by a professional opinion, a scientifically valid test such as urinalysis or blood analysis, and in some cases by the opinion of a layperson.

III.   Training and Education

A.   Supervisors and other management personnel are to be trained in the following areas:
1.   Detecting the signs and behavior of employees who may be using drugs or alcohol in violation of this policy
2.   Intervening in situations that may involve violations of this policy
3.   Recognizing the above activities as a direct job responsibility
B.   Employees (including supervisors) are to be informed of the following:
1.   The health and safety dangers associated with drug and alcohol use
2.   The provisions of this policy
3.   The provisions of FHWA and DOT testing requirements

IV.   Inspections and Searches

A.   The Company may conduct unannounced general inspections and searches for drugs or alcohol on Company premises or in Company vehicles or equipment wherever located. Employees are expected to cooperate.
B.   Search of an employee and his or her personal property may be made when there is reasonable cause to believe that the employee is in violation of this policy.
C.   An employee's consent to a search is required as a condition of employment, and the employee's refusal to consent may result in disciplinary action, including discharge, even for a first refusal.
D.   Illegal drugs, drugs believed to be illegal, and drug paraphernalia found on Company property may be turned over to the appropriate law enforcement agency, and full cooperation will be given to any subsequent investigation. Substances that cannot be identified as an illegal drug by a layperson's examination will be turned over to a drug-testing vendor for scientific analysis.
E.   Other forms of contraband, such as firearms, explosives, and lethal weapons, will be subject to seizure during an inspection or search. An employee who is found to possess contraband on Company property or while on Company business will be subject to discipline up to and including discharge.

V. Discipline

A. Any employee who possesses, distributes, sells, attempts to sell, or transfers illegal drugs on Company premises or on Company business will be discharged.

B. Any employee who tests positive for an illegal drug or alcohol in a biological test conducted under the provisions of this policy will be subject to discipline up to and including discharge.

C. Any employee who refuses to undergo a health evaluation and/or biological testing will be subject to discipline up to and including discharge.

D. Any employee who is found to be in possession of contraband in violation of this policy will be subject to discipline up to and including discharge.

E. Any employee who fails to cooperate with the MRO during the investigation of a positive test result will be subject to discipline up to and including discharge.

F. Any employee who attempts to substitute or contaminate his or her specimen to be presented for testing will be terminated.

G. If an employee is the subject of a drug-related investigation by the Company or by a law enforcement agency, the employee may be suspended without pay pending completion of the investigation.

VI. Affected Persons

A. This policy does not apply to any person for whom compliance would violate the domestic laws or policies of another country.

B. This policy applies to all employees.

C. Drug testing under this policy affects two broad classes: (1) employees who are not subject to DOT testing and (2) drivers who are subject to DOT testing.

    1. Employees who are not subject to DOT testing are subject to testing for drugs and alcohol independent of DOT testing.

    2. Drivers who are subject to DOT testing are subject to testing for drugs in accordance with DOT requirements and are subject to testing for alcohol that is conducted independent of DOT testing.

VII. Applicability to Persons Not Subject to DOT Testing

A. Prohibited Activities

    1. The undisclosed use of any legal drug by any employee while performing Company business or while on Company premises is prohibited. However, an employee may continue to work, even though using a legal drug, if Company management has determined, after consulting with appropriate health and/or human resources representatives, that such use does not pose a threat to safety and that the using employee's job performance will not be significantly affected. Otherwise, the employee may be required to take a leave of absence or comply with other appropriate action as determined by Company management.

    2. An employee whose medical therapy requires the use of a legal drug must report such use to his or her supervisor prior to the performance of Company business. The supervisor who is so informed will contact the appropriate health and/or human resources representative for guidance.

3. The Company at all times reserves the right to judge the effect that a legal drug may have on work performance and to restrict the using employee's work activity or presence at the workplace accordingly.
4. The use, sale, purchase, transfer, or possession in any detectable manner of an illegal drug or alcohol by any employee while on Company premises or while performing Company business is prohibited.

B. Testing of Job Applicants
1. All applicants for employment will be subject to biological testing. If evidence of the use of illegal drugs by an applicant is discovered, either through biological testing or other means, the employment process will be suspended.
2. If the applicant refuses to take a biological test, the employment process will be suspended.
3. If an applicant attempts to substitute or contaminate his or her specimen to be tested, the employment process will be suspended.

C. Testing of Current Employees
1. The Company may perform biological testing of an employee as follows:
   a. In reasonable cause situations
   b. In postaccident situations
   c. When random or periodic testing is determined appropriate to ensure safe operations
   d. When random or periodic testing is determined necessary to comply with contractual requirements
   e. Upon return of the employee to work following suspension, layoff, or extended leave of absence
   f. Anytime during or following medical rehabilitation
2. An employee's consent to submit to biological testing is required as a condition of employment, and the employee's refusal to consent may result in disciplinary action, including discharge, for a first refusal or any subsequent refusal.
3. An employee who is tested as the result of involvement in a reasonable cause situation may be suspended without pay pending completion of whatever inquiries may be required.

D. Responsibilities
1. Each individual required to submit to drug testing shall, as soon as practicable, provide the required biological specimens for testing. Failure to meet this responsibility is an offense punishable by termination.
2. Individuals in supervisory positions shall, as soon as practicable following an incident that requires drug testing, collect the required biological specimens for testing and arrange for their prompt delivery or transfer to the drug-testing laboratory. Failure to meet this responsibility is an offense punishable by termination.

E. Confidentiality
All employee information relating to biological testing will be protected by the Company as confidential unless otherwise required by law or overriding public health and safety concerns or authorized in writing by the employee.

F. Appeals
1. An employee whose biological test is reported positive for drug or alcohol will be asked in a confidential meeting or telephone conversation to offer an explanation. The purpose of the meeting or telephone conference will be

to determine whether there is any reason that a positive test could have resulted from some cause other than drug or alcohol use that is in violation of this policy. If the employee is desirous of a second opinion, he or she may request a retest by an alternate laboratory, approved by the Company, of the same specimen at the employee's expense.

2. An appeal that merits further inquiry may require that the employee be suspended without pay until the inquiry and the appeal process are completed.

VIII.   Applicability to Drivers Subject to DOT Testing

A.   Drug Use Prohibitions
1. No driver shall be on duty if the driver uses any controlled substances or tests positive for the use of controlled substances, except as provided in the section titled Prescribed Drugs.
2. A person who tests positive for the use of a controlled substance, as defined in 49 CFR Part 40, is medically unqualified to operate a motor vehicle.
3. A person who refuses to be tested will not be permitted to operate a commercial motor vehicle. Such refusal will be treated as a positive test and cause the driver to be considered medically unqualified to operate a motor vehicle.

B.   Prescribed Drugs
1. Any driver who is alleged to have violated the section of this policy titled Drug Use Prohibitions will have available as an affirmative defense, to be proven by the driver through clear and convincing evidence, that his or her use of a controlled substance (except for methadone) was prescribed by a licensed medical practitioner who is familiar with the driver's medical history and assigned duties. The MRO may provide an opportunity for a driver to discuss a positive test result and clarify if a prescribed medication was involved.
2. This section does not release a driver from the requirement to notify the Company of therapeutic drug use.

C.   Reasonable Cause Testing
1. The Company will require a driver to be tested, upon reasonable cause, for the use of controlled substances.
2. A driver will submit to testing, upon reasonable cause, for the use of controlled substances when requested to do so by the Company.
3. The conduct that forms the basis for reasonable cause should be witnessed by at least two supervisors if at all feasible. If only one supervisor is available, only one supervisor need witness the conduct. The witnesses must have received training in the detection of probable drug use.
4. The documentation of the driver's conduct will be prepared and signed by the witnesses within 24 hours of the observed behavior or before the results of the tests are released, whichever is earlier.
5. The Company will ensure that the driver is transported immediately to a collection site for the collection of a urine sample.
6. The Company will ensure that the controlled substance testing conforms with 49 CFR Part 40.

D. Preemployment Testing
1. The Company will require, as a prequalification condition, drug testing of any driver-applicant whom the Company intends to hire or use, and any driver-applicant will submit to controlled substance testing as a prequalification condition.
2. Prior to collection of a urine sample, a driver-applicant will be notified that the sample will be tested for the presence of controlled substances.
3. The Company may use a driver who is not employed and tested by the Company when the Company is sure that the driver participates in a controlled substance testing program that meets the DOT requirements. When a driver is used more than once a year, the Company will make such assurance every six months. The assurance will, as a minimum, consist of contacting the controlled substance testing program entity prior to using the driver and obtaining the following information:
    a. Name and address of the program
    b. Verification that the driver participates in the program
    c. Verification that the program conforms to 49 CFR Part 40
    d. Verification that the driver is qualified under DOT rules
    e. The date the driver was last tested for controlled substances
4. Drug-testing information pertaining to drivers who are not employed and tested by the Company will be maintained separately from drug-testing information pertaining to the Company's own antidrug program.
E. Biennial (Periodic) Testing
1. The Company will, as a minimum, require a driver to be drug tested during the first medical examination of the driver after implementation of the Company's drug-testing program.
2. The Company may discontinue entirely or may discontinue and later resume periodic testing after the first calendar year in which the Company has implemented its random drug-testing program.
3. The Company may use a driver who participates in a drug-testing program of another motor carrier or controlled substance test consortium.
4. The Company will ensure that its biennial testing procedures conform with 49 CFR Part 40.
F. Random Testing
1. During the first 12 months following implementation of random drug testing pursuant to this policy, the Company will ensure the following:
    a. The random drug testing is spread reasonably through the 12-month period
    b. The last test collection during the year is conducted at an annualized rate of 50 percent
    c. The total number of tests conducted during the 12 months is equal to at least 25 percent of the drivers subject to testing
2. The Company will use a random selection process to select and request a driver to be tested for the use of controlled substances.
3. A driver will submit to controlled substance testing when selected by a random selection process.
4. The sample shall consist of a urine specimen.
5. The Company will ensure that its drug-testing program conforms with 49 CFR Part 40.

G. Postaccident Testing
   1. A driver will provide a urine specimen to be tested for the use of controlled substances as soon as possible after a reportable accident but in no case later than 32 hours after the accident.
   2. A driver who is seriously injured and cannot provide a specimen at the time of the accident will provide the necessary authorization for obtaining hospital reports and other documents that would indicate whether there were any controlled substances in his or her system.
   3. The sample shall consist of a urine specimen.
   4. A driver shall ensure that the specimen is forwarded and processed by a laboratory that conforms with the 49 CFR Part 40 guidelines.
H. Disqualification
   1. A driver will be disqualified by issuance of a letter of disqualification for a period of one year following a refusal to give a urine sample when the driver has been involved in a fatal accident. An exception will be granted to a driver who is unable to provide a urine sample as the result of a serious injury as described in the section titled Postaccident Testing.
   2. A driver shall be disqualified by issuance of a letter of disqualification for a period of one year for a positive test of controlled substance use when the driver has been involved in a fatal accident.
I. Notification of Test Results
   1. The Company will notify each driver-applicant of the results of a preemployment controlled substance test provided the driver-applicant requests such results within 60 days of being notified of the disposition of the employment application.
   2. The Company will notify each driver of the results of periodic, random, or postaccident controlled substance tests when the test results are positive. The driver will also be advised what drug was discovered.
J. Record Keeping
   1. The Company will ensure that all records related to the administration and results of the drug-testing program for its drivers subject to the testing requirements are maintained for a minimum period of five years except that individual negative test results will be maintained for a minimum of one year.
   2. The MRO shall be the sole custodian of individual test results. The MRO will retain the reports of individual test results for a minimum of five years.
   3. The Company will retain in the employee's qualification file such information that will indicate only the following:
      a. That the employee submitted to a controlled substance test
      b. The date and location of such test
      c. The identity of the person or entity performing the test
      d. Whether the test finding was positive or negative
   4. The Company will produce upon demand, and will permit the FHWA administrator to examine, all records related to the administration and results of controlled substance testing performed under this part of the policy.
   5. The Company will maintain an annual (calendar year) summary of the records related to the administration and results of the controlled substance–testing program. This summary will include, at a minimum, the following:

   a. The total number of controlled substance tests administered
   b. The number of controlled substance tests administered in each category (i.e., prequalification, periodic, reasonable cause, and random)
   c. The total number of individuals who did not pass a controlled substance test
   d. The total number of individuals who did not pass a controlled substance test by testing category
   e. The disposition of each individual who did not pass a controlled substance test
   f. The number of controlled substance tests performed by a laboratory that indicated evidence of a prohibited controlled substance or metabolite in the screening test in a sufficient quantity to warrant a confirmatory test
   g. The number of controlled substance tests performed by a laboratory that indicated evidence of a prohibited controlled substance or metabolite in the confirmatory test in a sufficient quantity to be reported as a positive finding to the MRO
   h. The number of controlled substance tests that were performed by a laboratory that indicated evidence of a prohibited controlled substance or metabolite in the confirmatory test in a sufficient quantity to be reported as a positive finding by substance category (e.g., marijuana, cocaine, opium, PCP, or amphetamine)

K. Access to Individual Test Results
   1. The Company will ensure that no person will obtain the individual test results retained by the MRO and the MRO will not release the individual test results of any employee to any person without first obtaining written authorization from the tested employee. Nothing in this paragraph will prohibit the MRO from releasing to the Company the information delineated in the sections titled Notification of Test Results and Record Keeping.
   2. The Company will ensure that no person will obtain the drug-testing information entered into an employee's qualification file and will not release such information without first obtaining written authorization from the tested employee.

L. Employee Assistance Program (EAP)
   1. The Company will maintain an EAP that will, as a minimum, include the following:
      a. An education and training component for drivers that addresses controlled substances
      b. An education and training component for supervisory personnel that addresses controlled substances
      c. A written statement that outlines the EAP to be kept on file and available for inspection at the Company's principal place of business
   2. The EAP will include an effective training program for supervisory personnel and all drivers. The training program will address at least the following elements:
      a. The effects and consequences of controlled substance use on personal health, safety, and the work environment
      b. The manifestations and behavioral causes that may indicate controlled substance use or abuse
      c. Documentation of training given to drivers and supervisory personnel

M. Aftercare Monitoring
   After returning to work, drivers who test positive must continue in an aftercare
   program and be subject to follow-up testing for no longer than five years following
   return to work.

DRUG-TESTING POLICY FOR A PETROLEUM COMPANY

Statement of Policy

The purpose of this policy is to help, in a positive manner, employees from becoming ineffective, both on and off the job, due to the use of drugs or alcohol. The Company recognizes its obligation to protect the health and safety of its employees, to provide safe and effective operations for the public, and to protect the assets and image of the Company for its stockholders. Therefore, the Company is committed to achieving a safe work environment free of alcohol and drug abuse through education, intervention, and, if appropriate, disciplinary measures. Accordingly, the following policy will be enforced:

1. The use, sale, attempt to sell, possession, or distribution of illegal drugs, alcohol or controlled substances (unless prescribed by a licensed physician for medical reasons) and the paraphernalia associated with such on Company premises, including parking areas, are prohibited. Employees under the influence of alcohol, nonmedical controlled substances, or illegal drugs are prohibited from Company property. Employees under the influence of illegal drugs, alcohol, or controlled substances while at work will be subject to disciplinary action, including discharge. Employees selling, attempting to sell, transferring, or distributing illegal drugs or controlled substances will be discharged.

2. Entry onto Company property constitutes consent to and recognition of the right of the Company and its authorized agents to search persons, automobiles, lockers, and other property of individuals while entering, on, or leaving Company property.

3. If an employee becomes the victim of alcohol or drug use, the Company will cooperate with the employee in attempted rehabilitation, provided the employee fully cooperates with such rehabilitative efforts and provided rehabilitative efforts have not been attempted in the past. The Company will not attempt rehabilitation of employees who distribute, sell, or transfer illegal drugs or controlled substances. The medical information will be treated as confidential in accordance with existing Company policy.

Administration

All employees should take seriously the dangers inherent in the consumption of alcohol and drugs, not only from the standpoint of their personal health but also from the standpoint of the safety and potential property damage to themselves and others and the effects on their families.

The consistent and proper administration of the Company's policy is necessary to ensure its effectiveness and enforceability before any reviewing authorities. Set forth below are administrative guidelines to be used by all management personnel with regard to the alcohol and drug abuse policy of the Company.

Sale, Attempted Sale, Distribution, or Transfer of Illegal or Controlled Drugs

The sale, attempted sale, distribution, or transfer of illegal or controlled drugs is a serious offense and a violation of the state and federal laws. Furthermore, an employee who engages in such activities represents a potential danger in that he or she may involve other employees in the illegal use of drugs. Accordingly, any employee will be dismissed who engages in the sale, attempted sale, distribution, or transfer of illegal or controlled drugs on Company premises or while off Company premises whether or not on Company business. It is not the policy of the Company to attempt rehabilitation of employees who sell, attempt to sell, distribute, or transfer illegal or controlled drugs.

If an employee is suspected of engaging in the sale, attempted sale, transfer, or distribution of illegal or controlled drugs, the details should be reviewed with appropriate line management and the Human Resources Manager. If it appears that the suspicions reported have substance, the situation must be reviewed with the Legal Department and the Corporate Security Department. Cooperation should be given to appropriate law enforcement officers in connection with investigations they may undertake.

In those cases where our first knowledge of any illegal activity by the employee is as a result of an arrest, the matter should be referred to the appropriate line management and the Human Resources Manager, who must review the situation with the Legal Department and the Corporate Security Department before taking any action.

After all Company investigations have been completed and all available facts have been reviewed, the employee will be dismissed if the evidence substantiates that the employee has been involved in the distribution, sale, attempted sale, or transfer of illegal or controlled drugs. If the distribution, sale, attempted sale, or transfer occurred on Company property or on Company business, the employee's dismissal should not be delayed awaiting any court determination in the matter. If the distribution, sale, attempted sale, or transfer of illegal or controlled drugs occurred while off Company property and not on Company business, the employee should be placed on leave without pay pending the resolution of criminal proceedings. Upon resolution of the criminal proceedings, a determination will be made as to the employee's status, following a full review of all evidence with the Legal Department.

Use or Possession of Drugs or Alcohol in the Workplace or Reporting to Work Under the Influence

Any employee who is found drinking or in possession of alcoholic beverages on Company premises, including Company parking lots, or in Company operated vehicles, or coming or returning to work in an apparent intoxicated condition (e.g., stumbling, slurred speech, unusual behavior, bloodshot pupils, or alcohol smell on breath) is subject to disciplinary action up to and including dismissal. Such an employee must be removed from the job at once and required to undergo health evaluations and/or biological testing such as urinalysis, saliva testing, and blood analysis. The employee should not be returned to work until a determination of what disciplinary action, if any, is merited.

Where an employee is being required to undergo the health evaluations and/or biological testing, the supervisor must make sure the employee understands that the requirement to take the test is a direct and proper instruction from the supervisor with no other alternatives available except to refuse a direct instruction. The supervisor should advise the employee that a refusal to take the test as directed will be considered as a refusal of a direct order and such refusal may result in disciplinary action up to and including discharge.

If illegal or controlled drugs (unless prescribed by a licensed physician for medical reasons) are found in an employee's possession on Company premises, such drugs should be turned over to law enforcement officials. The employee should be disciplined upon satisfactory proof that the drug is an illegal drug or controlled substance (unless prescribed by a licensed doctor for medical reasons).

Any employee who is found receiving or purchasing illegal or controlled drugs on Company premises or while on Company business is subject to disciplinary action up to and including discharge.

Suspected Alcohol or Drug Abuse and Rehabilitation

Supervisors must be as knowledgeable as possible concerning the signs and symptoms of drug or alcohol dependence (including, but not limited to, things such as absenteeism, tardiness, change in physical appearance, disinterest in work, or change in personality). Suspected problems must be referred to appropriate line management and the Human Resources Manager before any action is taken. Since diagnosis is complex and a false accusation must be avoided, supervisors should not undertake the counseling or rehabilitation of an employee suspected of misusing drugs without the advice and assistance of health professionals but rather should report a suspected problem promptly, as a delay can be dangerous for the employee, other employees, and the Company.

When drug or alcohol misuse is suspected, the following steps should be followed carefully:

1. The employee's behavior and symptoms must be reported to appropriate line management and the Human Resources Manager.
2. It is important that each suspicion of drug of alcohol misuse be carefully investigated and documented. Therefore, line management, in conjunction with the Human Resources Manager, must conduct an immediate and thorough investigation before any action is taken.
3. If the investigation indicates a possible health-related problem and/or the presence of a work-related problem that has not been corrected, a meeting should be conducted between the employee and a supervisor. The supervisor should discuss with the employee any unsatisfactory behavior and performance, citing specific reasons, such as absenteeism, tardiness, physical appearance, disinterest in work, and failure to complete assignments. Following this discussion, the employee must be referred to a Company physician and/or a contract employee assistance program (EAP) for evaluation.

   The supervisor should make no suggestion of suspected drug or alcohol misuse during this discussion. If the employee refuses to agree to the referral to the company physician and/or a contract EAP, the supervisor should explain that such a refusal may be grounds for dismissal.

   Before the employee's visit to the Company physician and/or the contract EAP, the Human Resources Manager should give the physician and/or the contract EAP representative all the facts of the case and the employee should be told that the information has been made available to the physician and/or the contract EAP representative.
4. After the medical examination, if alcohol or drug abuse is indicated, the following steps should be taken:

a. The employee will be referred to a professionally recognized treatment program by the Company physician and/or the contract EAP representative. Rehabilitated employees will then be expected to achieve and maintain a standard level of productivity and remain substance-free when at work.

b. If rehabilitation has previously proved ineffective, or if the employee has not cooperated or refuses to participate in rehabilitation, disciplinary action should be taken. It may be desirable to suspend the employee as a warning concerning the seriousness of the offense, but the Company's position of refusing to retain habitual drug or alcohol abusers should be made quite clear to the employee.

c. Employees who have undergone substance abuse rehabilitation may be required to submit periodically, without prior notice, to test procedures. Under these circumstances, positive results may be a basis for termination.

Responsibility

Recognition of alcohol or drug abuse as a medical problem is not intended to inhibit or restrict disciplinary action that is clearly warranted. Reporting to work under the influence of such substances and use or possession of illicit drugs on the job cannot be condoned. However, alertness to these problems is the supervisor's responsibility, and it may be possible to help an employee, thereby salvaging an individual for family and community life and retaining an experienced worker for the Company.

DRUG-TESTING POLICY FOR A COMPANY
SUBJECT TO FEDERAL DRUG-TESTING RULES
ADMINISTERED BY THE U.S. COAST GUARD

I. Purpose

A. A primary purpose of this policy is to minimize the use of intoxicants by merchant marine personnel and to promote a drug-free and safe work environment.
B. This policy is also intended to promote overall a safe, healthful, and efficient working environment for all employees. Being under the influence of a controlled substance or alcohol on the job poses serious safety and health risks to the user and to all those who work with the user. The use, sale, purchase, transfer, or possession of an illegal drug in the workplace and the use, possession, or being under the influence of alcohol also pose unacceptable risks for safe, healthful, and efficient operations.
C. The Company recognizes its contractual obligations to its clients for the provision of services that are free of the influence of controlled substances and alcohol and will endeavor through this policy to provide such drug-free services.
D. Furthermore, the Company takes note of requirements to comply with U.S. Coast Guard (USCG) and Department of Transportation (DOT) regulations relating to the use of controlled substances and alcohol and will endeavor through this policy to maintain compliance.

II. Definitions

alcohol   Any beverage that contains ethyl alcohol (ethanol), including but not limited to beer, wine, and distilled spirits.
chemical test   A scientifically recognized test that analyzes an individual's breath, blood, urine, saliva, body fluids, or tissues for evidence of dangerous drug or alcohol use.
collection site   A place where individuals present themselves for the purpose of providing body fluid or tissue samples to be analyzed for specified controlled substances. A collection site will have all necessary personnel, materials, equipment, facilities, and supervision to provide for the collection, security, temporary storage, and transportation or shipment of the samples to a laboratory.
commitment of employment   The proof of employment required by CFR 12.25-5.
Company facilities   See *Company premises.*
Company premises   All property of the Company, including but not limited to buildings and surrounding areas on Company-owned or leased property, parking lots, and storage areas. The term also includes Company-owned or leased vessels, vehicles, and equipment wherever located. It also includes premises where the Company performs contract services.
contraband   Any article, the possession of which on Company premises or while on Company business, causes an employee to be in violation of a Company work rule. Contraband includes illegal drugs, alcoholic beverages, and drug paraphernalia.
controlled substances   Defined by 21 USC 802; includes all substances listed in Schedules I through V as they may be revised from time to time.

crew member   An individual who is (1) on board a vessel acting under the authority of a license, certificate of registry, or merchant mariner's document, whether or not the individual is a member of the vessel's crew; or (2) engaged or employed on board a vessel owned in the United States that is required by law or regulation to engage, employ, or be operated by an individual holding a license, certificate of registry, or merchant mariner's document.

   The term crewmember does not include (1) individuals primarily employed in the preparation of fish or fish products or in a support position not related to navigation on a fish-processing vessel; (2) scientific personnel on an oceanographic research vessel; and (3) individuals who have no duties that directly affect the safety of the vessel's navigation or operations.

dangerous drug   A narcotic drug, controlled substance, and marijuana, as defined in Section 102 of the Comprehensive Drug Abuse Prevention and Control Act of 1970 (21 USC 802).

dangerous drug level   The amount of traces of dangerous drugs or drug metabolites in an individual's breath, blood, urine, saliva, or body fluids or tissues.

drug   Any substance (other than alcohol) that is a controlled substance as defined in this policy.

drug test   A chemical test of an individual's urine for evidence of dangerous drug use.

employees subject to DOT testing   Those employees holding a license, certificate of registry, or merchant marine document who are subject to chemical testing in accordance with USCG and DOT regulations.

employer   A marine employer or sponsoring organization.

fails a chemical test for dangerous drugs   The test result is reported as positive for the presence of dangerous drugs or drug metabolites in an individual's system after an MRO's review in accordance with 49 CFR 40.27.

illegal drug   Any drug that is not legally obtainable; any drug that is legally obtainable but has not been legally obtained; any prescribed drug not legally obtained; any prescribed drug not being used for the prescribed purpose; any over-the-counter drug being used at a dosage level different from that recommended by the manufacturer or being used for a purpose other than that intended by the manufacturer; any drug being used for a purpose not in accordance with bona fide medical therapy. Examples of illegal drugs are Cannabis substances, such as marijuana and hashish, cocaine, heroin, phencyclidine (PCP), and so-called designer drugs and look-alike drugs.

individual directly involved in a serious marine incident   An individual whose order, action, or failure to act is determined to be, or cannot be ruled out as, a causative factor in the events leading to or causing a serious marine incident.

intoxicant   Any form of alcohol, dangerous drug, or combination thereof.

legal drug   Any prescribed drug or over-the-counter drug that has been legally obtained and is being used for the purpose for which it was prescribed or manufactured.

marine casualty   An injury that requires professional medical treatment beyond first aid and, in the case of a person engaged or employed on board a vessel in commercial service, that renders the individual unfit to perform routine vessel duties.

marine employer   The owner, managing operator, charterer, agent, master, or person in charge of a vessel other than a recreational vessel.

medical facility An American hospital, clinic, physician's office, or laboratory where blood and urine specimens can be collected according to recognized professional standards.

medical review officer (MRO) A licensed doctor of medicine designated by the Company to interpret and evaluate an individual's positive test result together with his or her medical history and any other relevant biomedical information.

possession Meant to also include the presence of any detectable amount of an illicit drug in the body system.

qualified medical personnel A physician, physician's assistant, nurse, emergency medical technician, or other person authorized under state or federal law or regulation to collect blood and urine specimens.

random testing A testing process in which selection for testing is made by a method using objective, neutral criteria ensuring that every person subject to testing has a substantially equal statistical chance of being selected. The method does not permit subjective factors to play a role in selection—that is, no person may be selected as a result of discretion.

reasonable cause A belief that the actions, appearance, or conduct of a person are indicative of the use of a controlled substance or alcohol. Such a belief is based on objective, articulable facts. A reasonable cause or for-cause situation is any situation in which an employee's job performance is in conflict with established job standards relating to safety and efficiency. The term includes accidents, near accidents, erratic conduct suggestive of drug or alcohol use, any unsafe performance behaviors, and unexplained deviations from productivity.

serious marine incident Any of the following events involving a vessel in commercial service:
1. Any marine casualty or accident as defined in 4.03-1 that is required by 4.05-1 to be reported to the Coast Guard and that results in any of the following:
   a. One or more deaths
   b. An injury to a crew member, passenger, or other person that requires professional medical treatment beyond first aid and, in the case of a person employed on board a vessel in commercial service, that renders the individual unfit to perform routine vessel duties
   c. Damage to property, as defined in 4.05-1(f) of this part, in excess of $100,000
   d. Actual or constructive total loss of any vessel subject to inspection under 46 USC 3301
   e. Actual or constructive total loss of any self-propelled vessel not subject to inspection under 46 USC 3301 and weighing 100 gross tons or more
2. A discharge of 10,000 or more gallons of oil into the navigable waters of the United States, as defined in 33 USC 1321, whether or not resulting from a marine casualty.
3. A discharge of a reportable quantity of a hazardous substance into the navigable waters of the United States or a release of a reportable quantity of a hazardous substance into the environment of the United States, whether or not resulting from a marine casualty.

sponsoring organization Any company, consortium, corporation, association, union, or other organization with which individuals serving in the marine industry or their employers are associated.

under the influence   A condition in which a person is affected by a drug or alcohol in any detectable manner. The symptoms of influence are not confined to those consistent with misbehavior or to obvious impairment of physical or mental ability, such as slurred speech or difficulty in maintaining balance. A determination of being under the influence can be established by a professional opinion, a scientifically valid test such as urinalysis or blood analysis, and in some cases by the opinion of a layperson.

vessel owned in the United States   Any vessel documented or numbered under the laws of the United States and any vessel owned by a citizen of the United States that is not documented or numbered by any nation.

III.   Training and Education

A.   Supervisors and other management personnel are to be trained in the following areas:
1.   Detecting the signs and behavior of employees who may be using drugs or alcohol in violation of this policy
2.   Intervening in situations that may involve violations of this policy
3.   Recognizing the above activities as a direct job responsibility

B.   Employees (including supervisors) are to be informed of the following:
1.   The health and safety dangers associated with drug and alcohol use
2.   The provisions of this policy
3.   The provisions of USCG and DOT testing requirements

IV.   Inspections and Searches

A.   The Company may conduct unannounced general inspections and searches for drugs or alcohol on vessels or on Company premises or equipment wherever located. Employees are expected to cooperate.

B.   Search of an employee and his or her personal property may be made when there is reasonable cause to believe that the employee is in violation of this policy.

C.   An employee's consent to a search is required as a condition of employment, and the employee's refusal to consent may result in disciplinary action, including discharge, even for a first refusal.

D.   Illegal drugs, drugs believed to be illegal, and drug paraphernalia found on Company property may be turned over to the appropriate law enforcement agency and full cooperation given to any subsequent investigation. Substances that cannot be identified as an illegal drug by a layperson's examination will be turned over to a drug-testing vendor for scientific analysis.

E.   Other forms of contraband, such as firearms, explosives, and lethal weapons, will be subject to seizure during an inspection or search. An employee who is found to possess contraband on Company property or while on Company business will be subject to discipline up to and including discharge.

V.   Discipline

A.   Any employee who possesses, distributes, sells, attempts to sell, or transfers illegal drugs on Company premises or on Company business will be discharged.

B. Any employee who tests positive for an illegal drug or alcohol in a chemical test conducted under the provisions of this policy will be subject to discipline up to and including discharge.

C. Any employee who refuses to undergo a health evaluation and/or chemical testing will be subject to discipline up to and including discharge.

D. Any employee who is found to be in possession of contraband in violation of this policy will be subject to discipline up to and including discharge.

E. Any employee who fails to cooperate with the MRO during the investigation of a positive test result will be subject to discipline up to and including discharge.

F. Any employee who attempts to substitute or contaminate his or her specimen to be presented for testing will be terminated.

G. If an employee is the subject of a drug-related investigation by the Company or by a law enforcement agency, the employee may be suspended without pay pending completion of the investigation.

VI. Affected Persons

A. This policy does not apply to any person for whom compliance would violate the domestic laws or policies of another country.

B. This policy applies to all employees.

C. Chemical testing under this policy affects two broad classes: (1) employees not subject to DOT testing, and (2) employees subject to DOT testing:
    1. Employees who are not subject to DOT testing are subject to testing for drugs and alcohol independent of DOT testing.
    2. Employees who are subject to DOT testing are subject to testing for drugs in accordance with USCG and DOT requirements and subject to testing for alcohol that is conducted independently of DOT testing.

VII. Applicability to Employees Not Subject to DOT Testing

A. Prohibited Activities
    1. The undisclosed use of any legal drug by any employee while performing Company business or while on Company premises is prohibited. However, an employee may continue to work, even though using a legal drug, if Company management has determined, after consulting with appropriate health and/or human resources representatives, that such use does not pose a threat to safety and that the using employee's job performance will not be significantly affected. Otherwise, the employee may be required to take a leave of absence or comply with other appropriate action as determined by Company management.
    2. An employee whose medical therapy requires the use of a legal drug must report such use to his or her supervisor prior to the performance of Company business. The supervisor who is so informed will contact the appropriate health and/or human resources representative for guidance.
    3. The Company at all times reserves the right to judge the effect that a legal drug may have on work performance and to restrict the using employee's work activity or presence at the workplace accordingly.

      4.   The use, sale, purchase, transfer, or possession in any detectable manner of an illegal drug or alcohol by any employee while on Company premises or while performing Company business is prohibited.

B. Testing of Job Applicants

     1. All applicants for employment will be subject to chemical testing. If evidence of the use of illegal drugs by an applicant is discovered, either through chemical testing or other means, the employment process will be suspended.

     2. If the applicant refuses to take a chemical test, the employment process will be suspended.

     3. If an applicant attempts to substitute or contaminate his or her specimen to be tested, the employment process will be suspended.

C. Testing of Current Employees

     1. The Company may perform chemical testing of an employee in the following cases:

        a. In reasonable cause situations

        b. In postaccident situations

        c. When random or periodic testing is determined appropriate to ensure safe operations

        d. When random or periodic testing is determined necessary to comply with contractual requirements

        e. Upon return of the employee to work following suspension, layoff, or extended leave of absence

        f. Anytime during or following medical rehabilitation

     2. An employee's consent to submit to chemical testing is required as a condition of employment, and the employee's refusal to consent may result in disciplinary action, including discharge, for a first refusal or any subsequent refusal.

     3. An employee who is tested as the result of involvement in a reasonable cause situation may be suspended without pay pending completion of whatever inquiries may be required.

     4. Each individual required to submit to drug testing shall, as soon as practicable, provide the required biological specimens for testing. Failure to meet this responsibility is an offense punishable by termination.

     5. Individuals in supervisory positions shall, as soon as practicable following an incident that requires drug testing, collect the required biological specimens for testing and arrange for their prompt delivery or transfer to the drug-testing laboratory. Failure to meet this responsibility is an offense punishable by termination.

D. Confidentiality

All employee information relating to chemical testing will be protected by the Company as confidential unless otherwise required by law or overriding public health and safety concerns or authorized in writing by the employee.

E. Appeals

     1. An employee whose chemical test is reported positive for drug or alcohol will be asked in a confidential meeting or telephone conference to offer an explanation. The purpose of the meeting or telephone conference will be to determine whether there is any reason that a positive test could have resulted from some other cause other than drug or alcohol use that is in violation of this policy. If the employee is desirous of a second opinion, he or she may

request a retest by an alternate laboratory, approved by the Company, of the
same specimen at the employee's expense.

2. An appeal that merits further inquiry may require that the employee be
   suspended without pay until the inquiry and the appeals process are completed.

VIII. Applicability to Employees
Subject to DOT Testing

A. Company Responsibilities in Serious Marine Incidents
   1. When the Company determines that a casualty or incident is, or is likely to
      become, a serious marine incident, the Company shall take all practicable
      steps to have each individual engaged or employed on board the vessel who
      is directly involved in the incident chemically tested for evidence of drug
      and alcohol use.
   2. The determination of which individuals are directly involved in a serious
      marine incident is to be made by the Company. A law enforcement officer
      may determine that additional individuals are directly involved in the se-
      rious marine incident. In such cases, the Company shall take all practicable
      steps to have these individuals chemically tested.
   3. The requirements for prompt chemical testing shall not prevent vessel per-
      sonnel who are required to be tested from performing duties in the aftermath
      of a serious marine incident when their performance is necessary for the
      preservation of life or property or the protection of the environment.
B. Individual Responsibilities in Serious Marine Incidents
   1. Any individual engaged or employed on board a vessel who is determined
      to be directly involved in a serious marine incident shall provide blood,
      breath, or urine specimens for chemical tests when directed to do so by the
      Company or a law enforcement officer.
   2. If the individual refuses to provide blood, breath, or urine specimens, this
      refusal shall be noted on Form CG-2692B and in the vessel's official logbook,
      if one is required.
   3. No individual may be forcibly compelled to provide specimens for chemical
      tests. However, refusal is considered a violation of regulation and will subject
      the individual to suspension and revocation proceedings and removal from
      any duties that affect the safety of the vessel's navigation or operations.
C. Specimen Collection Requirements
   1. The Company will ensure that all inspected vessels certificated for unre-
      stricted ocean routes and all inspected vessels certificated for restricted
      overseas routes have on board at all times a breath-testing device capable of
      determining the presence of alcohol in a person's system. The breath-testing
      device shall be used in accordance with procedures specified by the man-
      ufacturer.
   2. The Company shall ensure that urine specimen collection and shipping kits
      are readily available for use following serious marine incidents. The spec-
      imen collection and shipping kits need not be maintained aboard each vessel
      if they can otherwise be readily obtained within 24 hours of the time of the
      occurrence of the serious marine incident.

3. The Company shall ensure that specimens are collected as soon as practicable following the occurrence of a serious marine incident.

4. When obtaining blood, breath, and urine specimens, the Company shall ensure that the collection process is supervised by either qualified collection personnel, Company personnel, a law enforcement officer, or a representative of the Company.

5. Chemical tests of an individual's breath for the presence of alcohol using a breath-testing device may be conducted by any individual trained to conduct such tests. Blood specimens shall be taken only by qualified medical personnel.

D. Specimen Collection in Incidents Involving Fatalities

1. When an individual engaged or employed on board a vessel dies as a result of a serious marine incident, blood and urine specimens must be obtained from the remains of the individual for chemical testing if it is practicable to do so. The Company shall notify the appropriate local authority, such as the coroner or medical examiner, as soon as possible of the fatality and of DOT testing requirements. The Company shall provide the specimen collection and shipping kit and request that the local authority assist in obtaining the necessary specimens. When the custodian of the remains is a person other than the local authority, the Company shall request the custodian to cooperate in obtaining the required specimens.

2. If the local authority or custodian of the remains declines to cooperate in obtaining the necessary specimens, the Company shall provide an explanation of the circumstances on Form CG-2692B (Report of Required Chemical Drug and Alcohol Testing Following a Serious Marine Incident).

E. Specimen Handling and Shipping

1. The Company shall ensure that blood specimens collected are promptly shipped to a testing laboratory qualified to conduct tests on such specimens. A proper chain of custody must be maintained for each specimen from the time of collection through the authorized disposition of the specimen. Blood specimens must be shipped to the laboratory in a cooled condition by any means adequate to ensure delivery within 24 hours of receipt by the carrier.

2. The Company shall ensure that the urine specimen collection procedures and the chain-of-custody requirements are complied with. The Company shall ensure that urine specimens are promptly shipped to a laboratory complying with the requirements of 49 CFR Part 40. Urine specimens must be shipped by an expeditious means but need not be shipped in a cooled condition for overnight delivery.

F. Specimen Analysis

1. Each laboratory will provide prompt analysis of specimens collected consistent with the need to develop all relevant information and to produce a complete analysis report.

2. Laboratory reports shall be sent to the MRO. Whenever a urinalysis report indicates the presence of a dangerous drug or drug metabolite, the MRO shall review the report as required by CFR 40.27 and submit his or her findings to the Company. Blood test reports indicating the presence of alcohol shall be similarly reviewed to determine if there is a legitimate medical explanation.

3. Analysis results indicating the presence of alcohol, dangerous drugs, or drug

metabolites shall not be construed by themselves as constituting a finding that use of drugs or alcohol was the probable cause of a serious marine incident.

G. Reports and Test Results

1. Whenever an individual engaged or employed on a vessel is identified as being directly involved in a serious marine incident, the Company shall complete Form CG-2692B (Report of Required Chemical Drug and Alcohol Testing Following a Serious Marine Incident).

2. When the serious marine incident requires the submission of Form CG-2692 (Report of Marine Casualty, Injury or Death) to the Coast Guard, the report shall be appended to Form CG-2692.

3. In incidents involving discharges of oil or hazardous substances and when Form CG-2692 is not required to be submitted, Form CG-2692B shall be submitted to the Coast Guard Officer in Charge, Marine Inspection, having jurisdiction over the location where the discharge occurred or nearest the port of first arrival following the discharge.

4. Upon receipt of the report of chemical test results, the Company shall submit a copy of the test results for each person listed on the CG-2692B to the Coast Guard Officer in Charge, Marine Inspection, to whom the CG-2692B was submitted.

H. Chemical Testing

1. As part of a reasonable cause drug-testing program, the Company may test for drugs in addition to those specified in this policy when the Department of Health and Human Services (DHHS) has established an approved testing protocol and positive threshold for such substances and approval is granted by the Coast Guard under 49 CFR Part 40.

2. If an individual fails a chemical test for dangerous drugs, the individual will be presumed to be a user of dangerous drugs.

3. If an individual holding a license, certificate of registry, or merchant mariner's document fails a chemical test for dangerous drugs, the Company shall report the test results in writing to the nearest Coast Guard Officer in Charge, Marine Inspection. The individual shall be denied employment as a crew member or removed from duties that directly affect the safety of the vessel's navigation or operations as quickly as practicable and shall be subject to suspension and revocation proceedings against his or her license, certificate of registry, or merchant mariner's document under 46 CFR Part 5.

4. If an individual who does not hold a license, certificate of registry, or merchant mariner's document fails a chemical test for dangerous drugs, the individual shall be denied employment as a crew member or removed from duties that directly affect the vessel's navigation or operations as soon as practicable.

5. An individual who has failed a required chemical test for dangerous drugs may not be reemployed aboard a vessel until the requirements of this policy and 46 CFR Part 5, if applicable, have been satisfied.

I. Implementation of Chemical Testing

1. During the first 12 months following the institution of random drug testing pursuant to this section, the Company shall meet the following conditions:

   a. Random drug testing will be spread reasonably through the 12-month period

        b.   The last test collection during the year will be conducted at an annualized rate of 50 percent

        c.   The total number of tests conducted during the 12 months will be equal to at least 25 percent of the covered population

2. Periodic testing requirements will apply to physical examinations performed after December 21, 1990.

3. When a vessel owned in the United States is operating in waters that are not subject to the jurisdiction of the United States, the testing requirements do not apply to a citizen of a foreign country engaged or employed as a pilot in accordance with the laws or customs of that foreign country.

4. Testing shall not apply to any person for whom compliance with testing would violate the domestic laws or policies of another country.

J. Preemployment Testing

1. The Company shall not engage, employ, or otherwise give a commitment of employment to any individual to serve as a crew member unless the individual passes a chemical test for dangerous drugs.

2. An applicant is not required to undergo preemployment testing if the applicant provides satisfactory evidence that he or she has done either of the following:

        a.   Passed a preemployment test for the Company or another employer or a periodic chemical test for dangerous drugs within the previous six months

        b.   Been subject to a random testing program meeting USCG requirements during the previous 12 months, has not failed a chemical test for dangerous drugs, and has not refused to participate in required chemical tests

K. Periodic Testing

1. Whenever a physical examination is required for an individual, a chemical test for dangerous drugs must be included as a part of the physical examination. If a physical examination is required for a license or merchant mariner's document application, the applicant shall provide the results of a chemical test administered as part of the physical examination to the Coast Guard Regional Examination Center (REC). For those individuals required to receive physical examinations on a periodic basis, the individual shall provide the result of each required chemical test to the REC at the time the individual applies for a renewal of his or her license. Only the results of those chemical tests taken since the individual's most recent license renewal need be submitted.

2. The individual is not required to undergo periodic chemical testing if he or she provides satisfactory evidence that he or she has done one of the following:

        a.   Passed a preemployment or periodic chemical test for dangerous drugs within the previous six months

        b.   Been subject to a random testing program meeting USCG requirements during the previous 12 months, has not failed a chemical test for dangerous drugs, and has not refused to participate in required chemical tests

L. Random Testing

1. The Company shall provide for the selection of crew members for chemical testing for dangerous drugs on a random basis. Random selection of individ-

ual crew members means that every member of a given population has a substantially equal chance of selection on a scientifically valid basis. The testing frequency and the selection process shall be such that an employee's chance of selection continues to exist throughout his or her employment. Random selection may be accomplished by periodically selecting one or more vessels and testing all crew members aboard, provided each vessel subject to the Company's testing program remains equally subject to selection.

2. The Company may form or otherwise use sponsoring organizations or contractors to conduct random chemical-testing programs.
3. The Company shall ensure that crew members are tested on a random basis at an annual rate of not less than 50 percent.
4. An individual may not be engaged or employed, including self-employment, on a vessel in a position as master, operator, or person in charge for which a license or merchant mariner's document is required by law or regulation unless all crew members are subject to the random testing requirements.

M. Serious Marine Incident Testing

The Company shall ensure that all persons directly involved in a serious marine incident are chemically tested for evidence of dangerous drugs and alcohol in accordance with USCG requirements.

N. Reasonable Cause Testing

1. The Company shall require that any crew member who is engaged or employed on board a vessel owned in the United States that is required by law or regulation to engage, employ, or be operated by an individual holding a license, certificate of registry, or merchant mariner's document and who is reasonably suspected of using a dangerous drug be chemically tested for dangerous drugs.
2. The Company's decision to test must be based on a reasonable and articulable belief that the individual has used a dangerous drug based on direct observation of specific, contemporaneous physical, behavioral, or performance indicators of probable use. Where practicable, this belief should be based on the observation of the individual by two persons in supervisory positions.
3. When the Company requires testing of an individual under the provisions of this section, the individual must be informed of that fact and directed to provide a urine specimen as soon as practicable. This fact shall be entered in the vessel's official logbook, if one is required.
4. If an individual refuses to provide a urine specimen when directed to do so by the Company, this fact shall be entered in the vessel's official logbook, if one is required.

O. Records

1. The Company shall maintain records of chemical tests that the MRO reports as positive for a period of at least five years and shall make these records available to Coast Guard officials upon request. Records of tests reported as negative shall be retained for one year.
2. The records shall be sufficient to do the following:
   a. Satisfy the record-keeping requirements of the sections relating to Preemployment Testing and Periodic Testing
   b. Identify the total number of individuals chemically tested annually for dangerous drugs in each of the categories of testing, including the annual number of individuals failing chemical tests and the number and types of drugs for which individuals tested positive

IX.   Standards for Chemical Testing
of Employees Subject to DOT Testing

A.   Procedures
1.   Drug-testing programs shall be conducted in accordance with 49 CFR Part 40, Procedures for Transportation Workplace Drug Testing Programs. This section summarizes requirements for drug-testing programs contained in those regulations. Those regulations should be consulted to determine the specific procedures that must be established and used. Drug-testing programs required by this section shall use only drug-testing laboratories certified by the DHHS.
   a.   Collection site. The Company shall ensure that the collection site is adequate to provide for the collection, security, temporary storage, and shipping of specimens to a certified drug-testing laboratory.
   b.   Security. Procedures shall provide for the collection site to be secure. Collection sites dedicated solely to specimen collection must be secure at all times. Collection sites that are not dedicated solely to specimen collection must be secured during specimen collection.
   c.   Access to authorized personnel only. No unauthorized personnel shall be permitted in any part of a collection site when specimens are collected, nor shall unauthorized personnel be allowed access to specimens.
   d.   Privacy. Procedures for collecting urine specimens shall allow for individual privacy unless there is reason to believe that a particular individual may alter or substitute the specimen to be provided.
   e.   Integrity of specimens. Collection site personnel shall take precautions to ensure that each specimen is not adulterated or diluted during the collection process.
B.   Chain of Custody
1.   A chain of custody for each specimen to be chemically tested shall be established and maintained from the time of specimen collection through the testing of the specimen.
2.   If a specimen is not immediately prepared for shipment, it shall be safeguarded during temporary storage.
3.   Every effort shall be made to minimize the number of persons handling specimens.
C.   Specimen Handling and Shipping
1.   The Company shall obtain a specimen collection and shipping kit to be used to collect specimens and ship them to the certified drug-testing laboratory.
2.   The specimen collection and shipping kit, as required by 49 CFR Part 40, shall contain the following:
   a.   Plastic urine specimen bottles in a sufficient quantity to accommodate the people to be tested
   b.   Means for sealing and identifying specimen bottles
   c.   Chain-of-custody forms
   d.   A set of step-by-step instructions describing the proper procedures to be followed during specimen collection, handling, and shipping
   e.   Shipping materials
3.   The Company shall ensure that specimens are promptly shipped to a DHHS-certified testing laboratory. Chain-of-custody documents must accompany

each specimen from the time of collection through shipment to and testing by the laboratory.

    4. Specimens shall be shipped by an expeditious means.

D. Test Laboratory Requirements

    1. The Company shall ensure that all chemical testing for dangerous drugs required by this part is conducted by a DHHS-certified laboratory.

    2. The laboratory shall meet the requirements of 49 CFR Part 40.

E. Specimen Analysis

    1. Each specimen shall be analyzed in accordance with 49 CFR Part 40, which requires testing for marijuana, cocaine, opiates, PCP, and amphetamines.

    2. A specimen that indicates the presence of a dangerous drug at a level equal to or exceeding the levels established in 49 CFR 40.24 will be reported to the MRO as positive.

F. Specimen Analysis Reports

    1. The laboratory shall report all test results as required by 49 CFR 40.24(g). Reports are required to be made within an average of five days after receipt of a specimen by the laboratory.

    2. The laboratory will report as negative all specimens that are negative on the initial test or negative on the confirmatory test. Only specimens confirmed positive will be reported to the MRO for a specific drug or metabolite.

G. Medical Review Officer

    1. The Company shall designate or appoint an MRO meeting the qualifications of 49 CFR 40.27. The Company may choose to retain a qualified individual on staff to serve as MRO or contract for the provision of MRO services as part of the Company's drug-testing program.

    2. The MRO shall review and interpret each confirmed positive test result in accordance with 49 CFR 40.27.

    3. If the MRO verifies a laboratory confirmed positive report, the MRO shall report the positive test result to the designated Company official or to the Company's designated agent.

    4. Before an individual who has failed a required chemical test for dangerous drugs may return to work aboard a vessel, the MRO shall determine that the individual is drug-free and the risk of subsequent use of dangerous drugs by that person is sufficiently low to justify his or her return to work. In addition, the individual shall agree to be subject to increased, unannounced testing for a period as determined by the MRO of up to five years.

H. Release of Information

    1. Individual results from drug tests may be released if the individual tested signs a specific authorization for the release of the results to an identified person.

    2. Nothing in this section shall prevent an individual tested under this part from obtaining the results of that test.

X. Employee Assistance Program

The Company shall provide an Employee Assistance Program (EAP) for all crew members. The Company may choose to establish the EAP as a part of its internal personnel services or contract with an entity that will provide EAP services to a crew member. Each EAP must include education and training on drug use for crew members and the Company's supervisory personnel as provided below:

1. Each EAP education program must include at least the following elements:
   a. Display and distribution of informational materials
   b. Display and distribution of a community service hot-line telephone number for crew member assistance
   c. Display and distribution of the Company's policy regarding drug and alcohol use in the workplace
2. An EAP training program must be conducted for the Company's crew members and supervisory personnel. The training program must include at least the following elements:
   a. The effects and consequences of drug and alcohol use on personal health, safety, and the work environment
   b. The manifestations and behavioral cues that may indicate drug and alcohol use and abuse
   c. Documentation of training given to crew members and the Company's supervisory personnel; supervisory personnel must receive at least one hour of training

DRUG-TESTING POLICY FOR A MUNICIPAL GOVERNMENT

1. Policy

1.1 The City has a vital interest in maintaining a safe, healthful, and efficient working environment. Being under the influence of a drug or alcohol on the job poses serious safety and health risks to the user and to all those who work with the user. The use, sale, purchase, transfer, or possession of an illegal drug in the workplace and the use, possession, or being under the influence of alcohol also pose unacceptable risks for safe, healthful, and efficient operations.

1.2 The City believes it has the right and obligation to maintain a safe, healthful, and efficient workplace for all its employees and to protect the City's property, information, equipment, operations, and reputation.

1.3 The City recognizes its obligations to its citizens for the provision of services that are free of the influence of illegal drugs and alcohol and will endeavor through this policy to provide drug- and alcohol-free services.

1.4 The City further expresses its intent through this policy to comply with federal and state rules, regulations, or laws that relate to the maintenance of a workplace free from illegal drugs and alcohol.

2. Purpose

2.1 This policy outlines the goals and objectives of the City's drug- and alcohol-testing program and provides guidance to supervisors and employees concerning their responsibilities for carrying out the program.

3. Scope

3.1 This policy applies to all departments, all employees, and all job applicants, except that sworn employees of the Police and Fire departments may be governed by more restrictive policies that may be required by departmental rules and regulations.

4. Definitions

alcohol   Any beverage that contains ethyl alcohol (ethanol), including but not limited to beer, wine, and distilled spirits.

City facilities   See *City premises.*

City premises   All property of the City, including but not limited to the offices, facilities, and surrounding areas on City-owned or leased property, parking lots, and storage areas. The term also includes City-owned or leased vehicles and equipment wherever located.

contraband   Any article, the possession of which on City premises or while on City business, causes an employee to be in violation of a City work rule or law. Contraband includes illegal drugs and alcoholic beverages, drug paraphernalia, lethal weapons, firearms, explosives, incendiaries, stolen property, counterfeit money, untaxed whiskey, and pornographic materials.

drug testing   The scientific analysis of urine, blood, breath, saliva, hair, tissue, and other specimens of the human body for the purpose of detecting a drug or alcohol.

illegal drug   Any drug that is not legally obtainable; any drug that is legally obtainable but has not been legally obtained; any prescribed drug not legally obtained; any prescribed drug not being used for the prescribed purpose; any over-the-counter drug being used at a dosage level different from that recommended by the manufacturer or being used for a purpose other than that intended by the manufacturer; any drug being used for a purpose not in accordance with bona fide medical therapy. Examples of illegal drugs are Cannabis substances, such as marijuana and hashish, cocaine, heroin, phencyclidine (PCP), and so-called designer drugs and look-alike drugs.

legal drug   Any prescribed drug or over-the-counter drug that has been legally obtained and is being used for the purpose for which it was prescribed or manufactured.

reasonable belief   A belief based on objective facts sufficient to lead a prudent person to conclude that a particular employee is unable to satisfactorily perform his or her job duties due to drug or alcohol impairment. Such inability to perform may include, but is not limited to, decreases in the quality or quantity of the employee's productivity, judgment, reasoning, concentration, and psychomotor control, as well as marked changes in behavior. Accidents, deviations from safe working practices, and erratic conduct indicative of impairment are examples of reasonable belief situations.

safety-sensitive position   A position having any duty, the performance of which could cause injury to the incumbent or others or could cause serious damage to property.

under the influence   A condition in which a person is affected by a drug or alcohol in any detectable manner. The symptoms of influence are not confined to those consistent with misbehavior or to obvious impairment of physical or mental ability, such as slurred speech or difficulty in maintaining balance. A determination of being under the influence can be established by a professional opinion, a scientifically valid test such as urinalysis or blood analysis, and in some cases the opinion of a layperson.

5. Education

5.1   Supervisors and other management personnel are to be trained in the following areas:
   a.   Detecting the signs and behavior of employees who may be using drugs or alcohol in violation of this policy
   b.   Intervening in situations that may involve violations of this policy
   c.   Recognizing the above activities as a direct job responsibility

5.2   Employees are to be informed of the following:
   a.   The health and safety dangers associated with drug and alcohol use
   b.   The provisions of this policy

6. Prohibited Activities

6.1   Legal Drugs
   a.   The undisclosed use of any legal drug by any employee while performing City business or while on City premises is prohibited. However, an employee

may continue to work, even though using a legal drug, if City management has determined, after consulting with the City's health and/or human resources officials, that such use does not pose a threat to safety and that the using employee's job performance will not be significantly affected. Otherwise, the employee may be required to take a leave of absence or comply with other appropriate action as determined by City management.

b. An employee whose medical therapy requires the use of a legal drug must report such use to his or her supervisor prior to the performance of City business. The supervisor who is so informed will contact the City's designated human resources officials for guidance.

c. The City at all times reserves the right to judge the effect that a legal drug may have on work performance and to restrict the using employee's work activity or presence in the workplace accordingly.

6.2 Illegal Drugs and Alcohol

a. The use, sale, purchase, transfer, or possession of an illegal drug or alcohol by any employee while on City premises or while performing City business is prohibited.

7. Discipline

7.1 Any employee who possesses, distributes, sells, attempts to sell, or transfers illegal drugs on City premises or while on City business will be discharged.

7.2 Any employee who is found to be in possession of or under the influence of alcohol in violation of this policy will be subject to discipline up to and including discharge.

7.3 Any employee who is found to be in possession of contraband in violation of this policy will be subject to discipline up to and including discharge.

7.4 Any employee who is found through drug or alcohol testing to have in his or her body system a detectable amount of an illegal drug or alcohol will be subject to discipline up to and including discharge except that, depending on the circumstances of the case and the employee involved, the employee may be offered a one-time opportunity to enter and successfully complete a rehabilitation program that has been approved by the City. During rehabilitation, the employee will be subject to unannounced drug or alcohol testing. Upon return to work from rehabilitation, the employee will be subject to unannounced drug or alcohol testing for a period of five years. Any test that is confirmed as positive during or following rehabilitation will result in discharge.

8. Drug and Alcohol Testing of Job Applicants

8.1 All applicants for employment, including applicants for part-time and seasonal positions and applicants who are former employees, are subject to drug and alcohol testing.

8.2 An applicant must pass the drug test to be considered for employment.

8.3 An applicant will be notified of the City's drug- and alcohol-testing policy prior to being tested, will be informed in writing of his or her right to refuse to undergo such testing, and will be informed that the consequence of refusal is termination of the preemployment process.

8.4 An applicant will be provided written notice of this policy and will be required to acknowledge receipt and understanding of the policy by signature.

8.5   If an applicant refuses to take a drug or alcohol test, or if evidence of the use of illegal drugs or alcohol by an applicant is discovered through testing or other means, the preemployment process will be terminated.

9. Drug and Alcohol Testing of Employees

9.1   The City will notify employees of this policy by the following means:
   a. Providing to each employee a copy of the policy and obtaining a written acknowledgment from each employee that the policy has been received and read
   b. Announcing the policy in various written communications and making presentations at employee meetings

9.2   The City may perform drug or alcohol testing of the following persons:
   a. Any employee who manifests reasonable belief behavior
   b. Any employee who is involved in an accident that results or could result in the filing of a workmen's compensation claim
   c. On a random basis any employee who performs duties in a safety-sensitive position
   d. Any employee who is subject to drug or alcohol testing pursuant to federal or state rules, regulations, or laws

9.3   The City will conduct random drug and alcohol testing of a designated percentage of the work force at a frequency of once per month. Random selection will be performed through an unbiased computer-generated process.

9.4   An employee's consent to submit to drug or alcohol testing is required as a condition of employment, and the employee's refusal to consent may result in disciplinary action, including discharge, for a first refusal or any subsequent refusal.

9.5   An employee who is tested in a reasonable belief situation may be suspended pending receipt of written test results and whatever inquiries may be required.

10. Appeal of a Drug or Alcohol Test Result

10.1   An applicant or employee whose drug or alcohol test is reported positive will be offered the opportunity of a meeting to offer an explanation. The purpose of the meeting will be to determine whether there is any reason that a positive finding could have resulted from some cause other than drug or alcohol use. The City, through its health and/or human resources officials, will judge whether an offered explanation merits further inquiry.

10.2   An employee whose drug or alcohol test is reported positive will be offered the opportunity to do the following:
   a. Obtain and independently test, at the employee's expense, the remaining portion of the urine specimen that yielded the positive result
   b. Obtain the written test result and present it to an independent medical review at the employee's expense

10.3   The employee may use the City's medical benefits, to the extent that coverage may apply, for meeting the costs of 10.2(a) and (b).

10.4   During the period of an appeal and any resulting inquiries, the preemployment selection process for an applicant will be placed on hold and the employment status of an employee may be suspended. An employee who is suspended pending appeal will be permitted to use any available annual leave to remain in an active pay status. If the employee has no annual leave or chooses not to use it, the suspension will be without pay.

11. Rehabilitation and Employee Assistance

11.1 Rehabilitation assistance in lieu of discharge may be offered to the following persons:
    a. Any employee who has requested rehabilitation assistance, provided that the request is unrelated to an identification of the employee as a violator of this policy
    b. Any employee who has violated this policy, provided that the violation does not involve selling or transferring illegal drugs or serious misconduct

11.2 An employee who is in rehabilitation will be suspended, except that when indicated by the circumstances of the case and the written recommendation of a licensed physician or recognized rehabilitation professional, an employee may be permitted to work while undergoing rehabilitation on an outside-of-work basis. The written recommendation must include a statement to the effect that the employee's presence in the workplace will not constitute a safety hazard to the employee, coworkers, or others.

11.3 An employee whose rehabilitative therapy involves drug maintenance, hospitalization, or detoxification will not be considered for the exception from suspension described in 11.2.

11.4 An employee who is in rehabilitation or who has completed rehabilitation will be allowed to return to work upon presentation of a written release signed by a licensed physician or recognized rehabilitation professional. The release must include a statement to the effect that the employee's presence in the workplace will not constitute a safety hazard to the employee, coworkers, or others.

11.5 Rehabilitation assistance given by the City will be
    a. Limited to those medical benefits that may be available in the employee's medical benefits plan
    b. Obtained through a rehabilitation program that has been preapproved by the City
    c. Obtained by the employee during times that will not conflict with the employee's work time, except that the employee may use any available sick leave or annual leave to be absent from the job with pay

11.6 The City will provide to any employee, upon request and at no cost to the employee, information concerning local resources that are available for the treatment of drug- and alcohol-related problems.

12. Amnesty

12.1 Random drug testing will not be conducted during a period of 30 days immediately following the effective date of this policy. The purpose of an amnesty is to allow employees who are using drugs or alcohol to discontinue use without fear of detection by unannounced testing.

12.2 Amnesty will not apply to drug or alcohol testing of job applicants or to employees involved in reasonable belief situations.

13.   Inspections and Searches

13.1   The City may conduct unannounced general inspections and searches for drugs or alcohol on City premises or in City vehicles or equipment wherever located. Employees are expected to cooperate.

13.2   Search of an employee and his or her personal property may be made when there is reasonable belief to conclude that the employee is in violation of this policy.

13.3   An employee's consent to a search is required as a condition of employment, and the employee's refusal to consent may result in disciplinary action, including discharge, even for a first refusal.

13.4   Illegal drugs, drugs believed to be illegal, and drug paraphernalia found on City property will be turned over to the appropriate law enforcement agency, and full cooperation will be given to any subsequent investigation. Substances that cannot be identified as an illegal drug by a layperson's examination will be turned over to a forensic laboratory for scientific analysis.

13.5   Other forms of contraband, such as firearms, explosives, and lethal weapons, will be subject to seizure during an inspection or search. An employee who is found to possess contraband on City property or while on City business will be subject to discipline up to and including discharge.

13.6   If an employee is the subject of a drug-related investigation by the City or by a law enforcement agency, the employee may be suspended pending completion of the investigation.

14.   Confidentiality

14.1   All information relating to drug or alcohol testing or the identification of persons as users of drugs and alcohol will be protected by the City as confidential unless otherwise required by law or overriding public health and safety concerns or authorized in writing by the persons in question.

DRUG-TESTING POLICY PREPARED BY
REPRESENTATIVES OF THE BAKING INDUSTRY
IN CONCERT WITH TEAMSTER REPRESENTATIVES

WHEREAS, the Employer and the Union acknowledge that substance abuse is a serious and complex but treatable condition/disease that negatively affects the productive, personal, and family lives of employees and the stability of companies; and,

WHEREAS, the Employer and the Union are committed to addressing the problems of substance abuse to ensure the safety of the working environment, employees, and the public and to providing employees with access to necessary treatment and rehabilitation assistance; and

WHEREAS, the Employer and Union have defined a program of employee assistance and have provided coverage to ensure that employees requiring treatment and rehabilitation resulting from their substance abuse can receive such services without undue financial hardship;

NOW, THEREFORE, the Employer and the Union agree that,

1. Appropriate efforts will be undertaken by the Employer and the Union to establish employee understanding that the experience of alcohol or drug problems is not, of itself, grounds for adverse action. Employees will be strongly encouraged to seek and receive the services of the employee assistance program (EAP) prior to such problems' affecting job performance or resulting in on-the-job incidents.

    When the Employer has a reasonable suspicion based on objective criteria that an employee is under the influence of alcohol or drugs, hereinafter referred to as *substances*, the Employer may require that the employee immediately go to a medical facility to provide both urine and blood specimens for the purpose of testing and to receive a fitness-for-work examination by a licensed physician.

    Reasonable suspicion based on objective criteria means suspicion based on specific personal observations that the Employer's representative can describe concerning the appearance, behavior, speech, or breath odor of the employee. Suspicion is not reasonable, and thus not a basis for testing, if it is based solely on third-party observations and reports.

2. The requirement for this testing shall be implemented where practicable, in accordance with the following procedures:

    a. When the Supervisor has established suspicion that an employee may be under the influence of substance(s) based on specific, individualized observations, the Supervisor shall contact another Supervisor or management employee for purposes of confirming the reasonable suspicion. The Supervisor shall contact the Business Agent, Union Steward, or other bargaining unit employee for the purpose of informing and involving the appropriate and available Union representative in the immediate situation.

        In the presence of the employee and the Union representative, the Supervisor shall present the observations establishing the reasonable suspicion. The employee shall, upon hearing the Supervisor's confirmed observations, receive a written description of his or her rights, obligations, and options and shall be presented with the opportunity to self-refer to the EAP.

    b. While the observations of the Business Agent, Union Steward, or other bargaining unit employee may be solicited and are relevant in the context of the joint Employer/Union commitment to addressing the problem of substance abuse, Union representatives will not be expected to give their assent to the Supervisor's decision to require testing or to take other management action.

c. An employee who does not self-refer into the EAP and refuses to go to a medical facility after being informed of the observations establishing reasonable suspicion and of the requirement for immediate fitness for work examinations and provision of blood and urine samples will be discharged.

   If requested, the employee shall sign consent forms authorizing (1) the medical facility to withdraw a specimen of blood and urine; (2) the testing laboratory to release the results of the testing to the medical facility for physician review and to the Employer; and (3) at the employee's discretion, the same release as defined in (2) to the Union. By signing these consent forms, the employee does not waive any claim or cause of action under the law. An employee's refusal to sign the release shall constitute a refusal to be examined and tested, subject to Section 2d.

d. An employee who refuses to be examined and tested shall be encouraged to go to the medical facility for this purpose with the understanding that blood and urine samples drawn will not be tested unless that employee, within 24 hours, authorizes that these be tested.

   If, at the end of this period, the employee still refuses to have the samples tested, the employee will be discharged unless the employee agrees, within the same 24-hour period, to self-refer into the EAP.

e. The employee to be tested shall be taken to the medical facility by an Employer representative and at the request of the employee, the Business Agent, Union Steward, or other bargaining unit employee.

f. In an effort to protect individual privacy, employees will not be subject to direct observation while rendering urine samples. If the employee provides blood or urine samples that contain confirmed evidence of any form of tampering or substitution, the act shall constitute a refusal to be tested, and the employee shall be discharged.

g. Blood and urine samples shall be drawn subject to the provisions in Section 3 below. Upon receipt of the specimens by the laboratory, one of the two urine specimens will be placed immediately, unopened, in a locked freezer for storage for a period of six months. Employees may, within 24 hours of receipt of test results, request the presence of an approved, consulting toxicologist during the full conduct of a second, independent test to be conducted at the laboratory site. Employees requesting independent tests are liable for the costs of the second test and the consulting toxicologist unless the employee's second test results are negative.

   In cases of second tests, the urine specimen alone will be used, as this fluid better retains the integrity of its chemical contents. Because some drugs and drug metabolites deteriorate or are lost during freezing or storage, the retesting of specimens is not subject to the same testing level criteria as were used in the original analysis.

h. Employees subject to the requirement for testing shall be suspended, effective immediately after receipt of the fitness-for-work examination and rendering of samples, for the period of time required to process, screen, and confirm test results.

i. Employees whose test results are negative and who pass the fitness-for-work examination shall be reinstated with back pay for the period of suspension, except as provided in Section 4a. Employees whose test results are positive shall not be eligible for reinstatement with back pay but shall be given the opportunity to immediately self-refer into the EAP. In the absence of immediate self-referral, such employees will be discharged.

3. The examination and testing procedures and standards to be carried out by the medical facility personnel and testing laboratory shall be those adopted by the Employer and the Union, shall use the blood alcohol level established by state law for intoxication, shall rely in the testing for drugs other than alcohol on the urine specimen to test for the presence of drugs and/or their metabolites, shall consider presence only and not degree of intoxication or impairment, and shall include the following general components:

    a. Rigorous review, selection, and performance monitoring of medical facilities performing the examination and specimen collection of the laboratory facilities performing the tests

        (1) Medical facilities performing the examination and specimen collection must be under the direction of a licensed physician. The facility must employ at least one charge nurse who is a registered nurse.

            A licensed physician must perform the fitness-for-work examination and review the laboratory reports of drug tests. The physician must have knowledge of substance abuse disorders and must possess the appropriate medical training to interpret and evaluate all positive test results together with the employee's medical history, including medications used and any other relevant biomedical information.

            The medical facility must possess all necessary personnel, materials, equipment, facilities, and supervision to provide for the collection, security, temporary storage, and transportation (shipping) of blood and urine specimens to the drug laboratory. The medical facility must provide written assurances that the specimen collection space is secure; that chain-of-custody forms will be properly executed by authorized collection personnel upon receipt of specimens; that the handling and transportation of specimens from one authorized individual or place to another will be accomplished through the use of chain-of-custody procedures; and that no unauthorized personnel are permitted in any part of the specimen collection or storage spaces.

        (2) Laboratory facilities must comply with the applicable provisions of any state licensure requirements and must be approved by the union and/ or the parties to the agreement. Union approval of a laboratory shall be contingent on successful demonstration and on-site review establishing that the laboratory meets the standards for accreditation promulgated by the National Institute on Drug Abuse (NIDA) and on the laboratory's ongoing participation in a program of external quality assurance. These standards may be revised as recommended by the NIDA.

    b. Specific specimen collection procedures that include safeguards to ensure the employee's right to privacy

        Authorized specimen collection personnel shall request that the employee show positive identification by providing a pictured identification card such as a driver's license and shall ensure that the employee signs the waiver agreement that explains the procedures for testing and reporting results. These personnel shall remove all articles and items from the collection space or bathroom, shall make sure that toilet water is colored, shall turn off the hot-water valve under the sink, shall assume that the tamperproof specimen collection kit is intact, and shall instruct the employee to wash and dry his or her hands prior to entry. Employees shall remove all excess clothing and leave belongings outside the bathroom and shall provide urine samples in two containers. Employees will not be subject to direct observation while rendering samples. Authorized specimen collection personnel shall, however, be present outside the bathroom and shall receive containers, make sure that the quantity is sufficient for testing, check the color, and measure and record the temperature of each container. These personnel shall fill in specimen labels in the presence of the employee, cap and seal containers with evidence tape, and secure the employee's initials on the tape.

c. Flawless chain-of-custody procedures governing specimen handling throughout the testing process

Chain-of-custody procedures shall ensure that blood and urine samples not leave the sight of the employee until each vial has been sealed and initialed and that at least the following measures have been taken by medical facility and laboratory staff:

(1) Authorized medical facility personnel shall seal specimen tubes with evidence tape in the presence of the employee, and the employee shall initial the evidence tape. These personnel shall complete a chain-of-custody form and shall place the sealed and initialed specimen tubes, along with the chain-of-custody form and signed waiver, in the drug collection kit or box provided by the laboratory. The collection kit or box shall be sealed by authorized medical facility personnel, and this seal or tape shall be initialed by these personnel and by the employee.

The medical facility shall make prior arrangements for courier pickup of the specimens and ensure that all specimens are sent by courier or shipped to the testing laboratory as soon as possible. The medical facility shall ensure that no specimens will be shipped on a Friday or the day before a holiday and that any specimens held at the facility overnight shall be placed in a secured refrigerator until courier pickup.

(2) The testing laboratory shall ensure that personnel authorized to receive specimens open the package immediately, inspect the sealing tape for initials, and open the kit or box. These personnel shall examine and inspect the chain-of-custody form, the specimen tubes, and the kit or box to make sure that it conforms to the requirements of Subsection c(1). If these requirements are not met, the laboratory personnel shall immediately notify the laboratory's scientific director and document any and all inadequacies in the chain-of-custody requirements. The laboratory's scientific director shall immediately notify the medical facility, the Employer, and the Union of the inadequacies and retain the specimens in a locked freezer pending disposition directions.

If the requirements are met, authorized laboratory personnel shall sign on the appropriate line of the chain-of-custody form and deliver the specimen kit or box to authorized laboratory technologists for testing. Each technologist shall sign on the appropriate line of the chain-of-custody form.

All positive samples shall be resecured with evidence tape, signed, and dated by an authorized technologist. Upon completion of testing procedures, testing reports shall be prepared and signed by at least two authorized technologists for the review, approval, and signature of the scientific director.

d. Established levels below which specimens are deemed negative, as follows:

Drug Assay	Screening Cutoff Level
Blood alcohol*	100 mg/dl
Cocaine metabolite	300 ng/ml
Phencyclidine	25 ng/ml
Opiates	300 ng/ml
Amphetamines	1,000 ng/ml
Cannabinoids	100 ng/ml

*Subject to Section 3

e. Laboratory use of appropriate screening and confirmation procedures and technology

The laboratory shall ensure that each specimen will be screened by an immunoassay method—enzyme immunoassay (EIA), in this case EMIT; radioimmunoassay (RIA); or fluorescence polarization immunoassay (FPIA) for each drug or drug group. Each specimen also shall be analyzed for acid, neutral, and basic drugs by thin-layer chromatography (TLC). If either or both of these assays are positive, an intermediate screening procedure shall be performed by a second, authorized laboratory technologist using a more specific TLC procedure, an alternative second immunoassay method, or high-pressure liquid chromatography (HPLC).

Gas chromatography/mass spectrometry (GC/MS) must be used as the final confirmation method. All three tests must be positive before a specimen is reported as positive.

Blood and urine ethanol testing shall be performed by gas chromatography (GC). If the test is positive, a second GC column shall be used. If results are positive on both columns, an FPIA or EIA shall be used as the third and confirming test.

Final confirmation by GC/MS and/or FPIA shall be subject to the following levels, below which specimens are deemed negative:

Drug Assay	Confirmatory Cutoff Level
Blood alcohol*	100 mg/dl
Cocaine metabolite	150 ng/ml
Phencyclidine	25 ng/ml
Opiates	300 ng/ml
Amphetamines	300 ng/ml
Cannabinoids	300 ng/ml

*Subject to Section 3

Screening methods measure a group of drugs and/or their metabolites simultaneously. Confirmatory methods measure single and specific drugs and/or their metabolites. Cutoff levels for confirmatory methods may be lower than those for initial screening.

f. Procedures to ensure the confidentiality of test results and the treatment of these records as confidential health information or data

The laboratory shall ensure that testing reports, including the original chain-of-custody form, are mailed immediately to those personnel authorized by the medical facility, the Employer, and, if the employee so chooses, the Union and that, in the event that telephone reports of test results are required by the medical facility, the Employer, and the Union, a security code system be used to establish that results are being verbally reported only to those individuals authorized by the medical facility, the Employer, and the Union.

4. After examination and specimen testing results, the following shall apply:

a. If an employee is subject to discipline or termination under existing practices, he or she shall not use the substance abuse policy to circumvent the labor agreement or existing practices or to avoid discipline or termination.

b. In the cases not covered in Section 4a, the employee will have the opportunity for appropriate assistance, assessment, referral, treatment, and aftercare as provided in the EAP and as agreed in the EAP's individual treatment plan with the employee. Failure to seek and receive these services or failure to abide by the terms of the treatment plan shall be grounds for discharge.

c. An employee who seeks and receives assistance and who completes the defined EAP shall, upon return to work, be subject to random and mandatory tests for a period of nine months.

d. An employee who, on the basis of such random and mandatory tests defined in 4c, provides samples that contain positive and confirmed evidence of substances at or above the stipulated levels shall not be given a second opportunity to access the EAP as an alternative to discharge.

e. Employees who successfully complete the EAP and their individual treatment plan agreements and return to work will be encouraged to contact and avail themselves of the EAP's services on a self-referral basis whenever they desire ongoing assistance and support.

Employees who relapse, for whom reasonable suspicion of substance use is established a second time, and whose test results are positive will be subject to disciplinary procedures up to and including discharge. The Union and Employer may agree, however, to consider mitigating factors such as the employee's length of sobriety, job performance, and length of service in such situations.

5. The EAP shall include the following components:

a. Full clinical evaluation and appropriate assessment followed by a specific individual treatment plan and regimen for the receipt of counseling, treatment, aftercare, and related services subject to the ongoing monitoring of the EAP staff

b. Active encouragement and procedures for the voluntary self-referral of troubled employees to the EAP in cases in which reasonable suspicion has not been established and in which examination and testing procedures are not invoked

    c.   Assurances and procedures to protect the confidentiality of employees who voluntarily seek EAP services, as well as procedures governing the management of employee records such as medical information

6. Any disputes arising under this addendum shall be subject to the grievance procedure established in the labor agreement up to and including arbitration.

Appendix 3–B

A Checklist for Drafting a Policy

PERSONS AFFECTED BY THE POLICY

1. The policy will apply to

   [ ]   all employees.

   [ ]   some employees.
   If some employees, to which positions or classes of employees will it apply?

   _____

   _____

2. Is the rationale for making the policy applicable to some employees based on the fact that these employees perform safety-sensitive duties? If not, what is the reason for testing some but not all?

   _____

   _____

**CIRCUMSTANCES UNDER WHICH TESTING
WILL BE REQUIRED**

1. In which of the following situations do you want the policy to include drug screening?

   a.   Preemployment

   b.   Following an accident or near accident

   c.   When routine health evaluations are made

   d.   When behavior or performance suggests drug abuse

   e.   When employees are enrolled in drug rehabilitation

f. Periodically on a random selection basis

g. Periodically for all or selected employees

h. During or at the end of the probationary period

i. Upon return from a prolonged absence

j. During or following rehabilitation

k. Other _____

2. If you plan to conduct periodic screening, how frequently will you do it?

[ ] Monthly
[ ] Quarterly
[ ] Semiannually
[ ] Annually

3. What percent of the work force will be screened each time?

_____

EMPLOYEE RIGHTS

1. Will an employee's consent to drug testing be a condition of continued employment? _____

2. What disciplinary or adverse personnel action will result from the refusal to consent to a drug test by

a. a job applicant? _____

b. an employee? _____

c. a contractor employee? _____

3. The opportunities available for an employee to challenge or explain a positive drug test will include the right

a. to obtain a portion (that is, a split sample) of the urine so that it can be independently tested at the (employee's expense) (Company's expense).

b. to obtain the remaining portion of the urine specimen so that it can be independently tested at the (employee's expense) (Company's expense).

c. to a review of the test findings by a licensed physician with knowledge of substance abuse disorders at the (employee's expense) (Company's expense).

   d.   to a private meeting with designated Company officials.

   e.   Other _____

4.   If an employee's challenge or explanation of a positive drug test merits further inquiry, for the duration of the inquiry, the employee will be

   a.   suspended (with) (without) pay.

   b.   returned to work.

   c.   Other _____

NOTIFICATION TO EMPLOYEES

1.   The methods for notifying employees of the policy will include

   a.   giving to each employee a copy of the policy.

   b.   obtaining a written acknowledgment from each employee that the policy has been received and read.

   c.   sending memos, notices, and newsletters; posting notices on bulletin boards; performing other such services.

   d.   making presentations at employee meetings.

REHABILITATION

1.   Rehabilitation may be offered

   a.   when the employee has requested rehabilitation and the request is unrelated to an identification of the employee as a violator of the policy.

   b.   when the violation does not involve selling or distributing drugs or serious misconduct.

2.   The costs of rehabilitation will be

   a.   at no expense to the Company.

   b.   paid for by the Company only within the limits of the medical benefits provided in the employee's sick pay plan.

   c.   Other _____

3. Rehabilitation might be any of the following types. On the line to the right of each type, enter "Suspended" or "At work" to denote whether the employee will be suspended or will be allowed to work while undergoing that type of rehabilitation.

    a. Professional, nonmedical counseling on an outpatient basis

        _____

    b. Psychological or psychiatric counseling on an outpatient basis

        _____

    c. Daily outpatient drug maintenance _____

    d. Hospitalization _____

    e. Detoxification _____

4. The Company (has) (does not have) an employee assistance program (EAP) that provides

    a. information services only, such as the identity of local community resources available for the treatment of abuse-related problems.

    b. professional counseling on an in-house basis at no expense to the employee.

    c. professional counseling and treatment services that are linked to the medical benefits program.

    d. Other _____

ACTIVITIES PROHIBITED BY THE POLICY

Check or circle those activities that will be named in the policy as prohibited on the job or Company premises and will be subject to discipline. Also indicate the disciplinary action. Please use the verb *may* or *will* in each case.

1. Use of (illegal drugs) (alcohol)

        Discipline _____

2. Possession of (illegal drugs) (drug paraphernalia) (alcohol)

        Discipline _____

3. Sale of (illegal drugs) (drug paraphernalia) (alcohol)

    Discipline _____

4. Transfer or distribution of (illegal drugs) (drug paraphernalia) (alcohol)

    Discipline _____

5. Possession in the body system of any detectable amount of an illegal drug

    Discipline _____

6. Possession in the body system of alcohol at a level of (0.05) (0.10) as measured by a standard blood alcohol concentration test

    Discipline _____

AMNESTY PERIOD

An amnesty period allows employees who may be using drugs to discontinue use before a drug-testing program is put into effect. A 30-day period is standard.

1. The Company (wants) (does not want) to provide an amnesty period. The amnesty period desired is (30) (60) days.

INVESTIGATIONS

1. Under what circumstances will law enforcement be notified?

    _____

    _____

SEARCHES AND INSPECTIONS

1. Do you want the drug abuse policy to authorize searches of the workplace?

    _____

SPECIAL CONSIDERATIONS

1. Are you subject to the Federal Rehabilitation Act? _____

2. Are you subject to the Drug-Free Workplace Act of 1988? _____

3. Are any of your employees subject to federal drug testing? _____

4. Are any of your employees union workers? _____

MISCELLANEOUS

1. Will implementing procedures need to be developed? _____

2. Urine collections will be done

    a. by the direct observation method.

    b. by the dry bathroom method.

    c. by the modified dry bathroom method.

    d. using supplemental checks such as temperature measurement, color evaluation, and/or specific gravity. Specify. _____

3. What are the consequences if an applicant or employee refuses to provide a specimen or to cooperate?

    _____

4. What department in the Company will be assigned responsibility for administering the policy?

    _____

REVIEW

1. Does the policy provide clear guidelines to management, supervisors, and all employees? _____

2. Does the policy stress the importance of a safe and healthful working environment for all employees and make known the impact that drug abuse can have on job performance? _____

3. Does the policy require education of employees concerning the health and safety consequences of drug abuse? _____

4. Does the policy require training of supervisors and managers in how to recognize drug use and how to intervene? _____

5. Does the policy identify how and under what circumstances drug testing will be applied in enforcing the policy? _____

6. Does the policy inform contractors that they will be held accountable to following the same rules? _____

7. Does the policy identify any Company-paid medical benefits that are available for the treatment of drug abuse? _____

8. Does the policy identify any employee assistance benefits that may be provided by the Company? _____

Chapter 4

Educating Employees

This chapter examines the steps for developing a program to make employees aware of the specifics of the organization's drug policy and the general problem of drug use at work and in social settings. A variety of sample awareness materials appear as chapter appendixes.

Workplace drug abuse education is designed to develop or modify the attitudes and behaviors of employees concerning personal choices about using drugs. It encompasses a diverse spectrum of topics, activities, and media.

Many themes can be addressed in a drug abuse education program. Specific attention can be paid to the physiological and psychological effects of particular drugs. General themes can include the consequences of abuse on safety, the effects of drugs on fertility and pregnancy, the impact of drug abuse on the family unit, and the relationship between drugs and crime. A theme to be emphasized is the organization's drug abuse policy. The education program, together with a well-publicized policy announcement, will make clear the prohibited behaviors, the steps that will be taken to ensure that the policy is carried out, and the penalties that will be meted out to violators.

A punitive connotation is inescapably linked with explanations of policy. There is simply no way around the penalties, and any attempt to gloss over them will lead employees to believe that the policy will not be enforced. It does make good sense to counterbalance information about disciplinary action with positive information about management's concern for workers' safety and health and the well-being of their families.

The methods for developing employee awareness might include the following:

- Small conferences in which various employee groups view films, slides, and other audiovisual materials. Having an expert on hand to answer questions will add to the credibility of the presentation.
- Large group meetings. In addition to audiovisual materials and expert speakers, the agenda might include a message delivered personally by the chief executive officer (CEO) or a senior manager.
- Monthly bulletins distributed to employees at work or mailed to their homes. Each month the bulletin would feature a different drug-related

topic. There are several advantages to this approach: (1) it highlights management's concern over an extended period; (2) true learning or retention of knowledge is enhanced when information is presented in discrete, digestible portions; and (3) hard-copy materials that reach the home may help promote family involvement in preventing or resolving drug abuse problems.

- Distribution of an employee handbook on drug abuse.
- Wall posters, fliers placed inside paycheck envelopes, bumper stickers, display booths, and mobile display vans.

INITIAL PLANNING

A drug abuse education program requires a large measure of planning. It does not matter whether the program is big or small, new or old, or funded poorly or generously. Success and planning go hand in hand. A successful program will focus on real problems and identify measurable outcomes for evaluating program effectiveness.

Planning will take into account some important points about the nature of education in the workplace. The traditional methods of instruction to which we have all been exposed at school or college will have little value in educating adult workers.

Inherent in traditional methods of instruction is the notion that the student, presupposed to be a young person in compulsory attendance, should be provided with knowledge that will be useful throughout his or her lifetime. One problem with this approach is that the students in a drug abuse education program are not children; they are adults, and they need the information immediately. Traditional teaching methods continue to have substantial usefulness in teaching children, but they are simply not applicable to the learning needs of adults in a work setting.

BASIC ASSUMPTIONS

A successful drug education program is based on four main assumptions: self-concept, experience, readiness to learn, and orientation to learning.

Self-Concept

This assumption is that as a person grows older, he or she moves from a state of dependence on others to a state of increasing self-directedness. The point at which the individual achieves a self-concept of independence is the point at which childhood is psychologically cast aside. The individual sees himself or herself as being in control of his or her fate and will resist attempts by others to curtail that control.

We can observe that persons who enter the workplace are essentially self-directing. They know who they are, they know what they want, and they are in gainful employment because they made personal decisions that brought them there. In short, they are adults, and any attempt to treat them as children is certain to interfere with their learning.

Experience

This assumption is that as a person grows older, he or she collects a growing pool of personal experiences that serves as a valuable resource. At the same time, this pool of experiences provides the person with a reference point for new learning. Instructional techniques that build on experience are more likely to succeed than techniques that rely on blind-faith acceptance.

Readiness to Learn

This assumption is that as a person grows older, his or her readiness to learn undergoes a fundamental change. This readiness is no longer a function of parental demands and academic pressure but a function of what the person perceives as a requirement for achieving success in life. An adult wants to learn so that he or she can succeed in various roles, such as worker, spouse, and/or parent.

Orientation to Learning

This assumption holds that a child is conditioned to regard learning as something that will be applied later in life. An adult sees learning as an answer to a need that exists right now. The need in this case is to meet job responsibilities with respect to drug use, and the adult will regard such learning as a goal-directed activity.

Each of us follows or believes one or more theories about the process of learning. Ideas that seem to be based on common sense may get in the way of learning, and traditional methods may be ineffective in this context. Finding the correct combination of educational methods is a major challenge for the program administrator.

RESPONSIBILITY, AUTHORITY, AND SUPPORT

One of the first steps in developing a drug abuse education program is to identify the program's major functions and the cast of characters responsible for making it work. What will be the duties, and who will be designated to perform them? Which department will be responsible for managing the program? Who will be the accountable leader?

Responsibility can be assigned both generally and specifically. In the general sense, an organization might hold that a direct responsibility of all supervisors is to know the behavior cues of on-the-job impairment. A specific responsibility might require the safety manager to include a drug abuse prevention training module in the organization's accident-reduction efforts.

The assignment of specific responsibility needs to be done with care. In many instances, the program leaders and functionaries will see themselves as having a primary job, with the drug abuse education program as an added responsibility. This perception contributes to program failure. The preferred approach is to formalize program responsibilities by including them in job descriptions and performance rating schemes. When personal evaluation and reward are linked to program performance, individuals have a reason to invest a genuine effort in the program.

Accountability for program operations logically falls into one of four groups, with the other three playing support roles. These groups are the medical, human resources, safety, and security departments. The business necessity that justifies the existence of the program will be one factor in determining which department will have direct responsibility. Examples of business necessity are employee health, productivity, accident prevention, and protection of assets. No matter who is made responsible, it is important that the total organization be supportive. When program assignments are made by the senior executive, a strong commitment is demonstrated.

The actual and perceived authority of the program head will be determined by where the program fits in the organization's formal structure and to whom the program head reports. The program will be perceived as lacking authority if it is simply the appendage of a department or if the program head operates at several levels below the key decision makers. The degree of influence wielded by the program head also depends on his or her authority to spend and the amount of money allocated to the program budget.

The extent of support given to a drug abuse education program by employees is proportional to the program's official standing within the organization and the perceived value of the program to individuals. The first factor relates to formal responsibilities that designate the provision of support. The second factor operates in the context of personal benefit. Employees will support the program if they believe that it contributes to them personally. Examples of employee benefits are reduced fear of injury or death caused by drug-impaired coworkers and reduced conflict with coworkers whose personalities are negatively affected by drug use.

A PLANNING TEAM

A planning team can be very helpful in clarifying responsibilities and developing support within the organization. It also can serve in an evaluative and advisory capacity during program operation.

The core of the planning team should be representatives from departments that have direct and indirect (supportive) responsibilities for program operations. Other team members should be selected on the basis of functional disciplines related to drug abuse education, such as graphic arts and public affairs. Still other members may be chosen on the basis of interest. Large organizations that have substantial community interaction should include one or a few team members representing the local community.

A planning team can contribute creative ideas and objective opinions and can serve as a sounding board for program activities and projects. To the extent that members have been drawn from many groups, the team will be positioned to promote the program widely and garner support from a broad constituency. Perhaps the greatest contribution of a planning team is in identifying the kinds of problems that can and should be targeted by the drug abuse education program.

Targeting the Problems

It is easy to identify the general problems created by drug abuse in the workplace. Among these are increased accidents, low productivity, and absenteeism. It is not, however, easy to characterize the problems in terms of the organization's unique work processes, labor force, and culture. Is the problem related to the nature of the work? For example, is the work so boring or so demanding that employees find release in drugs? Are the workers drawn from neighborhoods where drug abuse is common? Has abuse been traditionally accepted or tolerated in the organization's industry?

Other information is needed as well. The planning team will want to know what kinds of drugs are being abused, which classes or groups of workers are involved, and where and when the abuse is occurring. The answers to these questions will help the team focus on targets that are meaningful to the organization.

Some of the answers can be found in the organization's own records and reports. Accident data, productivity numbers, and absentee rates are good indicators. Reports of incidents and disciplinary actions also can be revealing. A survey that guarantees the anonymity of responding employees can be an excellent information source.

Other sources might include local hospitals, community service agencies, law enforcement agencies, and the courts. These entities keep public records and deal with drug-related problems on a regular basis. Since the nature of the organization's drug abuse problem is likely to parallel that of the surrounding population, a drug use profile of the community can be very revealing.

Setting Goals and Objectives

Once the problems have been identified, the planning team can set goals and objectives. Specific steps in achieving those goals and objectives are developed later in the planning process.

A good way to differentiate between goals and objectives is to think of a goal as a place you want to get to and an objective as one stop along the route that will eventually take you to your destination. The goal is the outcome, and an objective is a step in the direction of the outcome.

The outcome, of course, is focused on problem solving. Let's assume that one of the problems identified by the planning team is the role of drugs in accidents in the assembly area of the plant. Since this is the problem, the goal or outcome would be to eliminate drug use by assembly workers. The objectives for achievement of this goal might include the following:

- Conduct drug abuse prevention classes for assembly workers.
- Conduct training sessions for assembly area supervisors that will teach them how to recognize impairment and how to intervene.
- Include in one issue of the newsletter a theme or major article dealing with drug abuse and assembly operations.
- Give an award to each assembly area workstation that maintains an accident-free record for one year.

Note that the objectives are tangible and measurable. For example, the first objective can be regarded as achieved when attendance records reflect that every assembly worker attended the class.

Each objective would have one or more action steps. The person charged with achieving the first objective might be expected to do the following:

1. Research the topic.
2. Develop a lesson plan.
3. Prepare transparencies for emphasizing key points.
4. Prepare handouts for distribution to attendees.
5. Show a film or videotape that supports the key points.
6. Prepare a record of attendance.
7. Prepare a critique form that will collect feedback from the attendees.

Action steps also can specify target dates and the persons who are responsible for completing the actions.

PROGRAM DESIGN

The program is still on the drawing board at this stage of development, but it is taking shape conceptually. Two main dimensions, utility and appeal, stand out. On the one hand, the program is intended to be a vehicle for reducing workplace drug problems, but on the other hand, it is meant to be appealing to employees and to motivate them.

In the design stage, information is collected concerning the attitudes, characteristics, learning abilities, and preferences of the people who are to be educated by the program. Too often, programs miss the mark because program content and the comprehension level of the audience are out of sync or the content message is at variance with the audience's preconceived notions. Young people, for example, may tune out messages that characterize marijuana use as being harmful to their health. Contrary messages are directed at them by their peers and in various media of the drug subculture. These kinds of problems must be anticipated and compensated for in the design of the program. The questions in Appendix 4–A can be used as a design checklist.

PROGRAM IMPLEMENTATION

Every organization has employee communication networks. The direction of transmission is both lateral and vertical—that is, from coworker to coworker and between supervisors and subordinates. Most networks are formal, such as the mechanisms for general memos and newsletters, but some are informal, such as the bowling team and Toastmasters group. The communication networks need to be identified and used for the benefit of the drug abuse education program. This is a practical and cost-effective approach, and it is certainly preferable to establishing a separate network.

The drug abuse message can be conveyed in many formats, including lectures, demonstrations, printed materials, employee service announcements, press releases, videotapes, newsletters, bulletin board notices, posters, general memos and letters, handbooks, guides, newspaper articles, displays, and speeches. The selection of a format or combination of formats will depend on the nature of the audience and the nature of the message. Size, age, composition, and knowledge level of the audience are important factors, along with topic length, production costs, and availability of resources.

Another important consideration is whether to produce program materials or acquire them from external sources. The advantage of having customized materials may be offset by significantly higher costs. The usual practice is to exploit in-house resources for materials that can be created inexpensively, to borrow and modify noncopyrighted materials from other organizations, and to purchase the remaining materials.

An approach growing in favor, especially in organizations subject to federal drug-testing regulations, is to engage the services of an outside consultant to deliver all or most of a drug abuse education program. The risk inherent in this approach is that the consultant's focus may not be on the organization's actual and important drug abuse problems.

INSTRUCTORS

Many program activities will involve presentations to groups, but not many programs will be blessed with a full complement of skilled speakers. In fact, the key players on the instructional staff will probably be volunteers from several departments and are not likely to be accomplished instructors.

The instructional staff is the backbone of an education program. If the instructors are incompetent, it will not matter whether the attending employees are bright and eager, the facilities first-rate, and the administration efficient.

Competency

An instructor's competency must be judged in two areas: (1) knowledge of subject and (2) ability to teach. If either area is deficient, the instructor's performance will be correspondingly deficient. Each of us at one time or another has been the victim of a knowledgeable instructor who, despite good intentions, was just not able to get the message across. An instructor who is weak in the subject but strong as a presenter is apt to be less noticeable. Through superior communication, a small amount of information can go a long way.

The exceptional instructor will be proficient in both subject matter and presentation. The average instructor will have a combination of strengths and weaknesses in each area, and the below average instructor will be significantly weak in at least one area. If the program administrator must use a below average instructor, the instructor's weakness should not be in topic knowledge. This problem cannot be corrected easily or quickly. Alternatively, the instructor who knows the topic but cannot teach very well will usually improve within a reasonable period of time. A certain amount of improvement will inevitably result from the teaching experience itself and from the process of instructors interacting with and learning from each other. But the most dramatic improvement will result from an instructor training course.

Training

An instructor training course is typically one or two weeks long and covers topics such as learning theory, instructional strategies and methods, learning aids, lesson plan writing, and development of practical exercises. A one-week course will provide only enough time to expose basic teaching concepts, whereas a two-week course will allow attendees to make one or more presentations using lesson plan materials, learning aids, and handouts developed while in the course.

There is nothing to prevent a program administrator from establishing instructor standards where none exist or from setting higher standards where minimums are demanded. An administrator who is satisfied with having no instructor standards or who chooses to operate at the minimum level will achieve mediocre results at best.

Preparation

Gathering material on the subject to be taught is the starting point for topic preparation. The sources include authoritative written references, ideas obtained from knowledgeable persons, and personal experience.

The instructor might begin by assembling all the personal knowledge he or she has concerning the topic. By writing this down on paper, the instructor can make a preliminary assessment of the material. This tentative grouping of ideas will help to reveal major gaps where research and collection of additional material are required.

The next move might be to draw on the experiences of others. A fruitful source is the subject matter specialist or expert who can provide up-to-date facts and firsthand testimony. Information obtained from knowledgeable persons will help the instructor clarify concepts and lead him or her toward an exploration of new sources.

The most abundant source is the library. Books, magazines, periodicals, journals, abstracts, microfilm, and other references can provide a large quantity of information. Note, however, that quantity is less important than quality. Accuracy and relevancy come first.

Once the information has been assembled, the next step is to evaluate it. Some ideas will need to be combined, while others can be reshaped or eliminated.

Topic preparation cannot be considered complete until a lesson plan or topic outline has been written. A well-constructed lesson plan will facilitate a good speaking presentation. By providing a structure for the delivery of ideas, the lesson plan helps the instructor make sure that the overall message is clear, each idea or teaching point supports the overall message, the teaching points flow smoothly and are in the correct order, and the topic can be presented in the allotted time. How well an instructor succeeds in presenting information will depend to a large extent on the fashion in which the information has been gathered and prepared.

PROGRAM EVALUATION

The purpose of evaluation is to ascertain whether the program is working. Evaluation is conducted along two lines: (1) to determine whether the goals and objectives established for the program are being achieved and (2) to determine whether the drug abuse problems addressed by the goals and objectives have lessened.

Recall the example given earlier about the drug abuse problem in the assembly area of the plant. The goal was to eliminate that problem, and the objectives were to give classes to the assembly workers, train the supervisors, prepare a newsletter article, and offer an incentive award. Were the objectives achieved? Were the action steps that composed each objective achieved?

These are documentable activities. The evaluation process will take note of what was done fully, partially, or not at all.

The critical answer comes in looking at the problem. Has drug abuse in the assembly area declined, stayed the same, or increased? This judgment can be reached by an examination of the same records that identified the problem.

It is instructive to observe that the first evaluation pathway measures efficiency and the second pathway measures effectiveness. Program efficiency is a reflection of how well the program functions according to plan. When objectives are met, the program is efficient but not necessarily effective. Program effectiveness is reflected by the extent of problem elimination.

This leads to another point. Although it is quite appropriate to apply education to the elimination of a drug-related problem, it is not appropriate to expect that education alone will solve the problem or even be helpful. The implication is that the evaluation process should encompass indicators that go beyond the parameters of education. It would not be correct to assume that a continued drug abuse problem in the assembly area is evidence of program failure. The problem may be too large or too entrenched to yield to a one-dimensional attack. In some circumstances, success may be impossible because of factors outside the program, such as management apathy or union resistance.

PROGRAM REVISION

Information gleaned from evaluation can be put to use in revising goals, objectives, and action steps. Change also might occur in response to the identification of new problems or the evolution of problems already targeted. In addition, revision might be dictated by resources. A drug abuse education program might expand or contract relative to financial and technological support and the availability of human expertise.

Programs that do not regularly undergo revision are not receiving the proper attention and are invariably unsuccessful. Dynamic programs are attuned to changing needs and adjust accordingly.

A drug abuse education program should be regarded as a long-range proposition. It would be a mistake to start a program with the intention of discontinuing it after the employees have been exposed to the program's main messages. Some programs begin with a flurry of activity and then quickly fade into oblivion. The starting point will always involve many activities, but they should be a foundation for follow-up education, not a one-shot effort.

ANNOUNCING THE POLICY

A policy can succeed only to the extent that it is understood by employees at every level. Announcement of the policy and its program for implementation is part of employee education and quite properly falls into that program area. The initial publicizing effort should be widespread, intense, and likely to involve a variety of forums and media. Long-term, ongoing policy education will be subdued in comparison but is equally important.

The usual avenues of publicity include internal memoranda, formal letters, bulletin board notices, newsletters, pamphlets, employee meetings, supervisor-subordinate conferences, orientation packets for new hires, and employee handbooks. Ultimately, the most effective means of making the policy known will be word-of-mouth communication among the employees.

A practical way of helping the grapevine to carry correct information is to provide each employee with his or her own information packet. Distribution can be through the company mail system, or the packets can be mailed with formal letters to employees at home. The latter approach provides an opportunity for the employee's family to be informed, which can be helpful, since drug abuse is frequently a family problem as well as a work problem.

The documentation used to announce a policy can include the policy itself, a letter from the CEO, a booklet that describes the policy, a guide for supervisors explaining how to enforce the policy, and factual information about the health and safety hazards of drug abuse, why management considers the policy necessary, and any employee assistance benefits that may be available.

Employees will view drug testing from many different perspectives. They may see it as illegal, intrusive, harsh, unnecessary, needed, long overdue, responsible, or caring. Management can gain greater acceptance of drug testing if it is presented as a safeguard for health and safety. The overall posture should be preventive rather than adversarial because the goal is for all employees to be safe, not for some employees to be caught and punished. The punitive aspects of drug testing cannot be ignored, but emphasizing management's concern for employees can facilitate the program's acceptance.

The objectives of announcing a policy are to make the employees aware of an important new rule and to obtain their cooperation. The controversial nature of drug testing is likely to stand in the way of efforts to make the policy understood. A technique for dealing with this problem is to distribute a list of questions and answers with the policy. The questions should be those that many employees are likely to ask. Appendix 4–B contains a sample list of some appropriate questions and answers about drug testing.

If you are concerned that a few employees will fail to get the message no matter how extensive the publicity, you can require that each employee return, through normal supervisory channels, a signed form acknowledging receipt and understanding of the policy. New employees can sign the form as part of the orientation process. The sample materials in Appendix 4–C can be used to make the policy known to employees and others.

If you want to include specific information about the effects of drug use, you might distribute one or more drug bulletins such as those contained in Appendix 4–D.

Appendix 4–A

A Program Design Checklist

LEARNING ABILITIES

1. In what form can the information be effectively presented? Written? Oral? Pictorial? Demonstration? Film?
2. Will learning be affected by the size or composition of the audience? Should particular topics be presented in small group meetings?
3. What is the maturity level of the audience? Should the same topic be presented in different ways for different audiences, such as line workers, supervisors, staff specialists, managers, and executives?

ATTITUDES AND BEHAVIORS

1. Will the audience be apathetic, hostile, friendly, curious, reserved, or supportive?
2. Would it be helpful to use outside presenters?
3. What can be designed into the program to counteract anticipated attitudinal problems?
4. What steps will be taken in response to disruptive behavior?

AUDIENCE ACCESSIBILITY

1. What is the best way to reach the audience? Should meetings be set up solely for the program, or should the program be put on the agendas of regularly scheduled meetings?
2. How many meetings will be needed to reach all members of the audience?
3. If accessibility is difficult, can the message be delivered through videotapes or some other medium?

KNOWLEDGE LEVEL

1. What does the audience already know about the topic? Is that knowledge likely to help or hinder the program?
2. At what level of understanding can a presentation begin without being repetitive?
3. Should lengthy or complex topics be taught in successive modules, each building on and interrelating with the others?

Appendix 4–B

Drug-Testing Questions and Answers for Employees

1. Will testing cover just drugs or drugs and alcohol?

   Depending on the circumstances, testing could include drugs, alcohol, or both.

2. Exactly what types of samples are involved?

   Drug testing will involve urine samples. Alcohol testing may involve breath, saliva, and/or blood samples.

3. How will the tests be made?

   For drug detection, a fully certified laboratory will do a two-step urinalysis. The first step is to examine the urine specimen using a highly sensitive screening technique. A positive test result on the first test will lead to a second test called a confirmation test that uses an even more accurate and reliable technique. Alcohol detection will be done by saliva or breath tests, with confirmation of positive results by blood analysis when possible.

4. How accurate are the drug tests?

   The screening technique will consist of an immunoassay test that has been found to be 96 to 98 percent accurate. The confirmation test is by gas chromatography/mass spectrometry (GC/MS), which is even more accurate. When both tests are used to examine a specimen, accuracy is as close to 100 percent as science permits.

5. What drugs may be looked for in the urinalysis?

   Cannabinoids (such as marijuana and hashish), cocaine, opiates (such as heroin, morphine, and codeine), amphetamines (called uppers), barbiturates (called downers), benzodiazepines (such as Valium and Librium), methaqualone, and phencyclidine (PCP).

6. Will a test show positive for a person who has been exposed to smoke from another person's marijuana cigarette?

   No. A person who has innocently inhaled someone else's marijuana smoke will not show traces of marijuana at a detectable level.

7. What about drugs that are prescribed by a physician?

    At the time you give a specimen, you will be asked to identify any over-the-counter or prescription medicines recently taken. The analytical procedure will take this information into account.

8. What does *for cause* mean?

    A for-cause situation is one in which an employee might be requested to take a drug test. Two examples of such a situation are (1) when an employee's behavior affects safety, is destructive to property, equipment, or the work environment, or is an immediate threat to the Company's reputation; and (2) when an employee demonstrates recurring behavior or performance problems and substance abuse is believed to be a factor.

    An employee will always be tested when involved in a reportable accident while operating company equipment or in an on-the-job accident. A near miss in which substance abuse is indicated also would require drug testing.

9. Will an individual be fired for refusing to be tested?

    Failure to cooperate with a properly authorized request for testing will be considered grounds for termination. The actual disciplinary action taken in a specific instance will depend on the circumstances and the seriousness of the situation that triggered the need for the test.

10. What happens to an employee who tests positive?

    The employee will be subject to disciplinary action, up to and including discharge.

11. Will the extent of employee testing be expanded in the future?

    Prior to developing this program, management carefully considered national statistics on drug use, the experience of other companies that have testing programs, and our own experience with incidences of drug use. We don't think we have an abnormal problem, but we are part of a society in which substance abuse is becoming more commonplace. We feel our program, as presently constituted, is sound and reasonable. If, over time, the level of substance abuse proves to be greater than first thought, consideration will be given to other options, including a more aggressive testing effort involving increased periodic sampling.

12. Why is there an amnesty period?

    The amnesty period will allow time for a drug-abusing employee to rid his or her body system of drugs prior to any testing the Company may choose to conduct.

13. Who will have access to drug test records and results?

    Drug test results will be treated as confidential information.

14. What is a medical review officer (MRO)?

    An MRO is a licensed physician who has knowledge of substance abuse disorders and has appropriate medical training to interpret and evaluate an individual's medical history and any other relevant biomedical information. The MRO receives laboratory results and makes sure that any positive result could not have occurred because of a legally prescribed medication or some other innocent explanation.

15. Could this policy be used to discriminate against employees?

We don't believe so, and we are committed to keeping that from happening.

Appendix 4–C

Sample Policy Announcements and Acknowledgment Forms

ANNOUNCEMENT OF POLICY BY MEMORANDUM

TO: All Employees

FROM: Office of the CEO

SUBJECT: Announcement of Drug and Alcohol Abuse Policies

As I am sure you are aware, the abuse of drugs and alcohol has become widespread in the United States and has received a great deal of recent publicity. The problem is no longer confined to a relative few but has expanded into all areas of our lives, including our schools and workplaces, both urban and rural. Substance abuse affects all of us. Its cost is staggering in terms of increased health risks, personal injury, property damage, family and social problems, and reduced productivity on the job. We would be naive to think that our Company is insulated from this problem.

Because of our concern for the safety of our employees, our property, and the public and our concern about the productivity of our work force, the Company has adopted two new corporate policies—one on drug abuse and one on alcohol abuse—that will be applicable to all U.S. dollar payroll employees. Our purpose in adopting these policies, which restate the Company's long-standing prohibition against the presence of drugs and alcohol in our offices and workplaces, is to further the Company's goal of establishing and maintaining a work environment free from the adverse effects of drug and alcohol abuse.

In connection with the above policies, a formal drug- and alcohol-testing program will begin 30 days from the date of this letter. Under this program, drug and alcohol tests will be included in all preemployment medical examinations. In addition, current employees who are required to take mandatory medical examinations will be tested for drugs and alcohol on an annual basis. Expatriate employees and their dependents will be tested for drugs and alcohol in connection with initial transfer outside the United States and during mandatory annual medical examinations because of the significant risks associated with drug use in many foreign countries and the detrimental consequences of drug and alcohol abuse to an expatriate community. Voluntary periodic medical examinations will not include testing for drugs and alcohol.

Annual drug and alcohol testing for employees required to take physical examinations has been adopted because these employees, by the nature of their jobs, could pose an immediate safety risk to themselves, fellow employees, property, and/or the general public by working under the influence of drugs and alcohol. In addition, employees who, in the judgment of management, may be working under the influence of drugs and alcohol will be subject to a medical examination that includes drug and alcohol testing without notice. This includes employees who are not part of the annual testing program. As in the past, if an employee's performance is deteriorating, management may require the employee to undergo a medical examination. Beginning 30 days from the date of this letter, such examinations will include drug and alcohol testing.

The policies also provide that the Company may conduct inspections, as well as medical examinations, at its discretion to determine whether an employee is in violation of the policies. Such actions will not be undertaken indiscriminately but only when there is a reasonable suspicion of a violation.

The Company has taken the position that all alcohol abuse and drug abuse is undesirable and not to be tolerated, whether or not that abuse/use results in impaired performance on the job.

We are aware that for those individuals who engage in the occasional use of illicit drugs on their own time, adoption of these policies may lead to positive test results and the consequences spelled out in the attachments, even though that occasional use may not appear to interfere with their work performance or safety on the job. We believe that the weight of available evidence suggests that the use of alcohol and/or drugs by employees will, over time, increase our risk of accidents and adversely affect our overall productivity. Neither of these potential consequences is acceptable to us.

The Company believes that this program addresses a legitimate business concern and is sensitive to the issue of employee privacy. One laboratory will analyze all samples Company-wide and will retain those that test positive. The laboratory uses state-of-the-art technology, ensuring the accuracy of test results. A sophisticated drug test with a 100 percent accuracy rate has been specifically chosen to avoid the false-positive error rate that has been described in many newspaper and magazine articles concerning industrial efforts to detect drug use in the work force. (A *false positive* refers to test results indicating the presence of drugs or alcohol when in fact the individual has not used illicit drugs or alcohol.)

Since the drug- and alcohol-testing programs are designed to detect use of those substances and positive results will be dealt with through the administration of appropriate disciplinary actions, I encourage any employee with a drug or alcohol problem to get help now rather than wait for a positive test result. If you have a problem, I urge you to contact the Medical Department now.

I hope you will join me in supporting the Company's objective of attaining a workplace free from the adverse effects of drug and alcohol abuse. We will all be well served when this objective is accomplished.

If you have any questions about this program, please contact your supervisor.

BULLETIN BOARD NOTICE

The use, transfer, possession, or sale of illegal or unauthorized materials on the premises of the Company or at any workplaces on which the Company has contracted to perform its work IS PROHIBITED. The intent is to maintain a safe and healthy work environment for employees and other personnel at the workplace and to protect Company property and other property for which the Company is liable. Searches of individuals and their personal effects, lockers, and vehicles may be conducted at such times and places as necessary to obtain compliance.

Prohibited articles include stolen and misappropriated Company property and materials, illegal and unauthorized drugs, alcoholic beverages, firearms, explosives, weapons, and hazardous substances or articles.

Illegal drugs include, but are not limited to, marijuana, heroin, cocaine, and prescription drugs (in the possession of the individual but not prescribed by a licensed physician for use by the individual). Unauthorized drugs include excessive quantities of prescribed drugs that may adversely influence performance or behavior.

If any of the above prohibited articles are found, the individual possessing the articles will be subject to disciplinary action. Any of the above articles discovered through searches will be taken into custody, when appropriate, and may be turned over to the proper law enforcement authorities.

Authorized personnel may conduct the searches without prior announcement and at such times and places on premises or work locations as considered appropriate by the Company. Urine samples may be requested in conjunction with the searches. Entry onto premises or work locations is consent to, and recognition of, the right of the Company and its authorized representatives to conduct the unannounced searches and to obtain urine samples for analysis.

Your cooperation and assistance are requested to help reduce accidents and pilferage and to make our workplaces as safe as possible.

LETTER TO CONTRACTOR CONCERNING DRUG ABUSE POLICY

Date

Contractor's name
Address
City, State, Zip

Dear Sir or Madam:

This is to inform you of our Company's drug abuse policy. The policy applies to contractor employees as well as our own employees.

The simple observance of the policy, as set forth below, will help ensure the continued well-being and safety of all personnel and property. Adherence is mandatory, and violation of it by any of your employees will not be tolerated. The policy states the following:

> The use, possession, sale, transfer, or being under the influence of illegal drugs or other intoxicants on Company premises or while conducting Company business is forbidden.

Violations of this policy by an employee of a contractor will be cause for immediately removing and barring that contractor's employee from any Company premises.

To enforce this policy, the Company may at any time conduct searches upon its premises. Searches may include but not be limited to persons, personal effects, and personal vehicles wherever located on Company premises. Refusal by persons in your employ to cooperate or submit to searches will be cause for immediately removing and barring such persons from any Company premises.

Entry by any person into Company premises constitutes consent to and recognition of the right of our Company and its authorized representatives to conduct searches.

We request that you inform your employees of this policy before they are assigned to our premises or facilities and require their strict compliance with it.

Please acknowledge acceptance of these conditions by signing and dating the original copy of this letter and returning it to us without delay. A duplicate copy is provided for your records.

Sincerely,

Signature of company official

Receipt and acceptance of the terms and conditions of this letter are acknowledged.

_____   _____

(Date)   (Signature of contractor official)

NOTICE TO JOB APPLICANTS CONCERNING DRUG TESTING

Why Do We Ask Job Applicants to Take Urine Tests?

Many people who work for us are assigned duties that if not properly performed, can result in serious consequences to the employee personally, fellow employees, and the Company. Among these serious consequences are injury or even death.

It is a well-known fact that drug abuse can severely impair a person's ability to perform properly. The Company has an obligation to provide a safe and efficient environment. Urine testing for drug abuse is one of the steps the Company is taking to meet that obligation.

If this is a new experience for you, you may be nervous and a little concerned. Please be assured that the persons who collect and test the urine specimens are professionals. They will respect you as a person and will reveal test results only to the Company. Giving a urine specimen is simple, takes little time, and involves no discomfort.

Your urine collection appointment is scheduled for:

Time _____   Date _____

Place _____

If you have taken any medication in the past 14 days, bring it to the collection appointment in its original container.

Also bring a form of personal identification that bears your photograph.

If an emergency prevents you from keeping the appointment, please call:

Name _____   Phone number _____

EMPLOYEE'S ACKNOWLEDGMENT OF POLICY BY MEMORANDUM

TO: (Employee's Supervisor)

FROM: (Employee)

SUBJECT: Acknowledgment of Policy

    I,_____, have read and understand the Company's policy concerning contraband such as firearms, alcoholic beverages, and illegal drugs. I also understand that this policy will be enforced and that personal searches, blood tests, urine tests, and/or polygraph tests may be used to enforce the policy.

    I understand completely that disciplinary action may be taken in the event I possess, use, or distribute contraband at a Company work location.

    I further understand that disciplinary action may be taken if I refuse to be searched or to cooperate with detection procedures.

_____   _____

Signature   Date

_____   _____

Witness   Date

ACKNOWLEDGMENT OF DRUG ABUSE POLICY BY AN EMPLOYEE

TO: (Employee's Name)

Please sign and return this form to your immediate supervisor.

Acknowledgment

By my signature below, I acknowledge that I have received, read, and understand the Company's policy concerning drug abuse.

_____   _____

(Date)   (Employee's signature)

ACKNOWLEDGMENT OF DRUG ABUSE POLICY BY A NONEMPLOYEE

I understand that in the interest of providing a safe and efficient environment for employees, contractors, and other nonemployees, the Company has and enforces a policy designed to control drug abuse on Company premises.

I understand that this policy is implemented from time to time by a variety of reasonable means. Such means include searches of persons, personal effects, and personal vehicles entering, on, or departing Company premises. The Company may also require nonemployees on Company premises to provide urine specimens for drug-testing purposes.

I understand that any nonemployee who declines to be searched or declines to provide a urine specimen may be escorted from the Company's premises, barred from reentry, and excluded from any future participation in Company operations.

I have read this policy (or it has been explained to me), and I understand the provisions of it that apply to me as a nonemployee on Company premises or engaged in Company business. I agree to comply with this policy and understand that compliance is a condition of my being permitted to be on the Company's premises or my participation in Company operations.

_____   _____
(Date)   (Signature of nonemployee)

_____   _____
(Employer of nonemployee)   (Printed name of nonemployee)

ACKNOWLEDGMENT OF DRUG TESTING BY
AN EMPLOYEE

I acknowledge receiving and reading the notice of the Company's drug-testing program. I understand the following points:

- I may be selected for drug testing.
- A refusal on my part to cooperate in the drug test or to provide a specimen for testing may subject me to discipline up to and including discharge.
- A confirmed positive drug test result will subject me to discipline up to and including discharge.

_____

(Printed or typed name)

_____

(Signature)

_____

(Date)

ACKNOWLEDGMENT OF SEARCH POLICY

In the interest of maintaining a safe and efficient environment for employees and nonemployees, including contractors, subcontractors, vendors, suppliers, visitors, and invitees, the Company has and enforces a policy designed to control drug abuse on Company premises and in connection with Company business.

The Company administers a search program to ensure compliance with its drug abuse policy. Accordingly, you may from time to time be asked to submit to a search of your person, personal effects, or personal vehicle while entering, on, or departing Company premises or while performing Company business. An employee who fails to cooperate or declines to submit to a search when requested may be subject to disciplinary action, including discharge. A nonemployee who fails to cooperate or declines to submit to a search may be escorted from Company premises, barred from reentry, and barred from future participation in Company business.

A written statement of this policy is attached or is prominently displayed at Company premises. You are urged to carefully read and gain a full understanding of it prior to signing this consent.

Employee or Nonemployee Response

I have read and understand the Company's policy provisions regarding searches. I agree to comply.

_____   _____

(Date)   (Signature)

_____   _____

(Signature of witness)   (Printed name of consenter)

[ ] Employee   Department _____

[ ] Nonemployee   Employer _____

Appendix 4–D

Sample Drug Bulletins

COCAINE

What Is It?

Cocaine is a stimulant drug extracted from the leaves of the coca plant. It appears in four forms. As a powder, cocaine is commonly inhaled (snorted), sometimes eaten, and sometimes dissolved to a liquid form and injected. In its so-called freebase form, cocaine is smoked or inhaled. As crack, it is usually added to tobacco, marijuana, or some other leafy substance and smoked in a pipe or as a cigarette. The fourth form is coca paste, a crude product that is used mostly in South America. It is smoked and may be especially dangerous because it almost always contains contaminants such as kerosene, which can cause lung damage.

What Does It Look Like?

Cocaine looks like a white crystalline powder and is often diluted with other ingredients. Crack looks like light brown or beige pellets or crystalline rocks that resemble coagulated soap. It is often packaged in small vials.

Powdered Cocaine

The most common form of this drug is cocaine hydrochloride, a fine white crystal-like powder. This form of cocaine is sometimes glamorized as a drug of the rich and famous.

Freebase

Freebase, or cocaine base, is a variant of cocaine hydrochloride. It is converted from the powder form to a highly concentrated purified form that can be smoked. The inhaled vapors enhance the effect because the drug's active ingredient moves directly and quickly to the brain. Since freebase is very potent, the risk of overdose is high. Another risk relates to the preparation method. The chemicals used to convert cocaine hydrochloride are highly volatile and flammable, creating hazards during the conversion process.

What Are the Effects?

Its effects are felt within ten seconds of administration. They include euphoria, restlessness, excitement, and a feeling of well-being. Because it stimulates the central nervous system, cocaine causes dilated pupils, increased pulse rate, elevated blood pressure, insomnia, and loss of appetite, in addition to tactile hallucinations, paranoia, and seizures. As with amphetamines, users tend to go on binges, and chronic heavy use can lead to a paranoid condition in which the user is highly suspicious or nervous. Cocaine use may lead to death through disruption of the brain's control of heart rate and respiration.

These drug bulletins were adapted with permission from a publication of Forward Edge, Inc., Houston, Texas.

CRACK

What Is It?

Crack is a purified form of cocaine that is smoked by inhaling the vapors that are given off as the drug is heated. Crack is processed and sold in small vials and is in the form of small chunks that can be smoked in a marijuana roach, a regular cigarette, or a special pipe usually made of glass. The drug gets its name from the crackling noise it makes when heated.

Purity

When ordinary cocaine is converted to crack, its purity increases greatly. Powdered cocaine—the type that is snorted—is generally 15 to 25 percent pure. Crack can be as much as 90 percent pure.

Method of Use

Smoking the drug magnifies the intensity of the user's reaction. Inhaling the crack vapors brings the drug directly into the lungs, where it is quickly absorbed into the bloodstream and carried to the brain in a highly concentrated form.

What Are the Effects?

Crack creates a reaction in 4 to 6 seconds and lasts 5 to 7 minutes. In contrast, snorted cocaine takes effect in 1 to 3 minutes and lasts 20 to 30 minutes. The short, intense high is followed fairly rapidly by depression. This seems to account for the many cases of users taking crack continuously until they run out of money or require medical help.

Dangers

The dangers of crack include the following:

- It enters the bloodstream in massive amounts, greatly increasing the risk of death by overdose.
- The anesthetic qualities of crack conceal serious lung damage.
- Repeated use of crack causes paranoia, hallucinations, and violence.
- Crack users have been found to lose weight, develop skin problems, experience convulsions, and have difficulty breathing.

CANNABIS (Marijuana)

THC

The chief psychoactive (mind-altering) ingredient in marijuana is tetrahydrocannabinol, or THC. In comparison to alcohol on a molecule-for-molecule basis, THC is 10,000 times stronger in its ability to produce intoxication. In recent years, the strength of marijuana has increased markedly. In 1975, samples exceeding 1 percent THC content were rare; by 1980 a 5 percent content was common; and today it is not unusual for street marijuana to contain 7 percent THC.

What Does It Look Like?

Marijuana looks like dried parsley mixed with stems and seeds.

What Are the Effects?

Most users of marijuana experience an increase in heart rate, reddening of the eyes, and dryness in the mouth and throat. Studies of marijuana's mental effects have revealed that the drug temporarily impairs short-term memory, alters the user's sense of time, and reduces the ability to perform tasks requiring concentration, swift reactions, and coordination. Many feel that their hearing, vision, and skin sensitivity are enhanced by the drug, although these reports have not been confirmed by research. The most commonly reported immediate adverse effect is acute panic anxiety reaction. This is usually described as an intense fear of losing control and going crazy.

Because users often inhale the unfiltered smoke deeply and then hold it in their lungs as long as possible, marijuana smoke is highly irritating and carcinogenic. Physical dependence on marijuana has been demonstrated in research subjects who ingested an amount equal to smoking 10 to 20 marijuana cigarettes a day. When the drug was discontinued, the subjects experienced withdrawal symptoms consisting of irritability, sleep disturbances, loss of appetite and weight, sweating, and stomach upset.

Research shows that the effects of marijuana can impair thinking, reading comprehension, verbal skills, and arithmetic skills. Researchers also believe that the drug may interfere with the development of social skills and may encourage escapism.

PHENCYCLIDINE (PCP)

What Is It?

Phencyclidine, or PCP, was developed in the late 1950s as a surgical anesthetic. Because of its unusual and unpleasant side effects in human patients (delirium, extreme excitement, and visual disturbances), PCP was restricted to use as a veterinary anesthetic and tranquilizer.

What Are the Effects?

The effects of PCP vary according to dosage levels. Low doses may provide the usual releasing effects of many psychoactive drugs, such as a floating euphoria and a feeling of numbness. Increased doses produce an excited, confused intoxication, which may include muscle rigidity, loss of concentration and memory, visual disturbances, delirium, feelings of isolation, convulsions, speech impairment, violent behavior, fear of death, and changes in perception.

Research shows that PCP seems to scramble the brain's ability to process external stimuli, altering how the user perceives and deals with the environment. Everyday activities, such as driving or even walking, can be an overwhelming task for the PCP user.

Is PCP Dangerous?

PCP intoxication can produce violent and bizarre behavior even in mild-mannered people. Violence may be directed at themselves or others and often accounts for serious injuries or death. Bizarre behavior by PCP users has produced deaths by drowning, burning, falling from high places, driving accidents, and overdoses.

A temporary, schizophrenic-like psychosis, which can last for days or weeks, also has occurred in users of moderate and higher doses. During a psychotic episode, the user may be excited, incoherent, and aggressive or exactly the opposite—uncommunicative, depressed, and withdrawn. Paranoia, a state in which a person feels persecuted, will often accompany a psychotic episode.

LSD

What Is It?

LSD is a man-made, or synthetic, hallucinogen. It is usually manufactured as a white, odorless powder and taken orally. LSD is an acronym for lysergic acid diethylamide. It is derived from ergot, a fungus.

Basically, LSD causes changes in sensation. Users have described changes in vision, depth perception, and the meanings of perceived objects. The person's sense of time and self are altered. The user may see music or hear color.

Physical reactions range from minor changes such as dilated pupils; a rise in body temperature, heartbeat, or blood pressure; tremors; and unconsciousness. The effects vary greatly according to the dosage, the personality of the user, and the conditions under which the drug is used.

What Does It Look Like?

LSD can be found as brightly colored tablets, impregnated blotter paper, thin squares of gelatin, and clear liquid.

Is It Mind-Expanding?

Although some users have claimed they feel more creative after taking LSD, these claims are not supported. In fact, LSD may reduce the motivation to work, thus reducing creativity.

What Are the Dangers?

After taking LSD, a person loses control over his or her normal thought processes. Although some perceptions are pleasant, others may cause panic or may make a person believe that he or she cannot be hurt. The long-term harmful reactions include anxiety, depression, and breaks from reality that may last from a few days to months.

The exact relationship between LSD and emotional disruption is not known, but it is suspected that when a person has suffered from an emotional disturbance prior to using LSD, the drug may cause a breakdown. Research has shown some changes in the mental functions of heavy users of LSD and some signs of organic brain damage.

PEYOTE, MESCALINE, AND PSILOCYBIN

What Are They?

These three substances are hallucinogens. They affect perception, sensation, thinking, self-awareness, and emotion. Changes in time and space perception, delusions, and hallucinations may be mild or overwhelming depending on dose and quality of the drug taken. Effects will vary from one person to another and from one occasion to another. Because hallucinogens affect the mind, they are sometimes called psychedelics.

What Do They Look Like?

Mescaline and peyote take the form of brown disks, tablets, or capsules that may be chewed, swallowed, or smoked. Psilocybin is always in its natural mushroom form and is taken orally.

Peyote

Peyote is a small cactus that grows wild in the northeastern part of Mexico and the Rio Grande valley of Texas. The dried bulb of the plant, called a peyote button, induces a psychedelic effect on the user. There has been very little illegal use of peyote because it has an obnoxious taste and causes nausea. It has been used by Mexican Indians for hundreds of years in ritual ceremonies.

Mescaline

Mescaline is a chemical extracted from peyote buttons, and its effects are similar to those of LSD. It is obtainable in gelatin capsules, as a powder to be mixed with water, or as a liquid.

Psilocybin

Psilocybin is an active ingredient of the psilocybin mushroom (grown in Mexico) and, like peyote and mescaline, is used in traditional Indian rites. When eaten, these sacred or magic mushrooms affect mood and perception in a manner similar to LSD. Another active ingredient of this mushroom is psilocyn, and both can be synthesized chemically.

INHALANTS

What Are They?

Inhalants are a group of diverse breathable substances that can be sniffed or inhaled. These are legal substances, and many of them are found in everyday household products.

Aerosols

Anything in an aerosol can, especially spray paint, is a likely product for abuse.

Other commonly abused spray products are vegetable oil and hair spray.

Toluenes

The compound toluene is found in gasoline, transmission fluid, model airplane glue and other glues, nail polish, nail polish remover, and a variety of ordinary substances found around the house.

Nitrites

Amyl nitrite is used for treating heart patients. When placed under the patient's nose, the blood vessels dilate and the heart beats faster. It is sold in a cloth-covered plastic bulb. When the bulb is broken, it makes a snapping sound (thus the nickname snapper or popper). Butyl nitrite also affects blood pressure and heart rate and is abused for the instant rush it gives.

Other Inhalants

Other inhalants include nitrous oxide (laughing gas), dry-cleaning fluids, anesthetics such as halothane, and room deodorizers.

What Are the Effects?

Although there is no single inhalant syndrome, there are common negative effects from using inhalants. They include nausea, sneezing, coughing, nose-bleeds, fatigue, lack of coordination, and loss of appetite. Solvents and aerosol sprays also may decrease the heart and respiratory rates and impair judgment. Amyl and butyl nitrite cause rapid pulse, headaches, and involuntary passing of urine and feces. Long-term use may result in weight loss, fatigue, electrolyte imbalance, and muscle weakness. Repeated sniffing of concentrated vapors over time can lead to permanent damage of the nervous system.

What Are the Risks?

There is a high risk of sudden death from spray inhalation because the spraying effect can either interfere directly with breathing or cause irregular heartbeats. The risk is increased when the fumes are sniffed from a paper bag. This is because they are in a highly concentrated form as a result of not being allowed to mix freely with the open air.

AMPHETAMINES

What Are They?

Amphetamines, or uppers, are drugs that stimulate the central nervous system, producing an increase in alertness and activity. Two trade names stand out: Dexedrine and Benzedrine.

Tolerance

Because tolerance often develops, the user will take increasingly large doses to achieve the desired result. Hallucinations can occur with excessive use. For example, a driver who takes Benzedrine to reduce sleepiness while driving runs the risk of an accident by reacting to something that is not there.

Dependence

A person who takes amphetamines on a regular basis develops a dependence that is extremely difficult to break. The user will often get caught up in a cycle of ups and downs in which alcohol or sleeping pills are consumed to relieve the insomnia that accompanies amphetamine use. Upon waking, the user will pop a few more pills in order to regain the high.

What Are the Health Risks?

Even small, infrequent doses can have toxic effects on some people. Restlessness, anxiety, mood swings, panic, circulatory and cardiac disturbances, paranoid thoughts, hallucinations, convulsions, and coma have been reported.

Heavy, frequent doses can cause brain damage, which results in speech problems and difficulty in turning thoughts into words. Taking amphetamines by injection greatly increases the risk, especially the risk of overdose.

Amphetamines can accumulate in the user's body over a period of time, resulting in a poisoning of the system. This toxic condition can cause amphetamine psychosis, an extremely paranoid and suspicious state of mind.

DEPRESSANTS

What Are They?

Barbiturates are depressant drugs. In small doses, they are effective in relieving anxiety and tension. In large doses, they are used to induce sleep. Certain barbiturates are used to treat epilepsy and for intravenous anesthesia. When large doses are not followed by sleep, signs of mental confusion, euphoria, and even stimulation similar to that produced by alcohol may occur.

Potentiation

Barbiturates are often used recreationally by persons seeking effects similar to those produced by alcohol. These persons often combine the two. Because alcohol potentiates, or increases, the barbiturate effects, this practice is extremely hazardous. Users also take them in combination with or as a substitute for other depressants, such as heroin. They are often taken alternately with amphetamines, as they tend to enhance the euphoric effects of amphetamines while calming the overwrought nervous states they produce. In large doses, barbiturates can cause severe poisoning, deep comas, respiratory and kidney failure, and death.

Dependence

How much and how often these drugs are taken determine how fast the user develops tolerance and whether physical withdrawal symptoms will occur. Barbiturate withdrawal is often more severe than heroin withdrawal. People who have difficulty dealing with stress or anxiety or who have trouble sleeping may overuse or become dependent on barbiturates.

Babies born to mothers who abuse depressants may be physically dependent on the drugs and show withdrawal symptoms shortly after they are born. Birth defects and behavioral problems have been associated with these children.

Barbiturates Kill

Barbiturate overdose is implicated in nearly one-third of all reported drug-induced deaths. Accidental deaths may occur when a user takes an unintended larger or repeated dose because of confusion or impairment in judgment caused by the initial intake of the drug.

NARCOTICS

What Are They?

Opiates, sometimes called narcotics, are a group of drugs that are used medically to relieve pain, but they also have a high potential for abuse. Some opiates come from a resin taken from the seed of the Asian poppy. This category of opiates includes opium, morphine, heroin, and codeine. Other types of opiates are synthetically or chemically manufactured.

What Do They Look Like?

Heroin is usually in the form of a white to dark brown powder. It also can be found as a tarlike substance. Codeine is found in tablets, capsules, and a dark liquid varying in thickness. It is sometimes in household medications such as cough medicines and pain relievers. Morphine can be found as white crystals, hypodermic tablets, and solutions. Opium is usually in the form of dark brown chunks or powder.

What Are the Effects?

Opiates tend to relax the user. When injected, the user feels an immediate rush. The user may go on the nod, moving back and forth from alertness to drowsiness. With very large doses, the user cannot be awakened, pupils become smaller, and the skin becomes cold, moist, and bluish in color. Breathing slows down, and death may occur.

Addiction

Dependence is very likely, especially when a person takes large doses or even small doses over an extended period. When a person becomes dependent, finding and taking the drug becomes the main focus in life. As more and more of the drug is taken over time, larger amounts are needed to get the same pleasant effects.

What Are the Dangers?

The physical dangers depend on the specific opiate used, its source, the dose, and the way it is used. Most of the dangers are caused by taking too much of the drug at one time, using unsterile needles, contamination of the drug itself, or combining the drug with other substances. Opiate users may eventually develop infections of the heart lining and valves, skin abscesses, and congested lungs. Infections from unsterile solutions, syringes, and needles can cause illnesses such as liver disease, hepatitis, and tetanus.

DRUG MYTHS

Drugs have been and probably always will be surrounded by myth. Many widely held beliefs about drugs and users have been proved untrue. Over the years, false claims have been made for many drugs. Heroin and cocaine have been called nonaddictive but are in fact highly addictive. LSD and peyote have been called mind expanders but work more like mind destroyers. Marijuana has been touted as a sex enhancer, but evidence shows that it reduces sexual desire and fertility. Marijuana is also commonly referred to as a benign or nondamaging drug even though it has been linked to a variety of medical problems.

What Is Known

The short-term effects of drugs on a user reflect both physical and physiological factors. These include the types and quantities of drugs consumed; the user's personal level of tolerance; the method of taking (swallowing, injecting, or inhaling); and the user's state of mind at the time of consumption. The immediate impact on a user will vary according to the factors. For example, a healthy individual who swallows a small amount of LSD at a party may experience no immediate health damage. If, however, the user is depressed or takes a larger dose, there is a risk of mental breakdown.

The immediate outcomes of drug use may include the user's passing out, experiencing mood changes, engaging in violence, suffering perceptual distortions, and losing control of body functions. These conditions make a person unable to judge time and distance, make sensible decisions, and operate vehicles or machinery. In such circumstances, a user poses a danger to himself or herself and those around him or her.

The long-term effects come with repeated and intensified use. Drug addiction is destructive and costly to the user, his or her family, and society.

MARIJUANA AND FERTILITY

Medical research found that female users of marijuana had defective menstrual cycles three times more frequently than a similar group of nonusers. The defective cycles involved either a failure to ovulate or a shortened period of fertility. These findings suggest that regular marijuana use may reduce fertility in women.

Laboratory tests using female monkeys, whose reproductive organs are very similar to those of humans, showed that THC-treated monkeys were four times more likely than untreated monkeys to abort or have stillborn infants. In addition, males born of the THC-treated monkeys weighed less than average at birth. Scientists believe that marijuana has a toxic effect on embryos and fetuses.

Studies of adult males have found that chronic users have lower levels of testosterone (the principal male sex hormone) than nonusers and that abstention after heavy use reversed the condition. Other research has shown that the sperm count diminishes as marijuana use increases and that some of the sperm of chronic users are defective and nonfunctional.

Other Dangers

Burnout is the term used to describe the effect of prolonged marijuana smoking. Burned-out users are dull, slow moving, and inattentive. They are sometimes so unaware of their surroundings that they do not respond to normal conversation. This form of mental impairment may not be completely reversible.

Marijuana use increases the heart rate as much as 50 percent depending on the amount of THC. It brings on chest pain in people who have a poor blood supply to the heart.

Marijuana can be particularly harmful to the lungs because users typically inhale the unfiltered smoke deeply and hold it for as long as possible, thereby keeping the smoke in contact with lung tissue.

DRUGS AND DRIVING

The effects of a drug vary greatly from one individual to another and even in the same individual at different times. A driver's age, sex, weight, and emotional state, as well as the amount of drug taken and when it was taken, are all factors that influence the ability to drive safely. Taking two drugs at a time is very dangerous because one drug can increase the effect of the other. This is especially true when one of the drugs is alcohol.

Alcohol and Caffeine
Alcohol works as a sedative. It affects judgment and coordination and is a factor in more than half of all U.S. highway deaths. Alcohol increases the sleep-inducing effects of tranquilizers and barbiturates. Mixing these drugs while driving is often fatal.

Caffeine, which is supposed to help the drowsy driver stay alert, cannot make a drunk driver sober. At best, it will change the person from a drowsy drunk to a wide-awake drunk.

Marijuana
This drug can greatly reduce a driver's ability to react, stay in the correct lane around curves, and maintain the proper speed and distance relative to other vehicles. A normal level of driving performance is not regained for at least 4 to 6 hours after smoking a single marijuana cigarette, and recent research has shown that this effect may last for up to 24 hours.

Depressants and Stimulants
Librium, Valium, Dalmane, and Quaaludes are examples of depressants that even in small doses will slow reaction time and interfere with hand-eye coordination and judgment. Mixing alcohol with a depressant can double the effect.

Amphetamines (such as Benzedrine and Dexadrine), cocaine, phenylpropanolamine, and ephedrine are examples of stimulants. Repeated use of stimulants to overcome fatigue will result in a loss of coordination.

Chapter 5

Training Supervisors

The kind of learning discussed in this chapter, as in the previous one, has no relevance to the formal systems of public and private education. I am not proposing that companies place supervisors in a formal classroom and engage them in a long-term program of learning. What I am proposing is a two-tiered approach. On one level, management would bring the supervisors into policy development by soliciting their ideas, involving them in the planning and design of the drug-testing program, using them as facilitators in the organization's drug awareness efforts, and placing them on committees or task forces charged with addressing drug abuse. On the second level, management would use formal training as a mechanism for providing supervisors with the knowledge and skills they need to work toward a drug-free workplace.

Supervisors who learn to carry out their drug policy responsibilities through active involvement in the shaping and implementation of policy will have a better understanding of, and a stronger commitment to, management's policy goals. This form of experience-based learning is produced through performance of the supervisory functions described elsewhere in this book. I will not discuss experiential learning in this chapter except to say that it is powerful, takes hold quickly, and lasts a long time. The primary focus here is on learning that is a product of planned and organized training.

Chapter 4 discusses drug abuse education for employees. Supervisors and managers also are employees and are included in the same target audience for promoting general awareness. But they have knowledge needs that go beyond general awareness. They are the leaders who provide the guidance and sanctions for ensuring policy adherence by others. The learning that results from the awareness program can serve as a foundation for training supervisors and managers.

THE NATURE OF LEARNING

Learning, which is the desired outcome of training, refers to behavioral changes that result from the student's exposure to knowledge and experience. In this case, the student is a supervisor, the knowledge is information concerning antidrug program responsibilities, and the experience is the opportunity to apply that knowledge in training and in a real-life working environment. Learning can be observed in changes in a person's thinking, action, and emotional response. These three types of behavior are generally called knowledge, skill, and attitude, respectively.

Knowledge is an awareness of facts, principles, meanings, concepts, ideas, and relationships. The pattern of an individual's thinking, performing, and responding emotionally are conditioned by knowledge. The probability that a supervisor will intervene when an indicator of drug use occurs is a function of whether the supervisor (1) recognizes the indicator, (2) knows the actions he or she is required to take, and (3) cares enough to act. Knowledge is, therefore, supportive of behavior. A conscious act by a supervisor to intervene can occur only if the supervisor knows what he or she is expected to do and has a willingness to do it.

Skill refers to both physical and mental abilities. Manipulating the hands, running, and jumping are physical skills. Mental skills include problem solving, analysis, critical thinking, judgment, and synthesis of ideas. Mental skills are more important in this context because the tasks that are assigned to supervisors are largely cognitive. These tasks include recognizing the drugs of abuse and the associated paraphernalia, recognizing the physiological and psychological effects of drugs on human performance, analyzing factual situations in which drug use may be involved, and making decisions. Counseling problem employees, making referrals to treatment, and conducting follow-up evaluations of employee performance also are mental skills.

Attitude refers to the manner in which behavior is carried out. Knowledge and skill may make it possible for a supervisor to perform a task in a prescribed way, but attitude influences whether the supervisor will perform it badly, well, or not at all. Negative attitudes reveal themselves in their interference with performance. For example, a supervisor who has a personal dislike of drug testing is likely to have an unfavorable attitude toward tasks related to drug testing.

THE TRANSFER OF KNOWLEDGE

A first step for the training administrator is to define the knowledge that must be imparted to the supervisors who will be responsible for carrying out the policy. One of the best ways to articulate such knowledge is through the use of training objectives. Following are some examples of training objectives:

- State the reasons for and the goals of the company's drug abuse policy.
- Name the responsibilities assigned to supervisors in the company's drug abuse policy and antidrug program.
- Recognize the physical appearance and characteristics of the major types of abused drugs and the paraphernalia associated with their use.

- Identify the performance and behavioral indicators of drug impairment.
- Identify the actions to take and not to take when intervening in an on-the-job situation that may involve a violation of the company's drug abuse policy.
- Explain the procedures required to be followed in reasonable cause and postaccident testing situations.
- Define the terms *reasonable cause, illegal drugs, under the influence, detectable amount,* and *consent required,* as well as other concepts related to the antidrug program.

Training objectives will vary from company to company. The above examples can serve as a good starting point in developing a curriculum for the training program.

Note that training objectives state clearly what is expected of the training administrator and the students. Note also that the objectives are amenable to evaluation. For example, if the objective is for the student to define *reasonable cause,* attainment is demonstrated when the student provides the definition. The mode of expression can be oral, in writing, or through a practical exercise that involves application of the concept.

THE BODY OF KNOWLEDGE

Training objectives also provide guidance as to the body of knowledge needed to support the training process. For the objectives listed previously, the training administrator would need to assemble materials relating to a body of knowledge that incorporates the company's drug abuse policy; procedures that support execution of the policy; antidrug program materials such as supervisor guides and employee handbooks; pictorial and written descriptions of the major types of abused drugs and drug paraphernalia; pictorial and written descriptions of the performance and behavioral indicators of drug impairment; and definitions of key concepts.

Drug-Testing Issues

Perhaps the most important and controversial issue is drug testing. The supervisor's instruction is not complete without imparting an understanding of the major issues in drug testing. Supervisors usually enter training with questions about why, when, and how testing will occur. Appendix 5–A addresses a number of drug-testing issues in a question and answer format. This material can be a valuable part of supervisory training.

Definition of Terms

The body of knowledge should include a definition of terms and concepts that may be unfamiliar to students. The training administrator should identify these early in the instruction process. Because learning depends on clear communication, the students must understand the basic terms of reference. The glossary at the end of this book can be helpful in preparing lesson plans and handouts. Following are some concepts that are particularly important to the training of supervisors.

Reasonable Cause

The terms *reasonable cause, reasonable belief, just cause, proper cause,* and *for cause* generally mean the same thing. The term *probable cause* is a law enforcement or legal term similar to reasonable cause but much more precise and demanding in its application.

The term *reasonable cause* is often used in the context of searching for evidence of an offense. A search is said to be reasonable when it is based on a good-faith belief, amounting to more than mere suspicion, that evidence of a certain offense can be found on a particular person or at a particular place.

The term *unreasonable cause* is often used to describe a search conducted when there are no facts that would lead a prudent person to believe that evidence of an offense will be found on a person or in a particular place. An example would be a search of an employee's locker for the purpose of finding anything that could be used against the employee.

In the context of drug testing, a reasonable cause situation involves observed actions that indicate an employee's use of a controlled substance. A decision-making model is applied to the observed action to help the intervening supervisor make the correct decision. The decision-making model takes the supervisor through a process of analysis that poses critical questions such as the following: Are the observed actions capable of explanation and substantiation? Are they specific, contemporaneous, and tangible? Are they associated with probable drug use? When all the answers are clearly yes, drug testing is the appropriate course of action.

Two Supervisors Rule

The purpose of this rule is to increase the level of confidence in a decision to test in a reasonable cause situation. The rule calls for two supervisors who have knowledge of the facts to decide whether to refer the employee for testing. Both or at least one of the supervisors should have received training in how to make a reasonable cause determination.

Consent to Test

Under this concept, which carries the force of law, no person may be forcibly compelled to provide biological specimens. An employer does, however, have the right to terminate an employee who refuses to provide a specimen when requested to do so. The employer's right must be supported by prior notice that a consent to test is a condition of employment.

Search with Implied Consent

A search with implied consent is a search conducted as a condition of employment or as part of an employment contract, such as a union contract. Conditions of employment and employment contracts frequently express or imply the consent to search employees and their belongings.

Implied consent searching is usually based on the belief that an injurious outcome can be reasonably expected to occur in the absence of a regularly conducted search program. For example, an injurious outcome could be an explosion or a fire in the workplace. The search program would be justified because of the need to ensure that ignition devices and impaired workers, whose judgment or lack of motor skills might contribute to an explosion or fire or might detract from the proper emergency response, are excluded from the workplace.

A search within an implied consent program is more along the lines of an inspection. Implied consent does not rely on the existence of reasonable belief. There need not be an incident or offense for an implied consent search.

Contraband

In the strict legal context, contraband is any item that is illegal to have in your possession. Untaxed whiskey, illegal drugs, stolen property, pornographic materials, military explosives, and counterfeit money are contraband. All of these are prohibited from the workplace because possession of them places the possessor in violation of the law. An employer will sometimes include in its definition of contraband other prohibited items, such as firearms and knives.

Amnesty

An amnesty provision usually accompanies the announcement of a drug abuse policy. The period of amnesty is typically not less than 30 and not more than 60 days. Essentially, management pledges to forgo drug testing for a period of time sufficient for any drug-abusing employee to get clean.

Amnesty does not usually apply in cases where the policy offense is other than merely having drugs in one's body system. Selling, possessing, and distributing drugs or drug paraphernalia would not qualify for amnesty.

Detectable Amount

This term relates to scientific studies that have shown lingering effects of drug impairment in persons who consumed drugs several days previously. An employer who adopts the detectable amount rule is saying that any employee who is found to have a detectable amount of an illegal drug in his or her body system is in violation of the company's policy and is subject to discipline.

Chain of Custody

A very important concept relates to the procedures that are followed to document how and by whom a specimen is handled from the time it is taken from the individual, processed in the laboratory, and placed in protective storage. This record is referred to as the chain of custody.

A failure to properly monitor the collection of a urine specimen can result in actions by the donor to substitute a false specimen, contaminate his or her fresh specimen, or switch specimens with another donor. Other problems related to chain of custody include mislabeling and cross-contamination of specimens due to carelessness and poor packaging.

THE PRINCIPLES OF SUPERVISION

A supervisory training program need not focus entirely on the specifics of the company's drug policy and practices. The specifics must be covered, but the training program also may include some general concepts about the nature of supervision. A broad approach that addresses leadership responsibilities may help supervisors to conceptualize management's goals for a drug-free workplace and to make the connection between those goals and day-to-day supervisory activities. Following are some examples of principles that can be included in the supervisors' training curriculum.

Seek Respect Rather Than Popularity

A supervisor should not accept favors from subordinates or perform special favors to be liked. A popular decision can be a resounding success when correct but an absolute disaster when wrong. Discipline should be applied when needed, and it should be applied fairly and evenly across the board. The supervisor should not socialize with subordinates, but he or she should show warmth, humor, and a concern for them as persons.

Involve Subordinates in Problem Solving

Subordinates should be made to feel that drug abuse problems manifested by a few members of the work group are problems for all members. They can be asked to give advice and help. By making it easy for subordinates to communicate their ideas, the supervisor will make them feel as though they are part of the solution. The ideas they contribute should be acted on to the extent they lead to a positive solution and conform with the company's rules.

Make Criticism Constructive

When something goes wrong, a supervisor should not automatically make assumptions about the cause and who is at fault. The best thing a supervisor can do is to bring his or her personal emotions under control, remain calm, and get all the facts before taking action. When criticism is appropriate, it should be used not as a punishment but as a learning tool to prevent recurrence of the problem.

Criticism combined with praise rarely offends and can be effective in achieving positive change without damaging a subordinate's personal dignity. Along this same line, a supervisor should never diminish the employee's worth in the eyes of his or her colleagues. This will make it harder for the employee to retain his or her status within the work group.

Consistency in the evaluation of employees is an absolute must. Any appearance of favoritism or discrimination in the manner of dealing with problems in work performance is unforgivable and can lead to a multitude of problems for the supervisor.

Pay Attention to Complaints

Employees should feel free to talk with their supervisors and not have to cut through a lot of red tape to air their complaints. A good supervisor will always grant a hearing, exercise patience, listen carefully, find out what the individual wants done, explain the grievance process, and get all the facts. In addition, the supervisor should not render a hasty judgment but should let the individual know his or her decision as soon as possible. The underlying concept is to show concern when subordinates are concerned.

Let People Know Where They Stand

People like to know what is expected of them, and they feel cheated when they are not told as early as possible of any changes that will affect them. A new drug abuse procedure can be a major source of worry for employees. A supervisor needs to communicate the need for drug abuse prevention procedures and how the procedures affect employees personally.

Enforce the Rules

Part of a supervisor's job is to see that policies and procedures are carried out. If a supervisor has reason to believe that an employee is in violation of the rules concerning drug abuse, the supervisor is obligated to take the specified action.

Know How to Obtain Help

A subordinate who appears to have a drug problem is in need of professional attention. The best service that a supervisor can provide for the employee and the company is to resolve the drug problem through early referral to medical diagnosis and treatment. Knowing how to obtain the appropriate medical help is the first step in moving the employee toward it.

A drug-abusing employee whose unacceptable performance has drawn supervisory attention often will want the supervisor to keep the abuse to himself or herself. The employee may admit abuse in the hope that the supervisor will agree to forgo action. The supervisor should never agree to this because the longer he or she puts off obtaining specialized help, the more difficult it will be for the employee to respond to treatment.

THE TRAINING PROCESS

When all the information has been gathered, the training administrator can develop one or more lesson plans, practical exercises, handouts, tests, and audiovisual presentations. The information also may lend itself to the use of commercially available slides, films, and demonstration devices such as drug identification kits. Then the actual instruction can begin.

Methods of Instruction

Broadly viewed, instruction is a three-stage operation that includes presentation of information, application by the student, and evaluation. Many approaches exist to present information and engage students in application activities. Presentation and application can occur as separate steps or as one step—that is, the presenter can provide all the required information first and then practice it later, or he or she can alternately present the information and practice it in small increments.

Formal evaluation requires that the instructor administer and grade an examination. Informal evaluation continues throughout the presentation and application processes and is directed toward enhancing learning rather than measuring it. A continuous, informal method of evaluation is usually more effective when teaching supervisors about drug use.

Key teaching points are addressed in the presentation stage. The number of teaching points should not exceed that which the students will be able to master. If a point is not expected to have substantial value on the job, there is little to be gained by presenting it. It is much better to select the critical concepts and teach them thoroughly than to touch lightly on a large number of concepts, many of which are certain to be forgotten if they are not put to use. For example, the history or origin of drugs may be interesting but is of no practical value to supervisors. Retention is facilitated when useful information is presented in a meaningful context.

Knowledge recently acquired or recently applied remains fresh in the mind of the learner. The presenter restates and emphasizes important information throughout and makes a point-by-point review at the conclusion. It certainly helps when the presentation includes techniques and media that excite and interest. Skilful use of displays, mock-ups, slides, transparencies, and films helps stimulate students. The techniques of presentation can include lectures, demonstrations, role playing, conferences, panels, and brainstorming.

In an application activity, the student applies the information received in the presentation stage. The newly acquired knowledge is transferred to a skill through practical application. The role of the presenter is now that of a facilitator or coach. The student is confronted with one or more simulated on-the-job situations that call for the application of what he or she has learned. The ultimate success or failure of an application activity is determined when the learner applies what he or she learned in training to real-life situations. Examples of application activities include students' involvement in case studies, role playing, and hypothetical situations.

Evaluation that occurs as part of the presentation and application activities will keep students from acquiring incorrect knowledge and skill. The essence of evaluation is to inform students of their mistakes when the mistakes happen. A small mistake that goes uncorrected in training may eventually lead to a large mistake on the job. The techniques of informal evaluation include posing questions to the group or to individuals, requiring each individual to demonstrate a task or skill, giving spot quizzes, and delivering critiques.

Helping Supervisors Develop the Necessary Skills

One of the great pitfalls of instruction is to present information without providing practice in applying that information. The reasons that presentation is often preferred over practice are usually stated as follows:

- A great deal of information can be delivered in a short time.
- A single presentation can reach many persons simultaneously.
- Presentation methods are less expensive than practice methods.

These apparent advantages are somewhat illusory because presentations are often made at such an abstract level or with such rapidity that students cannot grasp the essential points. Alternatively, the level of presentation may be so elementary that students are turned off. Some students do not pay attention even to an excellent presentation, and since the process is a one-way street, there is no surefire way to know whether or not the intended learning has occurred. Only when the students use the information in practical situations can the instructor determine whether transfer of knowledge is complete and whether that knowledge is being applied correctly.

A suitable exercise is to cue students with a document that describes a hypothetical situation. The situation presents details for analysis and requires the students to respond in a covert or overt manner. When making a covert response, the student thinks out the answer but does not verbalize it.

The instructor then gives the proper response so that students can compare their thinking with it. In the overt option, the student records a written response on the situation document. In addition to presenting the proper response, the presenter collects the situation sheets, examines them, and provides feedback to the students, especially those whose responses were inadequate.

A related method is case study. It is based on the proposition that a student who solves problems in the training environment increases his or her capacity to solve similar problems in the working environment. By confronting realistic cases, the student not only acquires new job-related skills but also practices applying those skills.

One type of case study is the presentation of an incident or problem in which the student analyzes a set of circumstances. The student is required to formulate action steps for intervening to solve the problem. The presenter may do some limited role playing by assuming the identity of one or more persons associated with the hypothetical case. The product of the student's analysis and the quality of the intervention will determine his or her score.

Helping Supervisors Develop the Proper Attitude

The main problem of training aimed at developing a particular attitude is the abstract nature of attitudes. The intended learning outcomes associated with acquiring skills and knowledge can be fairly easily evaluated, but this is not true of outcomes associated with acquiring attitudes. To be sure, attitudes can be taught, but the process is complex and requires time. Apart from the complexity and time required, I do not advocate trying to teach attitudes because positive attitudes will flow naturally from the learning experiences of the supervisors who undergo the training and supervisors generally share the same values and beliefs as management.

The training administrator should not rule out sending supervisors to related workshops and seminars, showing films, or providing reading materials, all of which affect the students' attitudes. But the main ingredients in promoting positive attitudes are the tone set by management and the on-the-job involvement of supervisors in dealing with drug use issues.

The attitudes of supervisors are profoundly affected by the attitudinal demonstrations of their superiors. Powerful messages are sent to supervisors when their superiors show an interest in and express concern about workplace drug use. No message is more powerful than for management to make drug abuse intervention part of the supervisor's job responsibility and a measure of his or her performance. Similar messages are conveyed by the employer's involvement in community antidrug programs and the appearance of antidrug posters, newsletters, and similar drug awareness materials in the workplace.

CONCLUSION

Supervisors are ideally positioned to help the organization maintain a drug-free workplace. Because supervisors are intimately involved in directing and evaluating the performance of their subordinates, they are able to intervene promptly when drug use is indicated.

Training initiatives should not be directed solely at first-line supervisors. Second-line supervisors, mid-level managers, and senior staffers also should be exposed to training because they too are in supervisory positions and need to know the same intervention strategies and tactics. The presence of senior persons in the training program offers the added benefit of giving supervisors an incentive to learn and the courage to intervene when drug use is indicated.

Supervisors are the enforcers of policy, and for all practical purposes, a drug-testing policy that is not enforced does not exist. Supervisors have to believe in the philosophy of a drug-free workplace and support management in working toward that goal. Supervisors bring their prelearned attitudes to the job, and although training can refine and nurture attitudes to some extent, for the most part they are resistive to major changes.

Attaining supervisory support of the drug-testing policy is only part of the picture. Supervisors need to know the part they play in carrying out the policy, and they need to have the skills for spotting drug abuse and intervening in the prescribed manner. Training is a process for developing the required knowledge and skills. Appendix 5–B contains some sample training materials. The drug bulletins in Appendix 4–D also could be included with the training materials.

Appendix 5–A

Drug-Testing Questions and Answers for Supervisors

Why do companies use drug testing?

Employers have traditionally evaluated employees to determine their fitness for duty. Within the context of occupational medicine programs, physical examinations were initially performed to ensure the selection of personnel free of medical conditions that would be likely to interfere with their ability to work safely and efficiently. In recent years, within the context of health promotion and wellness programs, an additional purpose of the medical evaluation has evolved—that is, to address risk factors that may impair employee health (such as poor nutrition, substance abuse, and hypertension). As drug abuse in the United States has risen, many companies have developed preemployment and in-service drug-testing programs. The primary purpose of these programs is to protect the health and safety of all employees through the early identification and referral for treatment of employees with drug and alcohol abuse problems. The integration of drug testing with programs of treatment, prevention, and drug education is proving to be an effective way of managing substance abuse problems in industry. Urinalysis is now being used as part of the preemployment screening process by many of the nation's largest employers, including major corporations, manufacturers, public utilities, and transportation companies, as well as by small businesses. In general, these companies will not hire individuals who present positive urine specimens indicating current use of illicit substances. However, many of these companies also counsel applicants who fail the drug test to seek treatment and to reapply.

Is drug testing legal?

At the present time, there is no federal or state constitutional provision that directly prohibits the use of drug detection programs. Issues of civil rights argue strongly for a well-thought-out policy based on the need for unbiased, accurate, and legally defensible testing for the job in question.

How often should employees be tested?

Company policy regarding the frequency of drug testing is usually based on risk factors associated with safety, security, and health. Drug testing is typically performed in preemployment evaluations, postaccident investigations, periodic medical examinations, and randomly, without announcement, as a preventive measure. The least intrusive method is incident-driven testing that occurs after an accident, incident, or reasonable cause event. High-risk or safety-sensitive occupations in which public safety is of special concern may require routine scheduled testing. In these cases, testing is often tied to evaluation of fitness for duty or to annual physical examinations. In extremely hazardous and high-risk occupations, periodic unannounced or random testing to ensure the health and safety of employees may be warranted.

What about individual rights, privacy, and confidentiality?

Principles of public safety, efficient performance, and optimal productivity must be balanced against reasonable expectations of privacy and confidentiality. Job situations in which there is a substantial risk to the public safety require more permissible intrusions than situations in which risks to the employee or community are perceived as minimal. On the one hand, an employer has the right to demand a drug-free workplace; on the other hand, an employee has reasonable rights to privacy and confidentiality. Since substance abuse is a diagnosable and treatable illness, policies and procedures should ensure the confidentiality of employee medical records, as in any other medical or health-related condition. Urinalysis test results, which could be part of such a diagnosis, should be treated with the same confidentiality.

Is a drug-testing program needed?

The decision to establish or not to establish a drug-testing program will depend on whether drug use is present and significant in the workplace and whether some other deterrent can work just as well. The decision also will depend to a large extent on the work setting. The initial question that management should consider is "What is the purpose of testing?" The key concerns must be for the health and safety of all employees (that is, early identification and referral for treatment) and the assurance that any drug detection or screening procedure would be carried out with reasonable regard for the personal privacy and dignity of the worker. The second critical question to consider is "What will be done when employees are identified as drug users?" Once these issues are clarified, a policy is drafted.

What level of drug in the urine indicates that an individual is impaired?

Although urine-screening technology is extremely effective in determining previous drug use, the positive results of a drug test cannot be used to prove intoxication or impaired performance. Inert drug metabolites may appear in urine for several days, even weeks (depending on the drug), without related impairment. However, a positive drug test does provide evidence of prior drug use.

How reliable are urinalysis methods?

A variety of methods are available for drug testing through urinalysis. Most of these are suitable for determining the presence or absence of a drug in a urine sample. The accuracy and reliability of these methods must be assessed in the context of the total laboratory system. If the laboratory uses well-trained and certified personnel who follow acceptable procedures, then the accuracy of the results should be very high. Laboratories should maintain good quality-control procedures, follow the manufacturer's protocols, and perform a confirmation assay on all positive tests using the gas chromatography/mass spectrometry (GC/MS) technique.

Equally important are the procedures followed to document how and by whom the sample is handled from the time it is taken from the individual, through the laboratory, until the final assay result is tabulated. This record is referred to as the chain of custody for the sample.

What does laboratory quality assurance mean?

Quality-assurance procedures are documented programs that the laboratory follows to ensure the highest possible reliability by controlling the way samples for analysis are handled and instruments are checked to be sure they are functioning correctly and by minimizing human error. It involves the analysis of standard samples and blank samples along with the unknown samples to ensure that the total laboratory system is producing the expected results. These known samples are referred to as quality-control samples.

Many reports have appeared in the news media about legal cases in which experts have questioned the validity of a drug-test result. Does this indicate that drug-testing methods are not sufficiently reliable for broad application?

No. Experts agree that high reliability and accuracy of drug test results are present when appropriate test methods are used, good laboratory procedures are followed, and adequately trained personnel carry out the analysis and interpretation.

What are the primary methods being used to screen a urine sample for drugs?

Two of the most widely used methods are the EMIT System, distributed by Syva Co., and the Abuscreen System, distributed by Roche Diagnostics, Inc. These are both based on immunoassay techniques.

What is a confirmation assay?

If an initial screening assay shows a sample as being positive, a second assay should be used to confirm the initial result. Using two different assays that operate on different chemical principles but both give a positive result greatly decreases the possibility that a cross-reacting substance or methodological problem could have created the positive result.

A confirmation assay is a test method that is more specific (or selective) than a screening assay. The only true confirmation assay is GC/MS. Other techniques that are used to examine a positive screen are more appropriately called verification assays. Verification assays do not match GC/MS in accuracy and reliability. Among the verification assays are thin-layer chromatography (TLC), high-performance liquid chromatography (HPLC), and fluorescence polarization immunoassay (FPIA).

Confirmation and verification assays are sophisticated instrumental methods that cost more than the screening methods, but they provide a greater margin of certainty when used in concert with the screening assay.

What is the method for confirmation of presumptive positives from initial urine screens?

GC/MS is the only true method for confirmation of a positive urine screening test.

What do *assay sensitivity* and *assay cutoff* mean?

The ability of an assay to detect low levels of drugs is inherently limited. The concentration of a drug below which the assay can no longer be considered reliable is the *sensitivity limit*. The *cutoff level* is the level below which any detection of a drug would be considered negative. Manufacturers of commercial urine screening systems set cutoff limits well above the sensitivity limits to minimize the possibility of a sample that is truly negative giving a positive result.

For example, although the immunoassay screens such as EMIT and Abuscreen are sufficiently sensitive to detect marijuana at levels below 20 ng/ml, the assays are usually used at cutoff levels of 50 or 100 ng/ml. This not only decreases the possibility of a false positive resulting from operating the assay too close to its level of sensitivity, but it also significantly decreases the possibility of a positive test caused by passive inhalation of marijuana smoke.

How can false-positive results occur?

It is theoretically possible for substances other than the drug in question to give a positive result in a screening assay. This is sometimes referred to as cross-reactivity. The test manufacturers know which substances can cause such a cross-reaction, and they have added controls to the tests to account for possible cross-reactivity. Generally, the screening assays available today are highly selective if they are properly used.

False-positive results also can result from human error. Chain-of-custody procedures, laboratory quality-assurance procedures, and confirmation by GC/MS are safeguards against false-positive test results.

How can false positives be eliminated?

Probably the two most important reasons for the occurrence of false positives are poor quality-assurance procedures in the laboratory and the absence of an appropriate confirmation assay to confirm presumptive positives arising from an initial screening procedure. A good laboratory will impose a stringent and well-documented quality-assurance system and will use GC/MS as the confirmation assay for all samples that test positive in a first screen.

Are rigorous and costly laboratory procedures always necessary?

The need to use assay systems that are based on state-of-the-art methods and rigorously controlled procedures is inherent in situations where the consequences of a positive result are great. Where reputation, livelihood, or the right to employment is an issue, maximum accuracy and reliability of the entire detection or deterrence system is imperative. In a case where the consequences are less severe, such as a counseling situation, it might be acceptable to use less rigorous systems. For instance, drug treatment professionals sometimes use portable screening systems to assist in the diagnosis and treatment of drug problems.

Can passive inhalation of marijuana smoke lead to a positive drug test even if the person did not smoke marijuana?

Passive inhalation of marijuana smoke does occur and can result in detectable levels of THC (tetrahydrocannabinol, the primary pharmacological component of marijuana) in blood and of its metabolites in urine. Clinical studies have shown, however, that it is highly unlikely that a nonsmoking individual could passively inhale sufficient smoke to result in a high enough drug concentration in urine for detection at the cutoff levels of currently used urinalysis methods.

Can the time of previous drug use be determined from urinalysis?

Not specifically. Urine specimens that test positive for cannabinoids, for instance, signify that a person has consumed marijuana or marijuana derivatives from within one hour to as much as three weeks or more before the specimen was collected. Generally, a single smoking session by a casual user of marijuana will result in a positive result for two to five days depending on the screening method and on the physiological factors that cause drug concentration to vary. Detection time increases significantly following a period of chronic use. Determination of a particular time of use is thus difficult. The same issues would hold for other drugs, although the time after use during which a positive analysis would be expected might be reduced to just a few days.

Can the level of intoxication due to marijuana use be gauged by urinalysis? Can use patterns be determined?

Impairment, intoxication, or time of last use cannot be judged from a single urine test. A true-positive urine test indicates only that the person used marijuana in the recent past, which could be hours, days, or weeks before, depending on the specific use pattern. Repeated analyses over time will, however, allow a better understanding of the past and current use patterns. An infrequent user should test negative in a few days. Repeated positive analyses over a period of more than two weeks probably indicate either continuing use or previous heavy chronic use.

How long after use can cocaine, heroin, or phencyclidine be detected by urinalysis?

Detection times depend on the sensitivity of the assay. The more sensitive the assay, the longer the drug can be detected. Drug concentrations are initially highest hours after drug use and decrease to undetectable levels over time. The time it takes to reach the point of undetectability depends on the particular drug and other factors such as an individual's metabolism. The sensitivity of urine assay methods generally available today allows detection of cocaine use for a period of one to three days and heroin or phencyclidine (PCP) use for two to four days. These detection times would be somewhat lengthened in cases of previous chronic drug use but probably to no more than double these times.

How long after marijuana is used can such use be detected?

Metabolites of the active ingredients of marijuana may be detectable in urine for up to ten days after a single smoking session. However, most individuals cease to excrete detectable drug concentrations in two to five days. Metabolites can sometimes be detected several weeks after a heavy chronic smoker (several cigarettes a day) has ceased smoking.

If a urine sample is negative one day after a positive sample has been obtained, does this mean the first result was wrong?

Not necessarily. The concentration of the drug in the urine can change considerably depending on the individual's liquid intake. The more an individual drinks, the more the drug is diluted in the urine. A negative result of a sample taken a few hours after drinking a significant amount of liquid is quite possible, even though a clearly positive sample might have been evident before the liquid intake. For this reason, a negative result does not mean that the person has not used the drug recently. As the excretion of marijuana metabolites reaches the approximate limit of detection by a given assay, repeated samples collected over several days may alternate between positive and negative before becoming all negative.

How are the results of a urine drug assay expressed?

Frequently the results of an assay are reported by the laboratory simply as positive or negative. If a sample is reported as positive, this means that the laboratory detected the drug in an amount exceeding the cutoff level it has set for that drug. Different laboratories using different procedures and methods may have different levels. For this reason, one laboratory could determine a sample to be positive and another determine the same sample to be negative if the amount of the drug in the sample fell between the cutoff levels used by the two laboratories.

Analyses also may be reported quantitatively. The concentration of the drug is expressed as a certain amount per volume of urine. Depending on the drug or the drug metabolite that is being analyzed, urine concentrations may be expressed either as nanograms per milliliter (ng/ml) or as micrograms per milliliter (μg/ml). (There are 28 million micrograms in an ounce and 1,000 nanograms in a microgram.) Cocaine metabolites may be detected in amounts as high as several micrograms in a heavy user, but the levels of metabolites from marijuana use rarely reach 1 μg/ml and are usually expressed in nanograms per milliliter.

What adverse health effects can be correlated with the presence of marijuana metabolites in urine?

No studies have attempted to correlate metabolites in urine with specific adverse health effects. The presence of metabolites in urine indicates previous use of marijuana, and use of marijuana, at least on a chronic basis, is likely to lead to adverse health effects. Specific effects, however, cannot be correlated with a single urine concentration of metabolites.

Appendix 5–B

Sample Training Materials

LESSON PLAN

TOPIC: Supervisor Training

PURPOSE: The purpose of this training is to prepare supervisors to meet the responsibilities charged to them in carrying out the Company's drug abuse policy.

LEARNING OBJECTIVES: As a result of this training, each supervisor will be able to do the following:

- State the reasons for and the goals of the Company's drug abuse policy
- Name the responsibilities assigned to supervisors in the Company's drug abuse policy and antidrug program
- Recognize the physical appearance and characteristics of the major types of abused drugs and the paraphernalia associated with their use
- Identify the performance and behavioral indicators of drug impairment
- Identify the actions to take and not to take when intervening in an on-the-job situation that may involve a violation of the Company's drug abuse policy
- Explain the procedures required to be followed in reasonable cause and post-accident testing situations
- Define the terms *reasonable cause, illegal drugs, under the influence, detectable amount,* and *consent required,* as well as other concepts related to the antidrug program

METHODS OF INSTRUCTION: Discussion, demonstrations, films, slides, transparencies, ungraded practical exercises, an ungraded spot quiz, and an ungraded final quiz.

INSTRUCTIONAL TIME: Total minimum time required is 200 minutes (4 instructional hours) arranged as follows: 150 minutes for spot quiz, discussion, demonstrations, audiovisuals, and written test; 25 minutes for a practical exercise in a hypothetical reasonable cause situation; and 25 minutes for a practical exercise in a hypothetical intervention situation.

OUTLINE OF KEY POINTS AND CHRONOLOGY OF LEARNING ACTIVITIES:
I. Introduction
    A. Gain attention
    B. State the learning objectives
    C. Relate the learning objectives to the supervisor's job

164

II. Body
  A. Knowledge that supports the learning objectives (Note: Administer the un-
     graded spot quiz.)
     1. The company's policy
        a. Policy reason
        b. Policy goals
        c. Assigned responsibilities
        d. Prohibited activities
        e. Methods for enforcement
        f. Sanctions
        g. Appeals
        h. Referral and treatment
        i. Return to duty
     2. Important concepts (Note: Use the 35mm slide set.)
        a. Reasonable cause
        b. Consent required
        c. Consequences of refusal
        d. Under the influence
        e. Detectable amount
        f. Illegal drugs
        g. Legal drugs
        h. Contraband
        i. Search limitations
        j. Use versus misuse
     3. Drug recognition (Note: Display the drug identification kit.)
        a. The major classes of abused drugs
        b. Methods of illegal drugs' administration
        c. Drug paraphernalia
     4. Indicators of drug abuse (Note: Show the film *The Drug File*.)
        a. Performance
        b. Behavior/conduct
        c. Physiological/psychological symptoms
        d. Cautions
     5. Drug-testing situations (Note: Show the film *The Straight Dope*.)
        a. Preemployment
        b. Reasonable cause
        c. Postaccident
        d. Periodic
        e. Rehabilitation
     6. Procedures in reasonable cause situations (Note: Use transparency set
        1.)
        a. Qualifying criteria
        b. Two supervisors rule
        c. Time requirements
        d. Transportation
     7. Procedures in postaccident testing (Note: Use transparency set 2.)
        a. Qualifying criteria
        b. Directly involved persons
        c. Good-faith determination

        d.   Time requirements

        e.   Transportation

    8.   Intervention

        a.   Dos and don'ts

        b.   Counseling

        c.   Referral/treatment

        d.   Suspension

        e.   Return to duty

    (Note: Administer the ungraded test.)

B.   Practice skills that support the learning objectives

    1.   Practical exercise 1 (Note: Pass out the hypothetical situation concerning a reasonable cause incident. Inform the attendees to follow the instructions on the situation form, analyze the situation for 15 minutes, and be prepared to participate in a 10-minute critique.)

    2.   Practical exercise 2 (Note: Pass out the hypothetical situation concerning an intervention incident. Inform the attendees to follow the instructions on the situation form, analyze the situation for 15 minutes, and be prepared to participate in a 10-minute critique.)

III.   Conclusion

   A.   Regain attention

   B.   Summarize major points

   C.   Closing statement

(Note: Distribute the student handouts pertaining to descriptions of the major classes of abused drugs.)

SPOT QUIZ

This short quiz is designed to help you clarify your own thoughts and feelings about some of the ideas that will be presented. It is not a test, and you will not turn it in. It is intended to enhance the discussions that follow. When you have finished, it is yours to use as you wish. You may want to look it over after the presentation to see if your thoughts and feelings changed.

Check the answer that best fits your personal understanding. Try to be frank and honest.

1. Is there a serious drug and alcohol problem in the United States?

    [ ]   Yes, but mainly among young people.

    [ ]   Yes. Some people turn to drugs or alcohol as a solution to pressures in life.

    [ ]   No. There is a problem, but it is not as serious as some people make it out to be.

2. Is there a serious drug and alcohol problem in the workplace in the United States?

    [ ]   No. The problem is mainly with students, unemployed persons, criminals, and undesirables.

    [ ]   No. We tend as a nation to focus on one problem at a time. Right now drug and alcohol abuse is getting a lot of attention, probably more than it deserves.

    [ ]   Yes. The problem exists in the workplace, just as it exists in other places in our society.

3. Is there a drug abuse or alcohol problem where you work?

    [ ]   No, but if it does exist where I work, it is so small as not to get excited about.

    [ ]   I'm not sure.

    [ ]   Yes. There is no reason to assume that my company is immune to this nationwide problem.

4. Should a supervisor, such as yourself, take action to deal with a subordinate who is a drug or alcohol abuser?

    [ ]   No. Problems of this type should be handled by top management or specialists from personnel.

    [ ]   No. I'm not trained to handle problems of this type.

    [ ]   Yes. I should be aware of and respond to drug and alcohol abuse by persons who work for me.

5. Is it part of your job to be looking for indications of drug and alcohol abuse by persons who work for you?

    [ ]   No. My job is not to be a detective but to meet productivity goals.

    [ ]   No. Drug or alcohol abuse is a private matter. If people want to ruin their lives, it is their business.

    [ ]   Yes. Drug or alcohol abuse affects job performance, and that is something I need to watch out for.

6. Is it possible to identify a heavy user of marijuana?

    [ ]   I'm not sure, but it is not my function to do so.

    [ ]   No. It is not something that is easily noticed, and the careful marijuana user can easily escape detection.

    [ ]   Yes. Heavy marijuana use can be seen if one knows what to look for.

7. Do you feel qualified to intervene in a case involving drug abuse by one of your subordinates?

    [ ]   No; but if I were trained, I could.

    [ ]   Yes, but I don't feel too confident about it.

    [ ]   Yes. I feel I know enough about drug abuse to intervene effectively and sensitively.

8. If you were required right now to counsel an employee who you believe is performing poorly due to a drug or alcohol problem, which of the following points should you keep in mind?

    [ ]   Try to diagnose the employee's problem so it can be dealt with before it gets worse.

    [ ]   Keep the emphasis of all discussions on job performance alone.

    [ ]   Develop a rapport with the employee so as to encourage him or her to confide in you and follow your guidance.

9. Place a check mark next to any of the following items that you feel can be related to alcohol or drug abuse.

    [ ]   Absenteeism   [ ]   Low productivity

    [ ]   Turnover   [ ]   Medical claims

[ ] Theft

[ ] Accidents

[ ] Customer goodwill

[ ] Insurance rates

[ ] Tardiness

[ ] Morale

[ ] Product loss/waste

[ ] Problems in supervision

PRACTICAL EXERCISE

Situation

Assume you are the supervisor of a warehouse where finished goods are stored before shipment. The foreman who coordinates the truck-loading operations has just entered your office to report that Tom Roberts, a forklift operator, had to be relieved of his duties as the result of getting into a fistfight with a truck driver. Two witnesses to the incident stated that Tom and the driver got into an argument concerning the way Tom was loading the driver's truck and that Tom dismounted his forklift and threw a punch at the driver. The foreman says that Tom is now sitting outside your office.

You know from records on file that Tom has been employed for three years. In his first two years, he received good performance reports, but about one year ago, his performance began to slip as a result of arriving late, leaving early, being absent from the warehouse during the day, and missing several workdays without notice or excuse. You have observed personally that Tom has mood and energy swings. One minute he is withdrawn and drowsy, and a short time later, he is extremely talkative and full of pep. About a week ago, when Tom was working at high speed, a pallet of finished goods fell from his forklift. The foreman reprimanded him for carrying a load larger than that permitted by safety rules.

You have just looked at Tom as he sits waiting outside your office, and your impression is that he is agitated, confused, and very nervous.

Requirements

Analyze the above situation. On a separate sheet of paper, jot down your answers to the following questions. Be prepared to explain and defend your answers in a general critique.

1. Based on Company policy and the concept of reasonable cause, answer the following questions:
   a. Can the facts of the fist fight be substantiated?
   b. Would the facts lead a reasonable person to conclude that Tom engaged in unacceptable behavior?
   c. Do the facts of the incident, Tom's record, and your personal observations over a period of time and at this instant indicate possible drug involvement?
   d. Is the totality of information sufficiently objective to be more than mere suspicion?
2. If you think drug use by Tom is possible, what class or classes of drugs do you think may be involved?
3. Should Tom be required to undergo drug testing? Whether you answered yes or no, what are the major facts that support your decision?
4. What other actions should you take? For example, consider actions with respect to the following:
   a. Transporting Tom to the drug-testing clinic or to his home
   b. Documenting the incident and your decision

c. Reporting the incident and your decision to a higher level of management
d. Counseling Tom
e. Referring Tom to the employee assistance program or to professional help

Chapter 6

Implementing a Drug-Testing Program

A SUPERVISOR'S INTERVENTION STRATEGY

The supervisor is the central player in an organization's game plan for a drug-free workplace. Execution of the game plan hinges on an understanding and acceptance of that role and on the level of effort expended. The supervisor's contribution as a key member of the organization's team will be limited or enhanced by management's efforts to prepare and condition the supervisor to enter the game at peak form. The more critical preparation and conditioning result from involving supervisors in the design and planning stages of the drug-testing program, educating them generally concerning the health and safety implications of drug use, and training them in their specific responsibilities for identifying job-related drug use and intervening in the manner prescribed by the game plan.

The supervisor is the person most likely to detect changes in the performance and behavior pattern of an abusing employee and is also the person responsible for initiating action to correct the problem. If the organization has referral or treatment programs, the supervisor is in the best position to make the referral and follow up to determine whether the treatment has been successful.

Look for Indicators of Drug Abuse

There are some common signs that point to the presence of drug abuse. Sometimes these signs appear to result from other causes, but when the supervisor examines them closely, they are frequently found to have roots in drug abuse. The following indicators often appear in the quality of an employee's work. They are generally called performance indicators because they are job-related forms of conduct.

- Frequent absences and lateness. Examples include not showing up for work on Fridays and Mondays and repeated lateness for work.

- Unexplained absences from the employee's assigned workstation. This may suggest that the employee is leaving work to meet with a supplier or to take a drug.
- Frequent telephone calls, perhaps for the purpose of arranging to meet with a supplier.
- Frequent and long visits to the rest room or locker room, perhaps to take a drug.
- Visits to the employee by strangers or other employees for matters unrelated to the job.

Another category of impairment indicators includes behavioral changes. The indicators are apparent in the manner in which an impaired employee acts or looks.

- An unexplained change in disposition in a short period of time. The employee may go from being uncooperative to cooperative, from quiet to talkative, or from sad to happy. The reason may be that the employee took a drug between the down mood and the up mood. If the mood swings in the opposite direction, it may indicate that the effects are wearing off.
- Weight loss and loss of appetite.
- Nervousness that might appear in the form of starting to smoke or increasing a smoking habit.
- Reluctance to show the arms or legs. If an employee is taking drugs intravenously, he or she will try to hide the injection marks by wearing long-sleeve garments and wearing slacks in place of skirts and dresses. Bloodstains on sleeves may appear.
- Withdrawal symptoms. The employee may show the physiological effects of a drug as it is wearing off. The common symptoms are a runny nose, sniffling, red eyes, trembling of the hands or mouth, an unsteady gait, and general fatigue.
- Active symptoms. The employee may show signs of being under the influence. Generally, a drug will either relax or excite. A person who has taken a relaxant (depressant) tends to be slow moving and dreamily happy and is likely to slur his or her words. A person who has taken an excitant (stimulant) tends to be energetic, twitchy, and fast moving and is likely to talk in a rapid, nonstop manner.

Some general indicators are even more suggestive of drug abuse:

- An admission by the individual.
- Possession of a prescription drug or an illegally manufactured drug without permission or reason. The drug may appear as a pill, tablet, capsule, powder, paste, leafy material, gumlike substance, or liquid. It also can be converted to an innocent-appearing object. For example, an opiate in a

liquid form can be soaked into a handkerchief and allowed to dry. When water is added, the handkerchief is wrung out into a small dish, drawn into a hypodermic syringe, and injected.

- Concealment on the body or in some place that is accessible to the user. A user will sometimes favor concealment in an area also used by other employees. If the concealed item is found, the user can then avoid being singled out.
- Possession or concealment of drug paraphernalia, such as a syringe, needle, cooker spoon, roach clip, or glass pipe.
- Needle marks, boil-like abscesses, scabs, or scars, especially on the arms, legs, or backs of the hands.
- Drowsiness or general lethargy, especially when accompanied by scratching of the body to relieve an itching sensation. This suggests a slight overdose of an opiate drug.
- A change in the size of a person's pupils. The pupils will constrict immediately after a person takes an opiate and dilate after he or she uses an amphetamine.
- A change in general conduct. An opiate user may stare vacantly and be generally unaware of his or her surroundings. A stimulant user may be excited, euphoric, and talkative. A user of marijuana, inhalants, and depressants may be sleepy. A user of hallucinogens such as PCP and LSD may engage in bizarre and possibly violent behavior.
- A change in diet. An abuser of stimulants will go for long periods of time without eating. A narcotics user may have a loss of appetite or consume candy, cookies, soda, and sweet food items.
- A variety of illness symptoms. For example, an opiate user in withdrawal may have the sniffles, flushed skin, muscular twitching, and nausea. A user of hallucinogens may experience an increase in blood pressure, heart rate, and blood sugar, as well as irregular breathing, sweating, trembling, dizziness, and nausea. A cocaine user may have inflamed nasal membranes.
- The use of drug jargon, awareness of how drugs are administered and their effects, and an attitude that excuses or defends drug use. The possession of magazines or literature that are marketed for persons interested in drug abuse is another indicator.
- Items that suggest drug use found in trash receptacles in rest rooms and public areas. Discarded paper and plastic bags, paint cans, aerosol containers, and bottles may have been left behind by drug users. The small vial that contained crack or the glassine envelope that contained heroin might be discarded, as well as metal bottle caps, eye droppers, syringes, and burnt matches used in the process of injecting heroin. Paper bags and glue containers suggest inhalant sniffing.
- Absence from the job for 15 to 30 minutes every 4 or 5 hours, especially in cases where the individual seeks absolute privacy.
- A discrepancy between income and expenditures for necessities. Addicts

will spend most of what they earn (and steal) on the substances they crave.

- A constant need for money. This may appear as borrowing from fellow workers, stealing, or writing bad checks.

A supervisor has to make a personal commitment to take action when he or she has observed a number of indicators. The supervisor should not, however, assume that every indicator is proof of drug abuse. He or she will have to weigh the facts present in each case before forming an opinion.

One thing the supervisor must not do is accuse an employee of abusing drugs based on observation alone. The indicators may be valid reasons to intervene, but the purpose of the intervention is to direct the employee's attention to the detrimental effects of his or her unsatisfactory performance or behavior and to bring an end to unacceptable work conduct.

For example, if the problem is absenteeism, the employee should be counseled in terms of the effects of his or her absenteeism on productivity. Absence from the job is a major source of loss to business. It drives up the cost of labor, drives productivity down, and places an unfair burden on employees who have to pick up the slack. For these reasons, it deserves special mention in any strategy designed to curb workplace drug abuse.

Here are some pointers for dealing with absenteeism:

- Insist on prompt notification when a subordinate is absent unexpectedly. Require subordinates to call in without fail and without delay when they must be absent without prior approval.
- Insist on prior discussions about necessary absences for personal reasons rather than after-the-fact explanations. Do not routinely accept vague stories and weak excuses.
- Keep a running record of absences that occur on Monday or the first day after a holiday. Compare this record with absences that occur on payday.
- Identify through well-kept records those employees who are absence-prone. Let it be known that this is a routine record-keeping practice.
- Have a heart-to-heart talk with each absence-prone employee. Obtain a commitment from the employee that he or she will take steps to correct the problem.
- Include mention of absenteeism at departmental meetings. Explain its seriousness in terms of higher costs, lost profits, and lower productivity and morale.
- Find out what other supervisors are doing to reduce absenteeism and act accordingly.

Avoid Enabling

An enabler is a person whose actions shield an abuser from suffering the disciplinary consequences of abuse. An enabler makes it possible, albeit unwittingly and with good intentions, for the drug abuser to continue his or her downward slide.

Enabling involves overlooking a pattern of absence from the job, accidents, or decreased productivity. It also might involve accepting excuses such as "I have a problem at home that is detracting from my work."

An enabler might get overly involved with an employee by trying to provide friendly advice and sympathetic counseling. A well-meaning supervisor may not be able to resist the temptation to judge the cause of an employee's problem and to formulate a cure. The cure will most likely result in less work for the employee, more time to do it in, less stringent standards for quality work, and more personal attention from the supervisor.

It is easy for a supervisor to fall into the pitfall of enabling. Dealing with a difficult employee is not fun. It creates tension in the supervisor, and just the thought of having to fill out incident reports and go through complicated disciplinary procedures is enough to keep a supervisor from taking action.

The supervisor's reluctance to act is only a small part of the enabling equation, however. The drug-abusing employee may be simultaneously feeling guilt, remorse, shame, fear, and defiance. Mixed in is likely to be a firmly held belief that he or she can stop using drugs whenever he or she wants. Thus, the employee is likely to become secretive and to avoid confronting the problem head-on. These symptoms are typical manifestations of drug abuse.

When unsatisfactory work eventually requires the supervisor to intervene, he or she may engage the employee in an informal conversation. Wanting to believe that the problem can be solved easily, the supervisor will accept the employee's explanations at face value. The supervisor will lend some validity to the explanations by reporting them to higher management. The enabling process has in effect caused the supervisor to make a commitment to the employee's skewed view of reality and to become a participant in his or her self-deception.

As the abuse progresses and performance deteriorates, the enabling supervisor and the abuser become more and more entwined in the process of denial. Intermittent instances of improvement may occur, but each will be quickly followed by a reversal. The supervisor may cover up, get others to pick up the increased workload, and make more elaborate excuses for the employee.

A supervisor's personal beliefs may contribute to the enabling process. He or she may believe that the employee could not possibly be a drug abuser because of the employee's intelligence, background, or other characteristics. The supervisor also may believe that taking action will be worse than not taking action, perhaps because doing so might damage the employee's career or because he or she does not trust the reporting procedure. This distrust may be based on perceptions that the established disciplinary procedures are complex, the union is uncaring or obstructive, performance standards are unclear or nonexistent, and management is unsupportive.

The enabling supervisor may progressively experience confusion, disappointment, exasperation, frustration, feeling of betrayal, and finally outright anger. An angry outburst is usually triggered as a reaction to an incident of unacceptable behavior by the problem employee.

After the explosion of anger, the supervisor may feel guilty about having lost control. The guilt also may spring from a feeling that he or she exerted too much pressure on the employee. To compensate, the supervisor will accept even more excuses and lower his or her expectations even further. The supervisor is now beginning to feel personally responsible for the employee, and if the employee picks up on this, he or she may begin to blame the supervisor, rather than the drugs, for his or her problems.

Ending the process of enabling is very difficult. It means finally recognizing drug abuse as the cause of unacceptable job performance, documenting performance problems, and confronting the affected employee with the evidence of the unacceptable performance. During this process, the supervisor must refuse to accept the employee's excuses and empty promises and refuse to defend or take responsibility for the employee's actions.

Document Performance Problems

When faced with declining or erratic employee performance, it is important for the supervisor to document observable, verifiable facts. Complete, accurate documentation is essential when dealing with an employee who has performance problems. Good documentation will show the job performance picture over a period of time and will emphasize to the employee the seriousness of the situation. If discipline is necessary, good documentation will support the corrective action.

It is extremely important to document every instance when a supervisor finds it necessary to intervene for the correction of an employee's improper performance, particularly performance that involves safety. Accurate and complete documentation will provide a true record of all discussions with the employee and with other involved persons, such as health and personnel representatives, and will form the basis and justification for a plan of action designed to eliminate the employee's unacceptable performance. This same documentation also can serve as a reference for preparing future performance reports.

Good documentation will reflect complete, objective, and accurate details of the employee's unsatisfactory performance, behavior, and unsafe actions and will provide a record of all the pertinent facts discussed at meetings about the employee. It will summarize comments by all involved persons and will outline the plan or action steps that were determined to be appropriate in resolving the problem.

The recorded facts also can facilitate a medical resolution of the employee's problems if that turns out to be the ultimate course of action. Good documentation will provide insight for diagnosticians, counselors, and other treatment professionals.

Confront the Employee

When the supervisor has observed deteriorating performance or unfavorable changes in personal or work patterns, there is no choice but to take some form of corrective action. Correction could start with a discussion of the performance difficulties with the employee, assuming that the difficulties are not so serious as to require notice to a higher level of supervision.

Confronting an employee whose job performance has deteriorated is never easy. It is especially hard when previous efforts have not worked, where tension has built up, or where communication has become strained or closed off entirely. It is possible, however, to conduct a constructive confrontation session, but the key lies in getting ready, setting the stage, and knowing what to expect.

Getting ready involves reviewing the facts of the case, preparing yourself mentally, and facing up to a task that may not be pleasant. Setting the stage involves creating a positive, constructive atmosphere by arranging an appointment with the employee, ensuring privacy for the meeting, and allowing sufficient time for it. Knowing what to expect means assessing the situation from the employee's perspective and being prepared for a defensive or even hostile reaction.

During the meeting, the supervisor should advise the employee that corrective steps must be taken by the employee to eliminate the unacceptable work behavior and that if the employee's performance does not improve within a reasonable period of time, some further action, including discipline, will be necessary. Although no-nonsense in tone, the conversation should be nonaccusatory, and the subject of drug abuse should be raised only by the employee.

It is important for the supervisor to be specific about the unacceptable behavior and to refer only to job performance. There should be no reference to what may be the underlying cause of the unacceptable performance. For example, no mention should be made of drug use even though the supervisor may have strong suspicions along this line.

If the employee mentions drug use or some other reason as the cause of the unacceptable performance, the supervisor should allow him or her to explain fully. Keep in mind, however, that the purpose of the meeting is to discuss the employee's performance, not to engage in drug abuse counseling.

The supervisor must be firm and clear about the nature and extent of the improvement that the employee is expected to make. The discussion might include performance targets and timetables that, if met, will restore the employee's performance to the expected standards.

The employee may attempt to deflect the supervisor's purposes by engaging in sympathy-evoking tactics. The supervisor cannot, however, allow the employee to distract him or her from insisting on improved performance. Allowing the employee to get off scot-free will only prolong the unacceptable performance and can prevent the employee from receiving the professional assistance he or she needs.

The supervisor cannot assume that drug abuse is the cause of an employee's improper performance. Very strong proof may exist to support such an assumption, including an admission by the employee, but the supervisor is not trained to make such a judgment and should look for guidance from qualified practitioners.

How will a supervisor know when it is appropriate for an employee to be referred to a treatment professional? At least three circumstances call for referral:

1.   When an employee expresses a desire for treatment of drug use
2.   When an obvious physical condition exists—for example, needle tracks or withdrawal symptoms
3.   When the employee's behavior strongly indicates drug dependence

When one or more of these circumstances occur, the supervisor should take immediate steps to bring the employee into contact with a designated professional. The employee should be told that a referral will be made and that the employee is expected to meet and cooperate with the professional. The supervisor needs to avoid saying or giving the impression that the employee will be disciplined for a failure to follow through with a treatment professional. However, the employee should know that discipline will be taken if the unsatisfactory job performance is not corrected within a specified period of time.

Make a Referral

When the supervisor concludes that the best course of action is to make a referral for diagnosis and treatment, the employee should be told of this decision, preferably during the meeting, and the meeting should be followed by a written notice to the employee.

The notice, which could be in the form of a letter or a memo, should review the job problem in terms of what the employee has done or not done. Specific, unambiguous language will leave no confusion as to the unacceptable conduct. Language that interprets the conduct or gives the supervisor's impression of the cause should be omitted.

The main purpose of the notice is to refer the employee to professional assistance. The source of assistance should be identified, and some encouragement should be given for following through. This could be accompanied by an expression of concern for the employee and a reminder that a failure to obtain assistance will be a factor if discipline becomes necessary. Following is an example of a written notice:

This memo is intended to identify significant deficiencies in your work performance that indicate a need for professional counseling. This memo does not constitute a disciplinary action, and it will not be placed in your personnel file.

You have repeatedly been late in reporting to work and have repeatedly left work early. You have been absent from your workstation without approval on several occasions, and you have not reported to work on at least three days in the past month. In addition to the problems created by your absence from work, you have interacted with your coworkers in an abrasive, irritable, and sometimes hostile manner. The conduct you have engaged in cannot be tolerated in an environment that relies on dependable appearance at work and cooperation among all employees.

I believe that this deterioration in your attendance and your ability to work well with others might arise from problems that are personal in nature. For that reason, I strongly urge you to set up an appointment to visit (name of EAP specialist, location, and phone number). This should be done without delay.

I have already made a contact on your behalf, and I have been told that any information relating to your use of the EAP will be confidential. No information can be released to me or anyone else without your consent.

During the next 30 days, I will be closely observing your attendance and personal interaction with coworkers. At the end of that time, I will evaluate your progress in correcting the deficiencies discussed above.

Because of my concern for you on a personal level and as an employee who can make a valuable contribution, I urge you to accept this offer of assistance.

In general, EAP representatives will not provide feedback to supervisors concerning the nature of an employee's participation or progress in counseling or other treatment. For discussions to occur, the employee would have to give a signed release. Obviously, it would not be proper for a supervisor to suggest that the employee sign such a release. The supervisor must rely on job performance in evaluating an employee's return to a fully productive status. Although it might be useful to know whether an employee is or is not trying to correct the underlying problem, the only decisive factor is quality of work.

If the employee shows improvement but less than the full improvement set by the supervisor, the supervisor may want to know something about the employee's treatment program. The supervisor may have underestimated the extent of the employee's problem, and although progress is being made in treatment, more time is needed to get the employee completely back on track. Appendix 6–A contains an example of a written release that would be signed by the employee and a cover memo from the treatment professional to the supervisor.

Monitor the Employee's Progress

In the days following the performance discussion, the supervisor should continue to observe and document the employee's performance. If the improvement that was specified in the meeting is not achieved within the specified time frame, a second interview may be appropriate. It is possible that the cause underlying the performance problem requires more specialized help or more time for improvement.

Monitoring of the employee's progress should continue until work performance becomes acceptable or until all reasonable efforts for improvement have failed. In the latter event, the supervisor will have to consult his or her supervisors concerning the situation.

IMPLEMENTING AN EMPLOYEE ASSISTANCE PROGRAM

Types of Program Referral

Referral to an EAP for help with any type of personal problem, including drug abuse, can come from a supervisor, as discussed in the previous section, a coworker, or the employee himself or herself.

Peer Referral

Workers as a group have the ability to promote a drug-free workplace through pressure on workers who choose to use drugs in defiance of workplace rules. Close ties among workers make it possible for them to spot drug abuse before job performance is seriously impaired. In many job situations, a worker is better positioned than a supervisor to notice the drug-abusing behaviors of a fellow worker, and a supervisor may be less effective in intervening than would one or a few coworkers using a friendly, concerned approach.

It is in the employer's interest to support, if not initiate, an informal peer network to make workers aware of the dangers of drugs, confront users with their unacceptable behaviors, encourage them to obtain treatment, and support those who enter into treatment. There is no reason why an informally operated peer referral network cannot exist in parallel with a company's formal mechanisms for supervisory referral and self-referral to an EAP.

The employer must be careful that official support of peer referral does not lead to antagonistic confrontations or to any activities of a disruptive nature. The appropriate activities of workers committed to peer referral include holding support sessions, posting antidrug notices, distributing news about the program, and offering to management new ideas for steering employees away from abuse.

Self-Referral

People with drug abuse problems typically do not self-refer. They are usually referred to an EAP by supervisors or coworkers. If an employee does refer himself or herself to an EAP, supervisors and fellow employees should be supportive, and procedures for self-referral and continued employment should be in place.

Professional Counseling

Counseling by a trained professional is usually the first step in processing a referred employee. The objectives of the counselor will be to diagnose the employee's problem, determine its severity, and detect the early signs of more serious problems to come. The employee may be free of a chemical dependence, marginally dependent, dependent and heading toward addiction, or fully addicted. The drugs being abused may be slightly toxic with a potential for moderate impairment, or they may be dangerously toxic with a potential for severe impairment, irrational behavior, and serious illness. The counselor needs to determine these factors because they are important in determining a treatment program for the employee. These factors also will have a bearing on whether the counselor will recommend that the employee be permitted to continue working, especially in a safety-sensitive job.

Counseling is aimed at helping the referred employee to gain an understanding of the problem and to face up to the task of overcoming it. There may be more than one treatment alternative, which can be outlined in counseling sessions. As much as anything, counseling can teach the employee skills that will help him or her avoid the patterns of social behavior that lead to contact with drugs and drug users.

When an employee enters counseling, the counselor conducts a thorough evaluation of the problem. This is called diagnostic counseling. During this phase, the counselor defines the dimensions of the problem and determines an appropriate treatment program. The prescribed treatment may consist of further counseling of a therapeutic nature.

Most referred employees can correct their behavior through counseling alone, but a very small number have severe problems that require treatment through hospitalization, detoxification, or drug maintenance. The latter cases are usually handled by a higher level of management and within the context of rules and benefits relating to suspension, sick leave, and return to duty.

If an employee is able to continue working while undergoing treatment, the supervisor should be supportive and allow a reasonable period of time for improvement. Follow-up meetings with the employee may be desirable to ensure consistency and to reinforce the expectation of a return to full productivity.

The Treatment Program

To a large extent, the type and duration of an individual's drug dependence determine the severity of his or her problem. In turn, the severity of the problem and the motivation of the individual to overcome the problem influence the duration of treatment. Some employees need to undergo treatment that will keep them off the job, while others are able to keep working while participating in outpatient forms of treatment such as counseling, psychotherapy, and group therapy.

An employer may elect to offer full treatment and rehabilitation benefits or limit benefits to those that are routinely provided in the medical benefits program. An employer might conclude that the investment already made to develop a productive employee is reason enough to provide assistance in lieu of termination. If an employer's economic situation does not allow for the provision of treatment benefits, it might provide for return to employment of individuals who undergo successful therapy at personal expense. At a minimum, the employer should provide information about drug treatment facilities in the local community.

Above all else, an EAP cannot be allowed to become a safe haven for employees to escape disciplinary action for violations of the drug policy. The employee should understand that he or she must show visible signs of improvement and abide by the company's drug-testing regulations.

DRUG-TESTING SITUATIONS

Safety in the workplace is an employer responsibility. The safety of the public can be endangered by drug abuse, and an employer who chooses to ignore this fact and take no action to eliminate the danger is at risk of being sued for negligence. This premise also applies to situations where the lives and well-being of drug-free employees are endangered by their drug-abusing co-workers.

The privacy expectations of an employee do not include freedom to endanger the lives of others, violate the law, or be exempt from reasonable examination, such as the taking of a urine specimen, to determine fitness for duty. The courts have consistently upheld employers that have used drug tests in cases where there was a convincing demonstration of changed employee behavior indicating probable drug use. The employer's position is enhanced when supervisors have been trained how to recognize drug abuse and respond to it. Following are discussions of situations that call for the administration of drug testing.

Preemployment Testing

By far, the most common form of situational drug testing is preemployment testing. The usual practice is to incorporate drug testing into the organization's selection and hiring process.

Prior to being tested, the applicant is informed in writing of (1) the employer's drug-testing policy, (2) the applicant's right to refuse to undergo the testing, (3) termination of the preemployment process as a consequence of refusal to undergo testing, and (4) ineligibility for employment if the applicant fails to pass the test. The applicant is asked to acknowledge in writing receipt and understanding of this notice.

In some companies, only those applicants who have cleared certain other screening mechanisms are referred to drug testing. This allows employers to avoid the cost of testing applicants who do not qualify for employment for other reasons.

The applicants who are referred to testing are provided with instructions for reporting to the designated company office or contract vendor's clinic for the collection of specimens. The instructions usually include a reminder of the need to produce at the collection site a form of photographic personal identification and to be prepared to name or describe any medication taken in the previous 30 days.

At the specimen collection site, the applicant is asked to acknowledge understanding of the prospective employer's drug-testing policy and to consent to the provision of a specimen for testing and the release of test results to the employer and/or designated agents.

The employer will instruct the drug-testing laboratory to release test results to designated employer officials or agents. All information related to drug testing or the identification of persons as users of drugs are protected by the employer as confidential unless otherwise required by law or over-riding public health and safety concerns or unless authorized in writing by the applicant in question.

A few employers provide an appeal provision for applicants. For example, an applicant whose drug test is reported positive may be given the opportunity for a private meeting to offer an explanation. The principal purpose of the meeting is to determine whether the positive finding could have resulted from a cause other than drug use. When this provision exists, the employer usually reserves the right to judge whether an applicant's explanation merits further inquiry. During the period of an appeal and any resulting inquiries, the preemployment process is placed on hold.

Random Testing

Random testing is the unannounced testing of a percentage of employees who have been selected for testing by a random selection method, such as an unbiased computer-generated technique. Random testing is usually conducted at a stated frequency—for example, once a month or once every other month. Advance notice is not given as to the date of testing or the employees selected for testing.

Random testing can include only employees who perform certain duties, such as safety-sensitive jobs, or it can include all employees. When some but not all employees are subject to being tested, the employer will identify those positions and inform the persons who hold those jobs in advance of any testing. On the day of testing, employees who were selected by the random selection method are told to report to the specimen collection site without delay.

Reasonable Cause Testing

A reasonable cause situation is a situation in which a supervisor is required to determine whether or not an employee whose on-duty conduct indicates impairment by a drug should be tested. The decision to test must be based on a reasonable and articulable belief that the employee is using a drug in violation of the employer's policy. The belief must be supported by specific, contemporaneous physical, behavioral, or performance indicators of probable drug use. Where possible, two supervisors, at least one of whom is trained in the detection of possible drug use, would substantiate and concur in the decision to test.

The supervisor(s) who makes a decision to conduct reasonable cause testing must make sure that the facts of the situation are (1) capable of explanation and substantiation; (2) specific, tangible, and contemporaneous; and (3) indicative of probable drug use by the employee. The evidence of probable drug use could include any of the common indicators of impairment, as defined earlier in this chapter.

Examples of conduct that suggests drug or alcohol impairment include being at fault in an accident, engaging in violent or disruptive behavior, being absent from the job excessively without explanation, engaging in erratic behavior, making mistakes in judgment or reasoning, and deviating from productivity norms and safe working practices. The conduct can take many forms but must be accompanied by indicators of impairment.

The reasonable cause determination and the collection of specimens should be made as soon as possible following the conduct that gave rise to the determination. *As soon as possible* means within 1 to 2 hours.

When alcohol use is indicated, either alone or in conjunction with drug use, the employee can be given a preliminary test based on the analysis of saliva or breath specimens for the presence of alcohol. The preliminary test can be conducted at the work location by someone trained in the administration of saliva or breath tests. If the preliminary test is positive, the employee would be transported without delay to a medical facility where a specimen of blood would be collected for analysis by a blood alcohol concentration (BAC) test.

An employee being tested in a reasonable cause situation would not be allowed to drive to or from the specimen collection location or from the place of work. If the employee refused to comply, the supervisor would be on solid ground in calling the police to prevent the operation of a motor vehicle by someone who was thought to be impaired.

Finally, the supervisor who makes the decision to administer reasonable cause testing prepares an after-action report that includes the facts that led to the decision to test, the steps taken to obtain testing, the names of persons who have knowledge of the situation, and other related details.

Postaccident Testing

Obviously, some accidents do not require either an investigation or drug testing. Generally, if an accident requires a formal investigation, it also requires drug testing, and the employer sets the criteria. Two criteria are most common: personal injury and property damage. The personal injury criterion might specify accidents that will result in the filing of a workmen's compensation claim or accidents that require professional medical treatment beyond first aid and render an employee unfit to perform routine duties. The property damage criterion might require drug testing in situations that result in a dollar loss above a certain amount.

The employees to be tested in a postaccident situation should include those who were directly involved in the accident and whose order, action, or failure to act was determined to be, or cannot be ruled out as, a causative factor in the events leading to or causing the accident. In other words, it is not necessary to test everyone involved in an accident, only those who could be at fault.

The supervisor having functional responsibility for investigation of an accident is obligated to make a timely, good-faith determination as to whether the accident meets the criteria and, if so, to take all practical steps to have each directly involved employee tested. As soon as possible following the accident, the supervisor should make arrangements for the employees to provide specimens. The time frame for obtaining specimens related to drug impairment is about 24 hours and for alcohol impairment 4 hours. Beyond those times, the specimens begin to deteriorate.

The supervisor responsible for conducting the accident investigation should make sure that the collected specimens are promptly shipped to the designated drug-testing laboratory. A chain of custody must be initiated and maintained for each specimen at the point of collection. Blood specimens must be shipped in a cooled condition and by a means that ensures delivery within 24 hours of receipt by the carrier. Urine specimens must be shipped by an expeditious means but need not be shipped in a cooled condition.

Periodic Testing

Periodic testing is conducted at established intervals, such as drug testing performed in conjunction with an employee's annual physical examination or fitness-for-duty evaluations performed in connection with the issuance or renewal of a license. The term also is used to describe unannounced or random testing that is conducted periodically, although not with precision as to the actual testing dates.

When a person knows that he or she will be tested on a certain date or within a narrow time frame, such as during a particular week, the deterring and detecting effects of drug testing are diminished. The person need only abstain from drug use shortly before the projected testing period. Only the cannabinoids (marijuana substances) have a long retention rate in the body system, but even in this case, a marijuana user could discontinue use 30 days prior to the testing period, switch to a drug that has a short retention rate, and continue use until a few days before the testing is scheduled. After the person has taken and passed the test, the former pattern of use could be resumed until the next testing period.

Testing of Contractors

A company that uses drug testing to help achieve a drug-free workplace will expect no less from contractors whose employees work on the company's premises. It would not make sense to conduct drug testing of regular employees and not require the same of contractor employees who work alongside them.

It is not unusual in an employer-contractor relationship for the employer to maintain a hands-off approach with respect to the contractor's employees. Little attention is generally given to personnel matters, and much attention is given to larger issues such as production quotas and cost containment. While safety may be a larger issue and the proper subject of managerial attention from both employer and contractor, the focus may not necessarily be on the steps taken by the contractor to ensure human reliability.

Some employers take the position that it is desirable not to know the details of contractors' activities because doing so means that the employer must assume liability for contractor errors. By looking too closely and providing too much guidance, the argument goes, an employer can be held accountable when something goes wrong. The problem with this argument, at least with respect to drug testing, is that when something goes wrong, the employer is going to be drawn into litigation no matter how distant or intimate the employer-contractor relationship is. The employer is going to be named as a defendant, if only because of a superior financial position.

Under these circumstances, the best course of action for the employer might be to pay close attention to a contractor's efforts to maintain a drug-free work force and to provide guidance when the efforts appear to be inconsistent with rules and practices set by the employer. A sensible approach is to provide contractor management with the company's drug-testing policy and obtain a commitment, either contractually or by letter of understanding, that the contractor will issue a complementary policy and enforce it. It is also sensible for the employer to monitor contractor compliance. Appendix 6–G contains a questionnaire that can be used to evaluate contractor compliance, and Appendix 6–H contains a document that can be used to inform a contractor of minimum drug-testing standards.

SUPPLEMENTS TO DRUG TESTING

Two other drug-detecting activities can be used as supplements to drug testing. The first is a drug recognition process for identifying impaired employees, and the second is searching for drugs and drug paraphernalia.

Drug Recognition Process

Nonmedical physical tests have been a traditional means of identifying persons who may be under the influence of drugs or alcohol. Roadside sobriety tests are widely used in traffic enforcement, and fitness-for-duty tests administered by health paraprofessionals are used in industrial work settings. The problem of recognizing drug-impaired workers and securing proof of impairment has led to the development of what has recently come to be called the drug recognition process.

The drug recognition process is a systematic method of examining a suspected drug-impaired employee to determine whether impairment is present and, if so, whether it is drug related. The process also seeks to identify the broad category of drugs, or their combinations, that is the likely cause of impairment.

The process is a postaccident or postincident procedure and is intended to provide reasonable cause for suspecting that drugs will be found in an employee's urine or blood specimen. The process is not a substitute for a drug test but a means of assembling proof of a belief that drugs are probably involved in a particular situation.

The process will point not only to drug involvement but also to a particular category of drugs. A person trained in drug recognition, for example, would be able to spot the involvement of a narcotic but might not be able to tell whether the narcotic was morphine, heroin, or codeine.

Why is it helpful to have the extra information that the drug recognition process can provide? Why not simply base a reasonable cause testing decision on the indicators of impairment? The answer is that a court may not agree that the observable impairment was sufficient to justify conducting a drug test. For example, it can be argued that the employee was ill and the indicators were related to a medical condition, not the ingestion of a drug.

Also, the employee may refuse to provide specimens for analysis and in so doing will deny the employer the opportunity to obtain scientific evidence. If the employee is disciplined in any way as a consequence of the refusal, a grievance or civil suit could follow. The employer's backup proof is the testimony of the trained person who made the evaluation.

In the context of immediacy, the key issue in a probable drug-impaired situation is the impairment itself. It may be helpful to learn the source of the impairment so that corrective action can be taken at a later time, but for the supervisor who is charged with making a decision to test or not test, the critical question is whether or not impairment is indicated. Remember that a positive drug test will not provide proof of impairment. The drug recognition process is an excellent way of providing such proof.

The evidence gleaned by the process will point to the presence, singly or in combination, of seven broad categories of drugs:

1. Depressants
2. Stimulants

3. Hallucinogens
4. Phencyclidine (PCP)
5. Inhalants
6. Narcotics
7. Cannabis

These categories distinguish between drugs that differ from one another in terms of their effects and the observable signs of impairment they produce.

The process becomes more complicated with polydrug use. Three different effects can occur from polydrug use: additive, antagonistic, and overlapping. These effects can occur separately or together.

The additive effect can be seen when a user takes two or more drugs that produce similar results. For example, a person in a stupor may have taken a depressant in addition to a narcotic analgesic. Both these drugs depress the central nervous system, and when taken together, they can produce exaggerated effects. The additive effect also might be seen with combinations of stimulants and PCP.

The antagonistic effect can be seen when a user takes drugs that produce opposite results. A person who has ingested a stimulant in combination with a depressant may exhibit alternately constricting and dilating pupils or pupils that are nearly normal because of the offsetting effects of the two drugs.

The overlapping effect is the occurrence of distinct effects in combination. For example, PCP causes nystagmus (involuntary oscillation of the eyeball) but does not affect pupil size. Narcotics constrict pupils but do not cause nystagmus. The presence of nystagmus and pupil constriction would be an overlapping effect that points to the use of these two drugs.

The drug recognition process involves the following 12 steps:

1. Administering a breath alcohol test
2. Making a preliminary interview of the individual
3. Asking questions, giving simple tests, and looking for the gross indicators of drug influence
4. Conducting an eye examination
5. Giving divided-attention psychophysical tests
6. Making a dark-room examination of the eyes
7. Checking the vital signs
8. Examining for muscle rigidity
9. Examining for hypodermic injection sites
10. Making a concluding interview of the individual
11. Making an evaluation based on the previous ten steps
12. If the evaluation in step 11 indicates impairment, collecting specimens for drug testing

The practitioners of the process, who are not necessarily health professionals, perform in a methodical, standardized fashion. Some of the steps include making judgments, while others rely on more objective measurements. For example, the steps involving interviews and opinions have an element of subjectivity, while steps involving tests are highly structured.

The accuracy and reliability of the drug recognition process relies mainly on the structured tests. A case in point is the eye examination. This test seeks to detect abnormal pupil constriction or dilation, strabismus, and nystagmus. Strabismus is the inability of one eye to attain binocular vision with the other due to an imbalance of eyeball muscles. The result is squinting. Pupil size and reaction can be readily determined by the use of a small flashlight and a pupilometer.

The person administering the test measures the diameter of the pupil and looks for strabismus and nystagmus. The pupil measurement is compared against a known standard—for instance, the standard adult pupil in normal room light will range from 2.9 to 6.5 millimeters in diameter. A measurement outside the standard range indicates constriction or dilation, both of which are physical characteristics known to be associated with impairment by particular categories of drugs.

Even though the tests rest on scientific principles, the problem with them is that they depend heavily on human interpretation. The bottom line conclusion is always a product of human intelligence and judgment. As a means for establishing reasonable cause, however, the drug recognition process has a great deal of value. A much higher level of confidence is attached to a reasonable cause determination when a supervisor or a company specialist who has been trained in the process examines an employee suspected of probable drug use and concludes that a drug is indicated as the impairing agent.

Searches for Drugs and Drug Paraphernalia

Are searches of the workplace appropriate? The question is not whether management has a right to conduct searches but whether searches will achieve the desired result. When it is the judgment of management that searches are needed and will help keep drugs out of the workplace, the next consideration should be how the searches will be conducted.

The search options consist of routine inspections, such as by a security officer at the point of entry to company premises; intermittent inspections, such as by a supervisor at selected workstations; and unannounced full searches, such as by a team of trained professionals at an entire job site.

Searches are justified on the ground that the employer has an obligation to provide a safe, healthful, and productive work environment. To meet that obligation, many employers will not allow the following on their premises or property:

- Illegal drugs and the paraphernalia associated with them
- Alcohol, except as may be specifically authorized for employer-approved purposes

- Firearms, explosive or incendiary devices or materials, weapons, and similar items having lethal characteristics
- Stolen property and similar materials whose possession constitutes a crime or violation of rules

The rules relating to prohibited materials usually apply to all persons on the employer's premises or property. The general practice is that all individuals entering or leaving the premises are subject to search of their persons, personal effects, handbags, luggage, or vehicles. Signs at the entry and exit points usually carry warnings such as the following:

> Possession of drugs, alcohol, firearms, explosives, weapons, and/or hazardous materials without proper authorization is not permitted on these premises. Entry is consent to and recognition of the right to search the person, the automobile, and other property of any and all individuals while entering, on, or departing the premises.

Searches are conducted from time to time as circumstances dictate to attain compliance with rules concerning prohibited materials and may be conducted anywhere on the employer's premises or property, not just at the entry and exit points. The practice is usually communicated to workers at the time of hire and periodically thereafter.

A person cannot be forced to submit to a search. Although an employer, by virtue of policy and prior notice, claims the right to conduct searches, people cannot be searched against their will. The employer can, however, require uncooperative persons to leave the premises immediately and ban them from returning. For an employee, this is the same as being terminated.

Searches of all persons or groups of persons can be conducted on an unannounced basis. The element of surprise is critical to the success of an unannounced search. Typically, the decision to conduct such a search is known only to a handful of senior managers.

A search team is usually designated in advance. A team consists of two or three persons from any of the following categories:

- A senior person at the facility or location where the search is to be conducted
- A representative of the security or human relations department
- A contract searcher

A contract searcher is a professional security person hired to conduct the search. The contract searcher may or may not, depending on the employer's preferences, use trained search dogs. When a contract searcher is used, the other team members participate as observers and intervene as necessary to deal with problems.

In advance of the search, the team develops a plan that takes into account details such as when and where to start, how to announce the search, how to close off the area(s) where the search will be conducted, which work operations will be suspended, and how to handle confiscated materials.

On the day of the search and when the team is ready to begin, a senior person at the facility assembles the affected persons into a convenient area where they are told that a search is to be conducted. The affected persons, who may be a combination of employees, contractors, and subcontractors, receive instructions that highlight the employer's policy and work rules regarding searches. An individual's right to withhold consent to a search, and the employer's right to remove a nonconsenter from the premises, also are highlighted.

Each person who agrees to the search is asked to signify consent by signing a written form. This consent often appears at the bottom of the same form used by the employer to inform persons of the search policy. The signification of consent should be obtained every time a search is conducted even though a signed consent may have been obtained when the person was first formally informed of the search policy.

After the consent is obtained, the search can begin. There are three places of interest to the searchers: the person, the person's workstation, and the person's private vehicle, if it is on the premises at the time the search is announced.

The search of the person should be done in a private place. The individual is asked to remove everything from his or her pockets, purse, billfold, and so on. When these have been checked, the person is asked to raise his or her trouser legs and roll down his or her socks. Under no circumstances should there be any touching of the person's body. If a female is to be searched, it is preferable to have a female conduct the search or be present as a witness. After the personal search is finished, the workstation and private vehicle can be searched.

Here are some guidelines for the searchers:

- Act courteously and do not subject anyone to accusations or defamatory remarks before, during, or after the search. Avoid any form of touching.
- Keep a written record of who was searched.
- Document in detail every incident that may lead to disciplinary action. This includes discovery of prohibited items, refusal to participate, suspicious actions, and disturbances.
- Photograph the prohibited items discovered. Mark the photographs as to what they show and make them a part of a written report.
- Place prohibited items in containers that are labeled or tagged to identify where they were found and by whom.

A written report of the search and its findings should be prepared. A good report will contain at least the following information:

- Date, time, and place of search
- Names of persons found to possess or own prohibited items, specific descriptions, and places where found
- Descriptions of incidents pertaining to search refusals, disturbances, and suspicious actions
- Photographs of materials seized
- Names of searchers

A full-scale unannounced search need not be scheduled if the search is limited to one or a few persons. Conversely, an unannounced search of all or a group of employees should not be used as an excuse to search one or a few persons whose conduct indicates use or possession of prohibited items.

Under the law, an employer cannot withhold illegal drugs found on company property, and a company official who makes such a decision is in violation of the law. Law enforcement authorities can be sensitive on this issue, particularly if contraband drugs such as cocaine, heroin, and marijuana are involved.

A policy provision that requires cooperation with and release of confiscated drugs to law enforcement authorities will keep the company on the right side of the law and at the same time send a message to employees who may be inclined to bring drugs to work.

SAMPLE PROGRAM MATERIALS

Appendixes 6–B through 6–H contain some sample materials that can be used in carrying out the activities described in this chapter.

Appendix 6–A

Consent for Release of Information and Release of Information Memorandum

CONSENT FOR RELEASE OF INFORMATION

I, (Name of employee), hereby consent to the disclosure of information concerning my progress in a treatment program I voluntarily entered with the encouragement of my employer.

I authorize (Name of treatment professional/facility) to disclose such information to (Name of supervisor) of (Name of company).

I understand that this consent is subject to revocation at any time, except to the extent that action has been taken in reliance of information released prior to revocation.

I affirm that this consent is freely given, without reservation, for the purpose set out above.

_____

(Printed or typed name of employee)

_____

(Signature of employee)

_____

(Date)

RELEASE OF INFORMATION MEMORANDUM

SUBJECT: Release of Patient Information

FROM: (Name of Treatment Professional/Facility)

TO: (Name of Supervisor and Company)

Enclosed please find information pertaining to (Name of employee), which is released in accordance with the attached copy of Consent for Release of Information.

The enclosed information is disclosed to you from confidential records. You should not disclose it further without the specific written consent of the person to whom it pertains.

_____

(Signature of treatment professional)

Appendix 6–B

Drug-Testing Program Procedures Developed for a Municipality

GENERAL

The following particulars will be in effect in all circumstances when drug or alcohol testing is performed.

1. Notification
   1.1 Prior to being tested, the applicant or employee to be tested will be informed in writing of the following:
      a. The City's drug- and alcohol-testing policy
      b. The individual's right to refuse to undergo testing
      c. The consequences of refusal to undergo testing
      d. The consequences of failure to pass testing
   1.2 The person to be tested will be asked to acknowledge receipt and understanding of the notice.
2. Consent
   2.1 No individual may be forcibly compelled to provide specimens for drug or alcohol testing.
   2.2 Refusal to provide specimens can, however, result in discipline, up to and including discharge, for employees and termination of the employment process for applicants.
   2.3 A failure to cooperate will be regarded as a refusal to provide a specimen and can result in discipline.
3. Training
   3.1 A supervisor may not make a decision to refer an employee for testing in a reasonable belief situation unless the supervisor has completed training in the following areas:
      a. Detecting the signs and behaviors of persons who may be using drugs or alcohol in violation of the City's drug and alcohol abuse policy
      b. Intervening in situations that may involve violations of the policy
      c. Recognizing these activities as a direct job responsibility
   3.2 It is the intention of the City that every supervisor will complete this training.
4. Two Supervisors Rule
   4.1 Two supervisors, both of whom are trained in drug and alcohol detection and intervention (as required by the City's policy), shall substantiate and concur in the decision to test an employee who is reasonably suspected of drug or alcohol use.

4.2   The decision to proceed with testing will be reported to a manager for approval. An exception to the manager approval requirement is granted when the approval cannot be obtained within the time parameters for testing, as explained elsewhere in these procedures.

5.   Detectable Amount

5.1   Any employee who is found through drug testing to have in his or her body system a detectable amount of an illegal drug will be subject to discipline up to and including discharge.

5.2   Any applicant who is found through drug testing to have in his or her body system a detectable amount of an illegal drug will be dropped from further consideration as a job candidate.

6.   Instructions to Report for Testing

6.1   Employees and applicants who are referred to testing will be provided instructions for reporting to the designated contract vendor's clinic for the collection of specimens.

6.2   The instructions will include the need to produce at the collection site a form of photographic personal identification (such as a State of Texas driving license) and to name or describe any medication taken in the previous 30 days.

7.   Declaration of Medication

7.1   At the collection site, the person to be tested will indicate on a form provided for that purpose the names of any medication taken in the previous 30 days.

8.   Release of Test Results

8.1   The drug-testing laboratory will be instructed to release test results to designated City officials and/or agents of the City.

8.2   All information relating to drug or alcohol testing or the identification of persons as users of drugs or alcohol will be protected by the City as confidential unless otherwise required by law or overriding public health and safety concerns or unless authorized in writing by the person in question.

9.   Appeal of a Positive Test Result

9.1   Any person whose drug or alcohol test is reported positive will be offered the opportunity of a private meeting to offer an explanation. The principal purpose of the meeting will be to determine whether there is any reason that a positive finding could have resulted from a cause other than drug or alcohol use.

9.2   The City, through its health and/or human resources officials, will judge whether an offered explanation merits further inquiry.

9.3   During the period of an appeal and any resulting inquiries, the preemployment process for applicants will be placed on hold and the employment status of an employee may be suspended. An employee who is suspended pending appeal will be permitted to use any available leave in order to remain in an active pay status. If the employee has no annual leave or chooses not to use it, the suspension will be without pay.

10.   Retesting of Urine Specimen

10.1   An employee whose drug or alcohol test is reported positive will be offered the opportunity to do the following:

a.   Obtain and independently test, at the employee's expense, the remaining portion of the urine specimen that yielded the positive result.

b.   Obtain the written test report of a positive urine test for the purpose of presenting it to an independent medical review at the employee's expense.

11.   Record Keeping
   11.1   Records pertaining to the City's drug-testing program will be maintained by the contract vendor that provides testing services.

PREEMPLOYMENT TESTING

1.   Persons Affected
   1.1   All applicants for employment, including applicants for part-time and seasonal positions and applicants who are former employees, are subject to drug and alcohol testing as part of the routine preemployment selection process.
2.   Refusal to Consent
   2.1   An applicant who declines to undergo testing or who declines to cooperate in the administration of testing will be dropped from consideration as a job candidate.
3.   Failure to Pass Testing
   3.1   An applicant who fails the preemployment drug or alcohol test will be dropped from consideration as a job candidate.
4.   Appeal of a Positive Test
   4.1   An applicant whose drug or alcohol test is reported positive will be offered the opportunity of a meeting to provide an explanation.
   4.2   The purpose of the meeting will be to determine whether there is any reason that a positive finding could have resulted from some cause other than drug or alcohol use.
   4.3   The City will make the final judgment as to whether an offered explanation merits further inquiry.
   4.4   During the period of an appeal and any resulting inquiries, the preemployment selection process for the applicant involved will be placed on hold.

RANDOM (UNANNOUNCED) TESTING

1.   Random Testing Defined
   1.1   Random testing is the unannounced testing of a percentage of employees who have been selected for testing randomly, such as by an unbiased computer-generated technique.
2.   Frequency
   2.1   Random testing will be conducted at a frequency of once a month with no advance notice as to the date of testing or the employees selected for testing.
3.   Persons Affected
   3.1   Random testing will be conducted only of employees who perform duties in safety-sensitive positions.
   3.2   The City will determine which positions are safety sensitive and will notify employees in those positions that they are subject to random testing.
4.   Notice of Selection
   4.1   An employee selected for random testing will be instructed to report to the specimen collection site without delay.

5. Failure to Appear
   5.1 Failure to appear promptly at the collection site will subject the employee to discipline. An exception to discipline will be granted only when the employee presents a valid reason in writing that is supported by a written report of the employee's supervisor.
6. Collection Site
   6.1 The collection site may be on City premises or at a contract vendor's clinic.

REASONABLE BELIEF TESTING

1. Reasonable Belief Defined
   1.1 A reasonable belief situation is a situation in which a supervisor is required by the City's Drug and Alcohol Abuse Policy to make a decision to administer a drug test to an employee whose on-duty conduct indicates impairment by a drug or alcohol.
   1.2 A reasonable and articulable belief that the employee is using a drug or alcohol in violation of the City's policy must be present.
   1.3 The belief must be supported by specific, contemporaneous physical, behavioral, or performance indicators of probable drug or alcohol use.
2. The Decision to Test
   2.1 The two supervisors rule, supported by management approval (where possible), will apply.
   2.2 A supervisor participating in the joint decision to conduct reasonable belief testing will make sure that the facts of the situation meet the following qualifications:
       a. They are capable of explanation and substantiation.
       b. They are specific, tangible, and contemporaneous.
       c. They are indicative of probable drug or alcohol use by the employee.
3. Indicators of Impairment
   3.1 The evidence of probable current drug or alcohol use could include any of the common indicators of impairment, including but not limited to stupor, excitation, slurred speech, staggering gait, loss of psychomotor control, marked changes in behavior, or the smell of alcohol.
4. Examples
   4.1 Examples of unacceptable conduct that suggests drug or alcohol impairment include but are not limited to the following:
       a. Being at fault in an accident
       b. Engaging in violent or disruptive behavior
       c. Being absent from the job excessively without explanation
       d. Engaging in unexplained erratic behavior
       e. Making mistakes in judgment or reasoning
       f. Deviating from productivity norms and safe working practices
   4.2 The unacceptable conduct can take many forms but must be accompanied by indicators of impairment for it to be considered indicative of drug or alcohol use.
5. Timing
   5.1 The reasonable belief determination will be made and the drug and/or alcohol tests will be conducted as soon as possible following the conduct that

gave rise to the reasonable belief and in no case longer than 24 hours for indicated drug use and no longer than 4 hours for indicated alcohol use.

6. Alcohol Testing Only
    6.1 When alcohol use but not drug use is indicated, the employee will be administered a preliminary test that is based on the analysis of saliva or breath specimens.
    6.2 The preliminary test will be conducted by a contract vendor employee who must be trained in the administration of preliminary alcohol tests.
    6.3 If the preliminary test is positive, a blood specimen will be drawn by a contract vendor employee who is trained and certified in the collection of blood specimens.

7. Drug and Alcohol Testing
    7.1 When drug use alone or use of drugs and alcohol together is an indicated possibility, the employee will be administered a preliminary alcohol test as described above and in addition will be required to provide a urine specimen for drug testing.

8. Safety Considerations
    8.1 An employee being processed for testing under these procedures will not be allowed to do the following:
        a. Operate a motor vehicle to or from the specimen collection site or from the place of work. Transportation for the employee will be provided by the City at the discretion of the supervisor involved.
        b. Engage in any safety-sensitive activities unless and until test results have been received.
    8.2 If the employee refuses to comply with the supervisor's prohibition against operation of a motor vehicle, the supervisor should call the police to report the employee as a possibly impaired driver.

9. Reporting
    9.1 The supervisors who jointly decide to administer reasonable belief testing will prepare an after-action report that includes the facts that led to the decision to test, the steps taken to obtain testing, the names of persons who have knowledge of the situation, and other related details.

POSTACCIDENT TESTING

1. Postaccident Testing Defined
    1.1 A postaccident testing situation is any situation in which an accident has resulted in an injury that could result in the filing of a workmen's compensation claim.
    1.2 Such an accident will typically require professional medical treatment beyond first aid and will render an employee unfit to perform routine duties.

2. Directly Involved Employees
    2.1 The employees to be tested in a postaccident situation include any employee directly involved in the accident whose order, action, or failure to act is determined to be, or cannot be ruled out as, a causative factor in the events leading to or causing the accident.

3. Supervisory Responsibilities
    3.1 The supervisor having functional responsibility for investigation of the ac-

cident shall make a timely, good-faith determination as to whether the accident meets the requirements of these procedures and, if so, to take all practical steps to have each directly involved employee tested for evidence of drug and alcohol use.

3.2 As soon as practical following the accident, the supervisor will make arrangements for the directly involved employees to provide specimens.

3.3 The time frame for obtaining specimens related to drug impairment is 24 hours and for alcohol impairment 4 hours.

4. Safety Considerations

4.1 An employee being processed for testing under these procedures will not be allowed to do the following:

a. Operate a motor vehicle to or from the specimen collection site or from the place of work. Transportation for the employee will be provided by the City at the direction of the supervisor involved.

b. Engage in any safety-sensitive activities unless and until negative test results have been received.

4.2 If the employee refuses to comply with the supervisor's prohibition against operation of a motor vehicle, the supervisor should call the police to report the employee as a possibly impaired driver.

5. Reporting

5.1 The supervisor having responsibility for investigating the accident will prepare an after-action report that includes the facts that led to the identification of the directly involved employees, the steps taken to obtain testing, the names of persons who have knowledge of the situation, and other related details.

COLLECTION AND ANALYSIS PROCEDURES

1. Definitions

1.1 For purposes of these procedures, the following definitions apply:

aliquot   A portion of a specimen used for testing.

chain of custody   Procedures to account for the integrity of each urine specimen by tracking its handling and storage from point of specimen collection to final disposition of the specimen. These procedures shall require that an approved chain-of-custody form be used from the time of collection to its receipt by the laboratory and that upon receipt by the laboratory, an appropriate laboratory chain-of-custody form(s) account for the sample or sample aliquots within the laboratory. Chain-of-custody forms shall, at a minimum, include an entry documenting the date and purpose each time a specimen or aliquot is handled or transferred and identifying every individual in the chain of custody.

collection site   A place designated by the City where individuals present themselves for the purpose of providing specimens to be analyzed for the presence of drugs or alcohol.

collection site person   A person who instructs and assists individuals at a collection site and who receives and makes an initial examination of the specimens provided by those individuals. A collection site person shall have successfully completed training to carry out this function.

confirmatory test   A second analytical procedure to identify the presence in a urine specimen of a specific drug or metabolite that is independent of the initial test and that uses a different technique and chemical principle from that of the initial test in order to ensure reliability and accuracy. Gas chromatography/mass spectrometry (GC/MS) is the only authorized confirmation method.

initial test   For drug testing, an immunoassay screen to eliminate negative urine specimens from further consideration. For alcohol testing, an analysis of breath or saliva specimens for the purpose of eliminating negative specimens from further consideration. Also known as *screening test* or *preliminary test*.

2. Specimen Collection
    2.1   The City's drug-testing program shall have one or more designated collection sites that have all the necessary personnel, materials, equipment, facilities, and supervision to provide for the collection, security, temporary storage, and shipping or transportation of specimens to a certified drug-testing laboratory.
    2.2   Procedures shall provide for the designated collection site to be secure. If a collection site facility is dedicated solely to urine collection, it shall be secure at all times. If a facility cannot be dedicated solely to drug testing, the portion of the facility used for testing shall be secured during drug testing.
    2.3   Chain-of-custody standardized forms shall be properly executed by the authorized collection site personnel upon receipt of specimens. Handling and transportation of urine specimens from one authorized individual or place to another shall always be accomplished through chain-of-custody procedures. Every effort shall be made to minimize the number of persons handling specimens.
    2.4   No unauthorized personnel shall be permitted in any part of the designated collection site when urine specimens are collected or stored.
    2.5   The City shall take precautions to ensure that a urine specimen not be adulterated or diluted during the collection procedure and that information on the urine bottle and in the records can identify the individual from whom the specimen was collected. The following minimum precautions shall be taken to ensure that unadulterated specimens are obtained and correctly identified:
          a.   To deter the dilution of specimens at the collection site, toilet bluing agents shall be placed in toilet tanks wherever possible, so the reservoir of water in the toilet bowl remains blue. There shall be no other source of water (e.g., no shower or sink) in the enclosure where urination occurs.
          b.   When an individual arrives at the collection site, the collection site person shall ask the individual to present photo identification. If the individual does not have proper photo identification, the collection site person shall contact the supervisor of the individual, the coordinator of the drug-testing program, or any other City official who can positively identify the individual. If the individual's identity cannot be established, the collection site person shall not proceed with the collection.
          c.   If the individual fails to arrive at the assigned time, the collection site

person shall contact the appropriate authority to obtain guidance on the action to be taken.

d. The collection site person shall ask the individual to remove any un-necessary outer garments, such as a coat or jacket, that might conceal items or substances that could be used to tamper with or adulterate the individual's urine specimen. The collection site person shall make sure that all personal belongings, such as a purse or briefcase, remain with the outer garments. The individual may retain his or her wallet.

e. The individual shall be instructed to wash and dry his or her hands prior to urination.

f. After washing his or her hands, the individual shall remain in the presence of the collection site person and shall not have access to any water fountain, faucet, soap dispenser, cleaning agent, or other mate-rials that could be used to adulterate the specimen.

g. The collection site person shall make written note of any unusual behavior or appearance.

h. Upon receiving the specimen from the individual, the collection site person shall determine that it contains at least 60 milliliters of urine. If there is less than 60 milliliters of urine in the container, the specimen will be discarded. The individual may be given a reasonable amount of liquid to drink (e.g., a glass of water) and will be asked to make a second attempt when ready. If the individual fails for any reason to provide 60 milliliters of urine, the collection site person shall contact the appropriate authority to obtain guidance on the action to be taken.

i. After the specimen has been provided and submitted to the collection site person, the individual shall be allowed to wash his or her hands.

j. Immediately after the specimen is collected, the collection site person shall measure the temperature of the specimen. The temperature-meas-uring device used must accurately reflect the temperature of the spec-imen and not contaminate the specimen. The time from urination to temperature measurement is critical and in no case shall exceed four minutes.

k. If the temperature of a specimen is outside the range of 32.5°C to 37.7°C, or 90.5°F to 99.8°F, that is reason to believe that the individual may have altered or substituted the specimen. An individual may volunteer to have his or her oral temperature taken to provide evidence to counter the reason to believe that the individual may have altered or substituted the specimen caused by the specimen's temperature falling outside the prescribed range.

l. Immediately after the specimen is collected, the collection site person shall inspect the specimen to determine its color and look for any signs of contaminants.

m. Specimens suspected of being adulterated shall be forwarded to the laboratory for testing.

n. Whenever there is reason to believe that a particular individual may have altered or substituted a specimen, a second specimen shall be obtained as soon as possible under the direct supervision of a same-gender collection site person.

o. Both the individual being tested and the collection site person shall keep the specimen in view at all times prior to its being sealed and labeled. The collection site person and individual shall be present at the same time during the collection procedures.

p. The collection site person shall place securely on the bottle an identification label that contains the date, the individual's specimen number, and any other identifying information.

q. The individual shall initial the identification label on the specimen bottle for the purpose of certifying that it is the specimen collected from him or her.

r. The collection site person shall record all information identifying the specimen.

s. The collection site person shall complete the chain-of-custody form.

t. The urine specimen and chain-of-custody form should be packaged for shipment. If the specimen is not immediately packaged for shipment, it shall be appropriately safeguarded.

u. While any part of the above chain-of-custody procedures is being performed, it is essential that the urine specimen and custody documents be under the control of the involved collection site person. If the involved collection site person leaves his or her workstation momentarily, the specimen and custody form shall be taken with him or her or shall be secured. After the collection site person returns to the workstation, the custody process will continue. If the collection site person is leaving for an extended period of time, the specimen shall be packaged for mailing before he or she leaves the site.

2.6 To the maximum extent possible, collection site personnel shall keep the individual's specimen bottle within sight both before and after the individual has urinated.

2.7 After the specimen is collected, it shall be properly sealed and labeled.

2.8 An approved chain-of-custody form shall be used for maintaining control and accountability of each specimen from the point of collection to final disposition of the specimen. The date and purpose shall be documented on an approved chain-of-custody form each time a specimen is handled or transferred, and every individual in the chain shall be identified. Every effort shall be made to minimize the number of persons handling specimens.

3. Transportation to Laboratory

3.1 Collection site personnel shall arrange to ship the collected specimens to the drug-testing laboratory.

3.2 The specimens shall be placed in containers designed to minimize the possibility of damage during shipment (for example, using specimen boxes or padded mailers), and those containers shall be sealed to eliminate the possibility of undetected tampering. On the tape sealing the container, the collection site supervisor shall sign and enter the date specimens were sealed in the containers for shipment.

3.3 The collection site personnel shall ensure that the chain-of-custody documentation is attached to each container sealed for shipment to the drug-testing laboratory.

3.4 Blood specimens must be shipped in a cooled condition by any means adequate to ensure delivery within 24 hours of receipt by the carrier. Urine specimens must be shipped by an expeditious means but need not be shipped in a cooled condition for overnight delivery.

4. Analysis at the Laboratory
   4.1 The laboratory shall test for the following eight major drug classes:
       a. Cannabinoids (marijuana)
       b. Cocaine
       c. Opiates
       d. Phencyclidine (PCP)
       e. Amphetamines
       f. Barbiturates
       g. Methaqualone
       h. Methadone
       i. Benzodiazepines
   4.2 The initial test shall use an enzyme immunoassay, such as the enzyme multiplied immunoassay technique (EMIT).
   4.3 All specimens identified as positive on the initial test shall be confirmed using GC/MS techniques.

5. Reporting Results
   5.1 The contract vendor shall report test results within an average of five working days after receipt of the specimen by the laboratory.
   5.2 The contract vendor will maintain records of test results on behalf of the City.
   5.3 The contract vendor shall report as negative all specimens that are negative on the initial test or negative on the confirmatory test. Only specimens confirmed positive shall be reported positive for a specific drug.

6. Long-Term Storage
   6.1 Unless otherwise authorized in writing by the City, the drug-testing laboratory shall retain and place in properly secured long-term frozen storage for a minimum of one year all specimens confirmed positive.
   6.2 Within this one-year period, the City may request the laboratory to retain the specimen for an additional period of time, but if no such request is received, the laboratory may discard the specimen after the end of one year, except that the laboratory shall be required to maintain any specimens under legal challenge for an indefinite period.

7. Retesting Specimens
   7.1 Because some analytes deteriorate or are lost during freezing and/or storage, quantitation for a retest is not subject to a specific cutoff requirement but must provide data sufficient to confirm the presence of the drug or metabolite.

8. Laboratory Facilities
   8.1 Laboratory facilities shall comply with applicable provisions of any state licensure requirements and shall have the capability, at the same laboratory premises, of performing initial and confirmatory tests.

Appendix 6–C

Notice of Legal Drug Use

In accordance with the Company's policy concerning safety on the job, please be advised that I am currently taking and possessing at work the following prescription drug, which has been prescribed for a valid medical purpose:

Name of drug _____

Prescription number _____   Prescription date _____

Prescribing physician's name _____

Prescribing physician's phone number _____

This drug produces the following side effects:

[ ] Dizziness   [ ] Drowsiness   [ ] Nausea

Other _____

My use of this drug is

[ ] temporary and is expected to end on or about _____.

[ ] indefinite.

[ ] permanent.

I hereby give my consent for the above-named prescribing physician to answer questions about my use of this drug.

_____   _____
(Employee's name)   (Employee's signature)

                                                    _____
                                                    (Date)

Appendix 6–D

Guidelines for Supervisors at an Oil and Gas Company

The following describes the procedures and responsibilities of supervisors in the implementation of the policy on use and possession of intoxicants, illegal drugs, deadly weapons, explosives, searches of Company property, and substance screening. The suspected need for a search or screening and all communication leading up to the search or screening are to be handled with extreme confidentiality.

IMPLEMENTATION

All District personnel will be notified of the policy by letter. Integral parts of the implementation plan include supervisor training, employee education, and contractor education.

Supervisor Training

Corporate Security, Company Medical, and Employee Relations will provide training to supervisors in the District. The training will include information on narcotics awareness; Company policy; how to determine whether there exists a reasonable need for a search for illegal drugs, intoxicants, deadly weapons, or explosives or for substance screening; and appropriate actions.

Employee Education

As notification of the policy is sent to all employees, literature on drug and alcohol abuse and the employee assistance program (EAP) shall be made available at all locations.

All District employees will attend group meetings for a review of the policy by Corporate Security, Company Medical, and Employee Relations. Every employee shall sign an acknowledgment form on receipt and understanding of the policy, which should be returned to the immediate supervisor. Each supervisor shall be responsible for forwarding acknowledgment forms for all employees to Employee Relations for filing. In addition, copies of the policy should be posted at all work locations. New hires should likewise receive a copy of the policy and acknowledgment form as part of the new employee orientation process.

Contractor Education

Contract employees shall be made aware of the policy through the following means: a letter outlining the policy, posted signs, and term agreements.

PREEMPLOYMENT SUBSTANCE SCREENING

Applicants for employment will be required to undergo urinalysis or other screening for illegal drugs. The job applicant will be informed of this drug screening prior to such screening. No preemployment screening is to take place without the applicant's permission. The applicant's permission is obtained by having the applicant sign a Preemployment Consent Form. Refusal by the applicant to sign such a consent form or to submit to a test will result in denial of employment.

When the presence of an illegal drug at any level is detected in the job applicant, employment will be denied.

The Company Medical Department will ensure that the chain of custody is maintained and that the samples are properly tested only at laboratories approved by the Company Medical Department.

SUBSTANCE SCREENING OF CURRENT EMPLOYEES

If a supervisor feels that there is a reasonable need for substance screening of an employee for illegal drugs or intoxicants, he or she will request screening through the appropriate organizational chain of command. The Department Manager, Company Medical Department, and District Employees Relations Manager will coordinate their actions as appropriate, including requesting support of legal or other staff groups as required. The Company Medical Department will be responsible for establishing the proper chain of custody and for arranging proper testing of samples and substances at approved laboratories.

No employee screening is to take place without the employee's permission. The employee's permission is obtained by having the employee sign an Employee Consent Form.

If an employee's actions, demeanor, or appearance leads a supervisor to reasonably suspect that the employee is under the influence of illegal drugs or intoxicants, the supervisor has the authority to initiate the substance-screening procedure regarding that employee without going through the chain of command if time is critical in assessing the situation. Management needs to be notified as soon as possible if screening was necessary without first going through the chain of command.

If an employee is unwilling to report to the Company Medical Department or a medical facility for evaluation and screening or such facility is unavailable, the supervisor should require the employee to report to an office area or, if not available, to a safe nonworking area.

In either of the above situations the supervisor is to contact Management for further guidance if its assistance is available. In the absence of such consultation and if the supervisor has a reasonable doubt about the employee's ability to meet job requirements satisfactorily and safely, the supervisor shall send the employee home pending results of testing or other administrative determination.

If the employee is to go to an approved medical facility outside the Company for substance screening or to go home, the supervisor is to arrange for the employee's safe transport.

Prior to initiating questioning relative to use or possession, the supervisor is to consult with Management if it is available. The supervisor is to have a witness present and, without other guidance, to limit his or her questioning to determining the employee's general condition (for instance, Does the employee feel sick? Does the employee know where he or she is? To whom is he or she talking? What is the reason for the employee's present condition?).

Where a represented employee is suspected of violating this policy, that employee may, upon request, have his or her Union Representative present during any employee questioning that may lead to disciplinary action. If a Union Representative is not immediately available, the questioning can continue.

If an employee refuses to report to a medical facility for evaluation or refuses to undergo substance screening in accordance with this policy or refuses to sign an Employee Consent Form, such employee shall immediately be sent home pending a review of the matter. Such an employee shall be subject to discipline up to and including termination of employment.

All substance screenings are to be documented by Company Medical and distributed to appropriate management.

SEARCHES

Searches of Company facilities and property can be conducted at any time and do not have to be based on reasonable suspicion, although the process normally begins with the supervisor. If a supervisor feels that there is reasonable need for a search for intoxicants, illegal drugs, deadly weapons, explosives, or any combination of these, he or she will obtain approval through the appropriate organizational chain of command. Corporate Security will arrange, conduct, and document the search. The appropriate Department Manager, Vice President, Employee Relations Manager, and Legal staff as necessary will be informed of the search as soon as possible.

If an employee's actions, demeanor, or appearance leads a supervisor to reasonably suspect that the employee is under the influence of illegal drugs or intoxicants, the supervisor has the authority to initiate the search procedure regarding that employee without going through the chain of command if time is critical in assessing the situation. Management needs to be notified as soon as possible if a search was necessary without first going through the steps to involve Corporate Security.

It will be the responsibility of Corporate Security to arrange and conduct the search. Corporate Security may, at its discretion, hire outside contract security services for the purpose of conducting a search. Corporate Security will handle and dispose of any illegal drugs, intoxicants, deadly weapons, or explosives found.

Corporate Security will promptly report the findings orally to the Vice President, the appropriate Department Manager, and the District Employee Relations Manager. Present at all searches will be a representative of Corporate Security, the ranking supervisor in the area, and, if reasonably available, the Department Manager or his or her alternate. If a represented employee requests that a Union Representative (Workmen's Committee or Steward) be present during a search of the Company facility or a personal search, District Employee Relations should be contacted prior to the search of that employee or his or her personal effects. If a Union Representative is not immediately available, the search can continue.

Company premises, the staging area, and items carried by a person who is subject to a search may be searched. Examples of these items are duffel bags, lunch boxes, jackets, lockers, toolboxes, desks, vehicles, and hats.

Personal physical searches of employees generally will not be conducted except in those cases when an employee is restrained because there exists reasonable need or reasonable belief that failure to do so might jeopardize safety, life, or property. In these cases, the ranking supervisor at the site will be responsible for making the decision to conduct such a personal physical search.

If an employee is suspected of being in violation of the policy concerning selling, purchasing, transferring, or possessing an illegal drug, the supervisor is to do the following:

1. Take possession of any suspected intoxicants or illegal drugs which are in plain sight
2. Secure any container or the like where alcohol or illegal drugs may be present for a subsequent search by appropriate personnel
3. Order the employee to report to an area in the facility where appropriate personnel, preferably more than one supervisor, can question the suspected employee or employees in private

If an employee claims that any drug in his or her possession is a medication prescribed by a doctor, the employee will be requested to sign an Authorization to Release Medical Information Form that is to be forwarded through Employee Relations to the Medical Department for verification by the employee's doctor. The employee also may be asked to provide any documentation that is necessary to assist the Medical Department in determining whether or not the medication is authorized.

If a search reveals that a contractor is in violation of the policy, the Company cannot fire the contractor's employee. Instead, the Company Supervisor in charge of the property or facility will notify the contractor's on-site representative or will call the contractor's office and ask the contractor to remove the offending employee from Company property. The contractor will be told by the responsible Company Supervisor that the subject employee will not be allowed to reenter Company property without specific written authority.

All searches are to be documented by Corporate Security, with assistance from supervisory personnel.

VIOLATIONS OF POLICY

Management and supervisors are to restrict conversations concerning possible violations of this policy to those persons who are participating in any questioning, evaluation, investigation, or disciplinary action and who need to know about the details of the investigation. This restriction includes not mentioning the name of the employee or employees suspected of violating this policy. Management, supervisors, and investigators are to instruct other employees, except as stated above, not to talk about such possible violations.

If illegal drugs, intoxicants, deadly weapons, or explosives are discovered in the possession or control of any employee, the apparent offending employee is to be sent home and told that he or she will be contacted as soon as the investigation is completed. Depending on the conclusions reached during such investigation, an employee may be subject to discipline up to and including termination of employment even for a first offense.

The following guidelines summarize actions for violations of the policy, recognizing that the supervisor should immediately consult an appropriate member of Management before final action is taken:

Findings	Anticipated Action
Detection of illegal drug in screening process	Termination or do not hire
Detection of legally obtained drug during screening process with symptoms of impairment on the job	Suspension
Use, possession, or selling of illegal drugs on Company property or while on company business	Termination
Unauthorized use or possession of alcoholic beverages in an operating area	Progressive discipline
Under the influence of intoxicants on Company property, including Company vehicles	Progressive discipline
Unopened alcoholic beverage in personal vehicle in parking lot but not in violation of state law	Progressive discipline
Firearm found in personal vehicle on Company parking lot but not in violation of state law	Progressive discipline
Possession of firearms on a lease	Progressive discipline
Use of firearms on Company property	Progressive discipline
Firearms in Company vehicle	Progressive discipline
Possession or use of unauthorized explosives on Company property, including in vehicle	Termination

Appendix 6–E

Search Consent

In the interest of maintaining a safe and efficient environment for employees and nonemployees, including contractors, subcontractors, vendors, suppliers, visitors, and invitees, the Company has and enforces a policy designed to control drug abuse on Company premises and in connection with Company business.

The Company administers a search program to ensure compliance with its drug abuse policy. Accordingly, you may from time to time be asked to submit to a search of your person, personal effects, or personal vehicle while entering, on, or departing Company premises or while performing Company business. An employee who fails to cooperate or declines to submit to a search when requested may be subject to disciplinary action, including discharge. A nonemployee who fails to cooperate or declines to submit to a search may be escorted from Company premises, barred from reentry, and barred from future participation in Company business.

A written statement of this policy is attached or is prominently displayed at Company premises. You are urged to carefully read and gain a full understanding of it prior to signing this consent.

EMPLOYEE OR NONEMPLOYEE RESPONSE

I have read and understand the Company's policy provisions regarding searches. I agree to comply.

_____   _____

(Date)   (Signature)

_____   _____

(Signature of witness)   (Printed name of consenter)

[ ]   Employee   Department _____

[ ]   Nonemployee   Employer _____

Appendix 6–F

Report of Performance or Behavior Incident

Date _____

Name of employee observed _____

Person who observed the incident _____

Length of time observed _____

Time and date of incident _____

Place of incident _____

Details of incident (Describe the employee's actions.)

_____

_____

_____

_____

_____

_____

_____

Names of witnesses

_____   _____

_____   _____

Action taken by supervisor or other responsible person

_____

_____

_____

Person preparing this report _____

Appendix 6–G

Questionnaire for Contractors

Yes No

[ ] [ ]   1. Do you have a written drug-testing policy? If yes, please attach a copy to this questionnaire.

[ ] [ ]   2. Have all the persons affected by the policy acknowledged understanding of it? If yes, explain how the acknowledgment was made.

_____

[ ] [ ]   3. Is the policy readily available at the collection site for reading by employees at the time urine specimens are collected?

[ ] [ ]   4. Is a written consent obtained from each specimen donor at the time the specimen is collected? If yes, please attach a sample copy to this questionnaire.

          5. Does your drug-testing policy allow and do you perform drug testing in the following situations?

[ ] [ ]   When evaluating job applicants
[ ] [ ]   When employee behavior suggests impairment (reasonable cause)
[ ] [ ]   Following an accident
[ ] [ ]   Periodically without announcement
[ ] [ ]   Randomly
[ ] [ ]   Incident to health evaluations
[ ] [ ]   Return to work following prolonged absence
[ ] [ ]   In connection with drug rehabilitation
[ ] [ ]   Other (describe)

[ ] [ ]   6. Does your written drug-testing policy cover your contractors and subcontractors?

[ ] [ ]   7. How frequently do you conduct unannounced testing?
[ ] [ ]   Monthly
[ ] [ ]   Every two months
[ ] [ ]   Quarterly
[ ] [ ]   Semiannually
[ ] [ ]   Annually
[ ] [ ]   Other (describe) _____

[ ] [ ]   8. When unannounced testing is conducted, are all employees present for duty required to provide a urine specimen? If some employees are treated differently, please explain why.

_____

_____

            9. Briefly describe the action you take when one of your contractor employees tests positive.

_____

_____

           10. During each 12-month period, what approximate percentage of your employees are tested for drugs? _____ percent

[ ] [ ]   11. Does your company do any of the drug testing?

[ ] [ ]   12. Is any drug testing done at a work location? If yes, please name the test technique and the agency conducting the testing.

_____

_____

[ ] [ ]   13. Does your company use a vendor to collect specimens? If yes, please identify the vendor and provide the vendor's address and phone number.

_____

_____

_____

          14. What precautions are taken to prevent contami-
nation or substitution of urine specimens at the
collection site?

[ ] [ ]   Observation during voiding
[ ] [ ]   "Clean bathroom" preparations
[ ] [ ]   Temperature check of specimens. If yes, how is
temperature measured?

_____

_____

[ ] [ ]   Other (describe)

_____

[ ] [ ]   15. Are the collected urine specimens accounted for
by strict chain-of-custody procedures? If yes, please
attach a sample copy of the chain-of-custody form.

[ ] [ ]   16. Are positive specimens tested a second time to
confirm the initial positive test results? If yes, identify the initial test technique and the confirmation
test technique.

          Initial _____

          Confirmation _____

          17. Briefly describe any action taken with respect to
an employee who tests positive in an initial, unconfirmed test.

_____

_____

18. What drug classes are looked for in the testing techniques?

[ ] [ ]   Cannabinoids (marijuana substances)
[ ] [ ]   Cocaine
[ ] [ ]   Opiates
[ ] [ ]   Amphetamines
[ ] [ ]   Phencyclidine (PCP)
[ ] [ ]   Barbiturates
[ ] [ ]   Benzodiazepines
[ ] [ ]   Methaqualone
[ ] [ ]   Other (identify) _____

[ ] [ ] 19. Do the cutoff levels for the various drug classes conform to the recommendations of the test system's manufacturer?

[ ] [ ] 20. Are positive, confirmed drug test results reviewed by a person knowledgeable in substance abuse disorders?

[ ] [ ] 21. Is the drug-testing laboratory certified by the U.S. Department of Health and Human Services? In the space below, please provide the name of the drug-testing laboratory and its address, phone number, and contact person.

_____

_____

_____

[ ] [ ] 22. Do you maintain at the work location a capability for administering blood alcohol concentration (BAC) tests, such as those based on the analysis of breath or saliva specimens?

[ ] [ ]   If yes, do you have supervisors or specialists who are trained in the administration of such tests?

[ ] [ ]   If yes, are these tests administered in reasonable cause and postaccident situations?

[ ] [ ]   If a test of this type is positive, is the person immediately transported to a facility where a blood specimen is drawn for confirmation testing?

[ ] [ ]   23. Have you received a copy of our Company's Drug and Alcohol Abuse Policy, which requires contractors to be free from illicit drugs and to be free from the influence of alcohol on our property?

[ ] [ ]   24. Are you aware of the contract language, which requires that contractors and third parties not possess, use, distribute, or sell illicit drugs or controlled substances in the workplace or when conducting business on behalf of our Company; requires employees and third parties to be free from illicit drugs and controlled substances and to be free from the influence of alcohol while on our Company's owned, leased, or operated premises; and requires contractors to agree to conduct periodic searches and testing for such substances?

            25. In the space below, identify the person in your company who serves as the principal contact concerning drug testing. Please include a telephone number.

_____

Appendix 6–H

Alcohol- and Drug-Testing Standards for Contractors

1. The contractor shall have a written policy on alcohol and drug abuse. The policy will include provisions for the following:
   a. Drug testing employees prior to their assignment to Company operations/facilities
   b. Reasonable cause testing
   c. Postaccident testing
   d. Random testing
2. During each 12-month period, the contractor shall drug test at least 50 percent of the number of employees who perform safety-sensitive work.
3. A copy of the contractor's policy must be available at the urine specimen collection point for reading by any contractor or subcontractor employee prior to giving a urine specimen.
4. The specimen donor will be required to provide positive identification at the collection point.
5. Written consent must be obtained from the donor at the collection point.
6. The chain of custody of the specimen must be preserved during each phase of the procedure as follows:
   a. The specimen container will be of the type that is packaged at the point of manufacture in a protective plastic envelope and affixed with a label.
   b. Nothing shall be introduced (such as a thermometer or litmus paper) into the specimen or its container at the collection point, and every reasonable effort will be made to prevent contamination.
   c. Direct observation of the voiding of the specimen is not mandatory, but the collector's position relative to the donor during the collection and voiding process will be uninterrupted and unobstructed, giving the collector the opportunity to detect any attempt to substitute, dilute, or contaminate the specimen.
   d. After the donor has voided into the container, the donor will place tape across the container cap, sign the label, place the container in a plastic envelope, place tape across the envelope sealing flap, and sign the tape.
7. Laboratory testing of the sample must include assays that test for amphetamines, barbiturates, benzodiazepines, cannabinoids, cocaine, methaqualone, opiates, and phencyclidine (PCP).
8. A laboratory certified by the U.S. Department of Health and Human Services must be used for the analysis of the specimens. The same laboratory must be

used in all phases of the specimen analysis, including screening and confirmation testing. Drug testing on-site or outside of the laboratory is not acceptable.

9.   The test methods shall consist of at least one preliminary screen using an enzyme immunoassay or a radioimmunoassay. All specimens preliminarily tested as positive must then be referred for confirmation to gas chromatography/mass spectrometry (GC/MS). The cutoff levels shall be those recommended by the test systems' manufacturers.

10.   All positive samples must be maintained by the laboratory in a frozen state for a 12-month period.

11.   Any donor whose test is confirmed positive for amphetamines, barbiturates, benzodiazepines, methaqualone, and opiates must be queried with respect to the use of prescription and over-the-counter medications. Any donor testing positive for these substances as a result of the legitimate use of prescribed medications should not be considered a user of illicit drugs.

12.   The contractor shall maintain at, or accessible to, work locations a capability for administering blood alcohol concentration (BAC) tests, such as those based on the analysis of breath or saliva specimens. These tests may be administered by the contractor's supervisors or specialists (who have been trained in the administration of such field tests) in reasonable cause and postaccident situations.

13.   All alcohol and drug test results must be maintained in a confidential manner and transmitted to Company officials on a need-to-know basis only.

Chapter 7

Collecting Specimens for Drug Testing

Obtaining an accurate and reliable drug test depends entirely on the provision of a fresh, uncontaminated specimen. More than this, the specimen must be linked beyond question to the individual who provided it. These are not easy tasks considering the motivations of some individuals to escape detection.

Mistakes are made in drug testing, but controls that detect most if not all mistakes exist. In the laboratory, where specimens are analyzed by highly sophisticated and automated testing instruments, very few mistakes occur because the opportunities for human error have been designed out of the process. When mistakes are discovered in the laboratory, they are almost always found to result from human activities.

Specimen collection is not a scientific process but an administrative process that relies on human labor. It is carried out with nothing more elaborate than a pen, some forms, and routine supplies. The people component is at the heart of the process and represents both its strength and weakness. The strength is the ability of the human mind to respond to different situations, and the weakness is the inevitability of error.

Specimen collection is often taken for granted. Employers tend to assume that because the function is administrative in nature, it will be correctly performed by people who operate according to simple, easy-to-follow procedures. This may be true in theory but not in practice.

Employers often fail to oversee specimen collection properly. They pay much more attention to the scientific process, in which mistakes are rarely made. The medical review officer (MRO), for example, is the employer's agent for ensuring the accuracy and reliability of test results, but no comparable oversight mechanism exists for ensuring the integrity of specimens.

Arbitrators, hearing officers, and judges, however, do not take specimen collection lightly. It also is foremost in the minds of labor representatives, plaintiffs' attorneys, and others who may be opposed to drug testing. The collection function can be the Achilles' heel of a company's drug-testing program.

What can be done to ensure quality collections? To start with, employers need to become more aware of their exposure to risk resulting from imperfect specimen collection. They should insist that the collectors be well trained and have sufficient experience; that the procedures for collecting conform to standards that guarantee the integrity of the specimens, strict chain of custody, and irrefutable linkage of each specimen to the donor; and that collections be attended by a system of controls, cross-checking, and close supervision. Appendixes 7–A through 7–D contain some sample materials that can be used in conducting a successful urine specimen collection program.

THE COLLECTION PROCESS

Obtaining Consents

Management may want to obtain from each employee a written consent in advance of testing. A consent can, however, be withdrawn at any time, and the only consent that counts is the one given at the time the urine specimen is collected for testing. Nonetheless, an advance consent has value, if only to underscore management's determination to conduct testing as authorized by policy. Appendix 7–B contains some sample consent forms.

The Collection Site

Specimens may be collected in one or several places. Collection sites could be on the employer's premises, such as in the regular bathroom facilities located in the employee's locker room, the medical station, portable toilet facilities set up outside, or a mobile van brought to the parking lot. Collection sites also can be away from the work location, such as at the offices of a collection vendor, a clinic or hospital, or a doctor's office. In exceptional cases, a public rest room may be used. An example of an exceptional case would be the need to make a collection following an accident at a location where there is no designated collection site.

The designated collection sites, whether located on or off company premises or operated by the company or a contractor, have a number of things in common:

- Each is staffed by personnel who are trained in the collection of specimens.
- Supervisory personnel are present to provide guidance to the collectors and ensure that established collection procedures are strictly followed.
- All the necessary forms, supplies, and equipment are on hand.
- The collection site is sufficient to accommodate donors being processed as well as donors waiting to be processed.

Whenever specimens are being collected, persons not properly engaged in the collection process should be prohibited from entering the collection site. If the site is dedicated solely to urine collection, it should be restricted and secure at all times. When the site is not dedicated solely to specimen collection, it should be made secure and designated a restricted area at those times when specimen collection is in progress.

Chain of Custody

The chain-of-custody form is usually a standard form developed by the drug-testing laboratory, the employer, or both. The form typically does the following:

- Identifies the drug-testing laboratory
- Identifies the type of test or tests to be made of the specimen
- Identifies the date of the collection
- Identifies the specimen donor
- Identifies the collector
- Identifies any other persons who have had access to the specimen, as well as the dates and reasons for access
- Includes a place for comments about medications taken by the donor that may be relevant to the testing scheme

The chain-of-custody form is executed by the specimen collector upon receipt of the specimen. The handling and transferring of a specimen from one person or place to another is documented by the form. The number of persons having access to a specimen is held to an absolute minimum.

Privacy

Many employers require witnessed collection of specimens. This approach need not be insensitive to privacy. A common practice is for the collector to take up a position 10 to 20 feet outside the bathroom stall, with the stall door partially open. The collector does not look directly at the donor but maintains a view from the rear or side that will allow the detection of any suspicious activity.

In the federal sector, the procedures for collecting urine specimens allow the individual privacy unless there is reason to believe that a particular individual may alter or substitute the specimen to be provided. Under the federal rules, a higher level supervisor must review and concur in advance with any decision by a collector to conduct a witnessed collection. Justifications for a witnessed collection include a prior or instant attempt to cheat on the test, a prior failure of a test, and a test of a person who is undergoing rehabilitation.

Bathroom Preparation

With or without a witness, precautions are taken to ensure that a urine specimen not be adulterated or diluted during the collection procedure. A bluing agent can be placed in the toilet tank so that the reservoir of water in the bowl remains blue. If the donor puts any of the blued water in the specimen bottle, this condition can be visually detected by the collector.

There should be no other source of water in the enclosure where urination occurs. In many facilities, this will mean the disconnection of water lines to sinks and showers. Another sensible preparation is to remove from the bathroom any materials, such as soap or air fresheners, that could be used to contaminate a specimen.

Positive Identification of the Donor

When an individual arrives at the collection site, the collector will ask the individual to present photo identification, such as a driver's license or company badge. If the individual does not have acceptable photo identification, the collector will contact the individual's supervisor, the coordinator of the drug-testing program, or any other company official who can positively identify the individual. If the individual's identity cannot be established, the collector will not proceed with the collection or will proceed only after noting this fact on the donor's chain-of-custody form.

Preparing the Donor

The collector will ask the individual to remove any unnecessary outer garments, such as a coat or jacket, that might conceal items or substances that could be used to tamper with or adulterate the urine specimen. Any hand-held personal belongings, such as a purse or briefcase, are placed with the outer garments in a secure place until the donor has been processed. The collector will allow the donor to keep his or her wallet, pocket watch, or other valuable items, but depending on the employer's instructions, the collector might ask the donor to allow an examination of them.

The donor is allowed to wash and dry his or her hands prior to urination. After this is done, the individual remains in the presence of the collector without access to water, soap, or any other materials that could be used to contaminate the specimen. Washing of the hands also should be permitted following urination.

Specimen Volume

Upon receiving the specimen from the individual, the collector will visually examine the specimen bottle to make sure that it contains at least 60 milliliters of urine. Markings on the side of the bottle indicate the volume. If the donor has trouble providing the necessary amount, additional urine can be collected in one or more other bottles in subsequent voiding attempts until the total amount reaches 60 milliliters. (The temperatures of the partial specimens are measured as they are collected.) An alternative procedure would be to collect nothing less than the required 60 milliliters in one voiding. Partial voids would be discarded.

The donor may be given a reasonable amount of liquid (preferably water) for the purpose of facilitating the production of a full specimen. If the individual fails to provide a full specimen within a reasonable period of time (about two hours), the usual practice is to terminate collection from that individual and document the circumstances.

Temperature Check

Immediately after the specimen is collected, the collector measures the temperature of the specimen. The temperature-measuring device must be accurate and not contaminate the specimen. Disposable, single-use thermometers can be used, but the collector can accidentally contaminate the specimen with these. A temperature patch, which is attached to the outside of the specimen bottle, is better for two reasons. First, it can be attached to a closed bottle, and second, it can be attached by the donor, meaning that the collector need not handle the specimen bottle at any time while it is open.

The time from urination to temperature measurement cannot exceed four minutes. If the temperature of a specimen is outside the range of 32.5°C to 37.7°C, or 90.5°F to 99.8°F, there is reason to be suspicious. The individual might be asked to allow the collector to take his or her oral temperature to help explain a suspiciously low specimen temperature.

Color Check

Immediately after the specimen is collected, the collector will inspect the specimen to determine its color and look for any signs of contaminants. A bluish color suggests dilution with water from the toilet bowl, while a clear or very pale yellow suggests dilution with water or some other source. Particles or cloudiness indicate contamination.

Suspect Specimens

Any unusual findings that result from the temperature or visual check are noted on a form designed for this purpose, and the collector will immediately report the findings and any particular suspicions to a supervisor. The supervisor will decide, on the basis of the facts presented, whether there is reason to believe that the donor has submitted a bogus or adulterated specimen.

If the supervisor concludes that the evidence is insufficient, the specimen is processed routinely except that a written record of the suspicions and the supervisor's decision is prepared and retained for possible use later. For instance, if the drug-testing laboratory reported that the specimen contained contaminants, the laboratory report and the collector's notes would provide a strong justification for conducting a follow-up unannounced and witnessed specimen collection.

If the collection site supervisor concludes that there is sufficient evidence to suspect cheating by a donor, the donor will be asked before leaving the collection site to provide a second specimen under more controlled conditions, such as with a witness present. The second specimen and the suspect specimen are both forwarded to the laboratory for testing.

Sealing and Marking

The individual being tested and the collector should keep the specimen in view at all times prior to its being sealed and labeled. The purpose of this procedure is to remove any later charge that the specimen was contaminated while the bottle was open and out of the immediate custody of the donor. Collection procedures that require the donor to perform all specimen-handling activities can be a safeguard against this type of accusation. The sample set of collection procedures in Appendix 7–A provide guidance in how to collect specimens without touching the specimen bottles. Holding the bottle upside down and shaking it gently ensures that the cap is tight.

The collector will ask or instruct the donor to observe the transfer of the specimen and the placement of a tamperproof seal over the bottle cap and down the sides of the bottle. The collection site person will securely place an identification label on the bottle with the date, the individual's specimen number, and any other identifying information. In some cases, the donor will write the identifying information on a label that was attached to the bottle during the manufacturing process. The individual will initial the label for the purpose of certifying that the bottle contains the specimen collected from him or her.

The collection site person will record all information identifying the specimen and sign his or her name beside the identifying information. Adjacent to this entry is a short preprinted statement to the effect that the donor acknowledges that the specimen identified on the form is the same specimen given by him or her. The collector will ask the donor to read and sign the statement.

Controlling Specimens

The collection site person also will complete the chain-of-custody form. The urine specimen and the form are now ready for shipment. If the specimen is not immediately prepared for shipment, it must be appropriately safeguarded during temporary storage.

While the chain-of-custody procedures are being performed, it is essential that the urine specimen and custody documents be under the collector's control. If the collector leaves the workstation even momentarily, the specimen and custody form must be secured. After he or she returns to the workstation, the custody process can continue.

The collector must keep the individual's specimen bottle in sight both before and after the individual has urinated. The chain-of-custody form is used to account for each specimen from the point of collection to final disposition. Each time a specimen is handled or transferred, the date and purpose are documented on the form, and every individual in the chain is identified.

The number of persons handling specimens is held to a minimum. This is done for more than administrative convenience. Even the smallest deviation from the established chain-of-custody procedures can be sufficient reason to reject a positive test result. The opportunities for deviation increase significantly when specimens are accessible to too many persons.

Transferring Specimens to the Laboratory

The collector will then arrange to ship the collected specimens to the drug-testing laboratory. The specimens and the chain-of-custody forms are placed in a larger specimen box or padded mailer designed to minimize the possibility of damage during shipment. The box or mailer is sealed to eliminate the possibility of undetected tampering. The collection site supervisor signs the sealing tape and enters the date the specimens were sealed for shipment.

At the Laboratory

A competent drug-testing laboratory will be secure at all times and have in place sufficient security measures to control access to the premises. Access is limited to specifically named individuals whose authorization is documented. With the exception of persons authorized to conduct inspections, all authorized visitors and maintenance and service personnel are escorted at all times. Documentation of each individual accessing these areas, the date and time of entry, and the purpose of entry is maintained.

When a shipment of specimens is received, laboratory employees routinely inspect each package for evidence of tampering and compare the information on the specimen bottles with that on the chain-of-custody forms. Any direct evidence of tampering or discrepancy in information is reported to the employer, and notes are made on the laboratory's chain-of-custody form (which accompanies the specimens while they are in the laboratory's possession).

Specimen bottles are normally retained in the laboratory's accession area until all analyses have been completed. Aliquots and the laboratory's chain-of-custody forms are used by laboratory personnel for conducting initial and confirmation tests.

Laboratories follow chain-of-custody procedures to maintain control and accountability of specimens from receipt through completion of testing, reporting of results, storage, and final disposition. Each time a specimen is handled or transferred, the date and purpose are documented and every individual in the chain is identified. Authorized technicians are responsible for each urine specimen or aliquot in their possession, and they must account for the chain of custody.

The chain-of-custody form used by the laboratory is often different from that used by the collector. Once a specimen has come into the laboratory, as documented on the collector's chain-of-custody form, an in-house laboratory form is initiated. This form documents the movement of the specimen through the various testing steps.

BLIND PROFICIENCY TESTING

Blind proficiency testing is one of the critical means for ensuring that a drug-testing laboratory is delivering high-quality services. Blind proficiency testing also is critical to employee acceptance of an employer's drug-testing program. Employees are reassured to know that test results are subject to the employer's careful and ongoing scrutiny.

Blind proficiency testing, which involves some added cost and logistical preparation, usually can be better performed by a contractor with expertise in this area. When an employer cannot afford blind performance testing, the alternative would be to engage a laboratory that is subject to blind testing by another employer or a federal agency. Although the employer will not have the assurance that its specimens are being afforded the highest quality processing, it is somewhat comforting to know that other clients are evaluating the laboratory's services.

DELAY IN COLLECTING A SPECIMEN

An extended delay in the collection of a urine specimen in a postaccident testing situation may result in deterioration or elimination of a drug or its metabolite from the body system. The determination as to whether a person involved in an accident is subject to testing should be made as soon as possible, particularly in cases where there is little uncertainty that the individual's action was a contributing factor in the accident.

The time-sensitive nature of urinalysis dictates that a specimen be collected with the least possible delay following an accident. The federal government uses 32 hours as the maximum period, which is probably too long.

The maximum period for making a good test is closer to 24 hours. With a blood sample the maximum period is considerably shorter, around 4 hours.

SPLIT SPECIMENS

The split-specimen method involves the splitting of a urine specimen or the taking of two specimens at the time of collection. The split portion, or the second specimen, is intended to serve as a backup in case something happens to the first specimen. This increases the chances that at least one specimen will be available for testing.

There is no scientific advantage to collecting two specimens. Rather, this method seeks to address administrative problems created by human error, such as mislabeling and improper packaging that leads to in-transit spillage. By doubling the administrative workload, however, the method increases the chances of human error and therefore is, in a sense, self-defeating.

Since the two specimens are identical, the second specimen could be used to verify or nullify the results obtained when the first specimen was tested. This is a desirable feature for both the employer and the employee. The employer has the potential for proving the accuracy of a contested test result, and the employee has the potential for proving that a positive test result was false. Given the massive volume of testing, however, this method is rarely used for either of these purposes.

Perhaps the best use of the split-specimen method is to alleviate concern about possible specimen mixup, contamination, or loss. Although this consideration may not be great enough to offset the added cost and effort, much can be said for any method that projects an image of caring and concern by the employer.

ON-SITE SCREENING OF SPECIMENS

The practice of conducting screening tests at an employer's work location is predicated on the premise that most of the collected specimens can be expected to be negative and that some savings can be realized by filtering out the negative specimens at the collection site and sending only the positive specimens to the laboratory for further testing. Some employers see another advantage to identifying a drug user at the collection site in that immediate action can be taken to remove the individual from the job for reasons of safety. This also sends a strong message to all employees that drug use will not be tolerated.

The employer may have all the right motives but is making all the wrong moves. First, on-site screening can be done for only one or two drugs. There simply is not enough time to test for five to nine drugs using portable equipment. Is every specimen that tests negative for one or two drugs not sent to the laboratory for further testing? In most cases, the answer is no. The specimens must be tested further, so the employer will not save any money by sending only positive specimens to the laboratory. Does the employer save money by having a one- or two-drug screen done on-site and the remaining screens done at the laboratory? No, because the laboratory is set up for routine, multiple testing on a volume basis. In fact, not testing for one or two drugs may represent an increased cost if the testing routine has to be modified.

Second, there is a great risk of accidental contamination whenever testing is done in uncontrolled conditions outside a laboratory environment. Even if the testing conditions are believed to guard against contamination, an employee could charge that a positive test result was caused by something at the worksite getting into the specimen while it was open during the screening test.

Third, under no circumstances is it a good idea to take any action against an employee on the basis of an unconfirmed positive test result. An employee who is removed from the job, especially in sight of coworkers, and who is later exonerated by a negative confirmation test has grounds for a good lawsuit.

Appendix 7–A

Sample Urine Specimen Collection Procedures

PART 1: GETTING SET UP

Obtain Details

When a client makes a request for a urine specimen collection session to be scheduled, the first thing you will want to do is find out who and how many persons will be giving specimens and then set a time and date that is convenient for the client.

Check Supplies

The next thing to do is make sure you have everything you will need when the collection takes place. The necessary materials consist of the following:

Forms

Notice to Employee Form
Consent Form
Urine Custody and Control Form
Permanent Record

Equipment

Specimen bottles
Plastic envelopes
Evidence tape
Shipping containers
Thumbprint labels
Thumbprint ink pad
Temperature patches
A chest or box for holding specimens
Disposable gloves

These procedures are provided courtesy of Forward Edge, Inc., Houston, Texas.

Other Items

A copy of the client's drug abuse policy
A felt-tip pen
A stapler
Rubber bands
Notepaper
Bluing agent

The Collection Site

Ideally, the collection location will consist of a clean bathroom situated within or near a quiet area away from other people. This private zone will allow the collection process to operate with minimum distraction to you and the urine donors.

One at a Time

An important consideration is for you to be able to process one donor at a time, with other donors waiting nearby but not in a position to observe or interrupt.

Male and Female

Collections from females must be made by a female, and collections from males must be made by a male.

Bathroom Preparation

Ensure that the bathroom has a toilet stall. Remove from the area around the commode any soap, cleaning materials, or substances that could be added to a specimen to contaminate it.

Place a bluing dye canister in the water tank of the commode. Flush the toilet several times to ensure that the water in the commode consistently takes on the characteristic blue color.

Higher Level Supervision

You will have at least two higher level supervisors to turn to for guidance during the collection: your own work supervisor and a supervisor representing the client. One or both of these persons will be present or readily accessible during the collection session.

PART 2: FILLING OUT THE FORMS

Prepare the Donors

While the bathroom is being made ready, meet briefly with the donors waiting nearby. Give them the Notice Form, which explains how the collection process works. This will help ease their apprehensions and make the process go smoothly.

Start the process by bringing one donor into the private zone. Introduce yourself and explain that you are going to ask the person to read and sign some forms and then to urinate into a bottle. Encourage the person to ask questions at this point or at any time during the process.

Reassure the Person

Assure the person that the process will be simple and not discomforting in any way.

Cover the Employer's Drug Policy

Ask the person if he or she understands the employer's drug abuse policy. If the answer is yes, hand the person the Consent Form and ask him or her to read and sign it.

If the person says he or she does not know about or understand the drug abuse policy, hand the person the policy and ask him or her to read it.

After the person has read the policy, or after you have read it to him or her (if needed), ask the person to acknowledge that he or she understands the policy. When the person tells you that he or she understands, hand him or her the Consent Form for signing. You will sign on this form as a witness.

Refusal to Sign

If a person will not acknowledge understanding or refuses to sign the Consent Form or other forms, discontinue processing that person and instruct him or her to wait at the collection area until a higher level supervisor can be contacted for further instructions.

Abusive Attitude

What do you do when a person is uncooperative or abusive? The answer is to stop processing that person, tell him or her to wait, contact a higher level supervisor, and then make some notes in case you are asked later to provide details.

Picture Identification

The donor will have been told to bring some form of picture identification, such as a driver's license. Information concerning the donor's identity will be needed in filling out the next form, the Urine Custody and Control Form.

Urine Custody and Control Form

Note that this form is laid out in steps that are explained on the form.

The specimen donor will first fill out Step 1. After the donor has filled out Step 1, ask him or her to present an identity card that bears both a picture and a serial number. Most driver's licenses have a picture and a number. A Social Security card does not and is therefore not an acceptable form of identification.

If the donor cannot produce acceptable identification, you can establish his or her identity by verifying it with another person. That person could be you if you know the donor personally, or it could be someone who works for the donor's company.

If your best efforts cannot verify the donor's identity, continue processing the person, and in the space beneath "Employer Name" in Step 1, enter the words "Identity could not be verified."

Identity Card Information

Most people will produce acceptable identification. In the space beneath "Employer Name" in Step 1, enter the type of identity card—for example, Texas driver's license—and then write in the license number.

Medication Information

Now ask the donor to fill out Step 5. This is where the donor can identify any medication that he or she has taken within the past 30 days. This information will be considered when the test results are reviewed.

You should now fill out Step 2 and put this form to the side while you fill out the Permanent Record.

Permanent Record

The Permanent Record provides information that will assist the Medical Review Officer should any questions arise concerning a collected specimen. The Permanent Record has these sections:

- Date of collection
- Donor's name
- Donor's Social Security number (This number will be obtained from the employer in advance of the collection. The donor will be asked to verify the number. If for some reason the Social Security number is not available and the donor refuses to furnish it, make a note to this effect in the Remarks section and contact a higher level supervisor for guidance. The supervisor may direct you to use a unique substitute number.)
- Specimen number (This number is the same number that will later be written on the label of the specimen bottle. Like the Social Security number, it links the specimen to the donor.)
- Type of test (Enter AT for applicant or preemployment testing; RT for random testing; RS for reasonable suspicion testing; FU for follow-up testing; AU for accident or unsafe practices testing; or VT for voluntary testing.)

Note: All the above items should be filled out now. All the following items on this form should be filled out after the specimen has been collected.

- Temperature of collected specimen
- Remarks—for example, any unusual occurrence such as the need to collect the specimen under observation
- Collector's signature

- Donor's signature, which certifies that the specimen identified as having been collected from him or her is in fact the specimen that he or she provided

Important Note

At this point, you have completely filled out one form (the Consent Form) and you have partially filled out two other forms (the Urine Custody and Control Form and the Permanent Record). A little later, after the specimen has been collected, you will fill out the remaining portions of the forms.

PART 3: OBTAINING THE SPECIMEN

Three Objectives

Keep your mind on three things as you collect a specimen:

1. Do not let the specimen bottle out of your sight. It may be necessary at a later time to show that no one else had access to the specimen while it was in your custody. Tell the donor to do the same. If you have to leave the collection area momentarily during the collection process, take the specimen bottle and its corresponding Urine Custody and Control Form with you. Explain to the donor what you are going to do and why so that there will be no suspicion of tampering on your part.
2. Do not touch the bottle directly. If you make it a practice not to touch the specimen bottle, you can never be accused of having contaminated the specimen.
3. Do not give the donor any chance to add a foreign substance to the bottle or to switch bottles.

All these objectives can be achieved by following some simple steps, which are outlined below.

Remove Outer Garments

Ask the donor to remove outer garments such as a coat, jacket, or bulky sweater. Also ask that any packages, briefcases, or purses be placed with the garments. The donor may keep his or her wallet.

No Smoking

If the donor is smoking, ask him or her to stop until the collection is finished. This will keep ashes from getting into the specimen bottle.

Handling the Bottle

Hand the donor a sealed plastic bag containing a sterile specimen bottle. Ask the donor to remove the bottle from the bag, discard the bag, and unscrew the bottle cap. Tell the donor to go into the bathroom and void into the bottle.

Follow the donor into the bathroom, keeping yourself positioned to maintain visual contact at all times except when the donor is inside the bathroom stall.

Freeze-up

Sometimes a donor cannot void or cannot provide at least 60 milliliters of urine. Refer to Part 5 for guidance on what to do when this occurs.

Be Discreet

Try to be as discreet as you can. By your presence nearby, you will be a very effective deterrent against attempts to cheat.

Do not allow the donor to have access to the bathroom's faucets, soap dispensers, or materials that could be used to adulterate the specimen.

Do not use any method that would cause the specimen to be left in the bathroom, placed somewhere even temporarily, or given to someone else. Also, do not cause the processing to be delayed at this point because as soon as possible, you will need to measure the specimen's temperature to ensure that its heat is consistent with a freshly voided specimen.

60 Milliliters

Make sure the donor fills the bottle with at least 60 milliliters of urine.

Leakage Check

Tell the donor to cap the bottle tightly, turn it upside down, and gently shake it to check for leakage.

Temperature Check

Hand the donor a temperature patch. Tell him or her to apply it to the side of the bottle. Wait 30 seconds and read the temperature. This check must be done within 4 minutes after the voiding.

Enter the temperature reading in Step 3 of the Urine Custody and Control Form and in the Temperature section of the Permanent Record.

If the temperature falls outside the range of 90.5°F to 99.8°F, there is reason to believe that the individual may have adulterated the specimen or made a substitution. When this happens, contact a higher level supervisor, report the situation, and ask for authorization to collect another specimen under direct observation by a same-gender collection site person. Further guidance is provided in Part 5.

Both specimens must be sent to the laboratory for testing.

Color Check

Ask the donor to hold the specimen bottle up to the light so that you can examine its color. Look for any signs of contamination, such as the presence of a bluing agent, or of dilution, such as color ranging from clear to pale yellow.

Do not take or handle the bottle.

Evidence Tape on Bottle Cap

Hand the donor a strip of evidence tape. Tell him or her to place it on the bottle so that the ends of the tape are on the sides with the middle part of the tape running across the top of the cap.

Label

Give the donor a felt-tip pen and tell him or her to fill out the label. The label at a minimum will require entries as to the following:

- The date
- The specimen number as shown in the Permanent Record
- The donor's initials

Also instruct the donor to initial the tape on the cap.

Thumbprint

The purpose of taking a thumbprint is to provide one more positive means of removing any doubt as to the identity of the person who gave the specimen.

Place the inked pad and a blank label on the table or desk. Ask the donor to press his or her right thumb on the pad and then onto the label. The pressure should be straight down and not heavy.

Now ask the donor to stick the label on the back of the specimen bottle without covering the bottle's label.

Putting the Bottle into the Protective Container

The bottle is now ready to go into a protective container. The protective container will vary according to the mode of shipment and/or the laboratory that has been designated to perform the testing. The container could be a specially constructed envelope that has a tamper-detecting seal, a zip-lock envelope, or a Styrofoam mailer.

Generally, the tamper-detecting and zip-lock envelopes are used for specimens that will be picked up, locally delivered, or packed in a larger box for shipment. The Styrofoam mailers are for specimens that will be individually mailed to the lab.

Hand the donor the protective container and tell him or her to put the bottle inside and close it.

Sealing the Protective Container

In order for the laboratory to detect any tampering with the container after it leaves your custody, the container will have a built-in tamper-detecting seal or you will seal the container with a strip of evidence tape.

Tell the donor to sign his or her name on the tamper-detecting seal or the strip of evidence tape in such a way that the signature overlaps the seal and the container.

Finish Filling Out the Forms

On the Permanent Record, place your signature in the Collector's Signature section and ask the donor to place a signature and date in the section where the donor certifies that the urine specimen identified on the form is his or hers, that it is fresh and has not been adulterated, and that the identifying information on the Permanent Record and on the specimen bottle is correct.

Now fill out Step 4 and Step 6 of the Urine Custody and Control Form, date it at the bottom, and ask the donor to sign on the signature line at the bottom. Note in Step 4 that you must sign and print your name to signify that you received the specimen directly from the donor. You also must sign and print your name on the line below to signify that you released the specimen. When the lab receives the specimen, the Received By line will be filled out and dated. The purpose of the change of custody should be entered by you as "Transfer to lab."

This form consists of five copies.

- Staple Copy 1 to the outside of the protective container. This copy will accompany the specimen to the lab.
- Retain Copy 2. Your work supervisor will ensure that this copy is given to the Medical Review Officer.
- Give Copy 3 to the donor.
- Retain Copy 4. Your work supervisor will place this copy on file.
- Retain Copy 5. Your work supervisor will ensure that this copy is given to the donor's employer.

Place the Specimen out of Reach

Put the donor's specimen and forms off to the side, out of the reach of anyone except yourself. A closed chest or box is provided for this.

Process the Next Donor

Thank the donor for being cooperative and ask him or her to send in the next donor for processing.

Final Check

After the last person has been processed, check to make sure that all of the persons scheduled for processing have been processed or accounted for. If a scheduled donor failed to appear for processing, refer to Part 5 for guidance.

For each person processed, you should have the following:

- One protective container that has been sealed with evidence tape. Inside the container will be the specimen bottle. Copy 1 of the Urine Custody and Control Form will be stapled to the outside of the protective container.
- One set of forms consisting of a Consent Form; Copies 2, 4, and 5 of the Urine Custody and Control Form; and an entry in the Permanent Record.

At this juncture, it is a good idea to look at the paperwork to make sure everything has been filled out and signed. It will help to have a fellow collection site person double-check the paperwork.

If necessary, call a donor on the phone to get missing information or arrange to bring the donor back if a signature is needed.

PART 4: GETTING THE SPECIMENS TO THE LABORATORY

Delivery and/or Pickup

In some localities, a laboratory will be so conveniently located that specimens can be taken to the lab by the collection site person or the lab will provide a pickup service.

Shipping the Specimens

If the laboratory is not located nearby, the specimens will need to be shipped. Shipping is done in one of two ways:

1. By mail. If mail is the method of shipment, the samples you have collected should be in a Styrofoam container. The outside surface of the Styrofoam container bears the lab's address.
2. By a commercial courier service. If shipment is to be by Federal Express or a similar rapid express service (overnight delivery is preferred), the specimens should be placed inside a bag or container provided by the shipping service.

Important Notes

Always try to ship within a few hours following collection. Under no circumstances should specimens be held more than one working day.

If specimens cannot be transferred immediately to the lab, place them in protected storage. This means under lock and key at the Forward Edge office.

When the specimens are given to a shipping/mailing service, enter the date on the outside of the shipping box and sign next to the date. Obtain a receipt from the lab or the mailing/shipping service.

The forms are not sent to the lab. They go to your work supervisor.

Hold to an absolute minimum the number of persons who take custody of the specimens.

Performance Test Specimens

To ensure the reliability and accuracy of drug-testing results, blind performance test (PT) specimens will be regularly sent to the lab along with specimens collected from donors. About 80 percent of the PT specimens contain no drugs, while the others contain known levels of one or more drugs. This is a means of monitoring laboratory performance. When PT specimens are to be included with a shipment of regularly collected specimens, you will be informed and directly supervised by your work supervisor.

The procedures for doing this are as follows:

1. Treat the PT specimens exactly the way you treat the other specimens.
2. Transfer the PT specimens into containers that are exactly like those used for the other specimens.
3. Use the same labeling and sealing and make entries on the forms in the same manner used for the other specimens.
4. Place the PT specimens and the other specimens together in the shipping box so that they all appear to be regularly collected specimens.

PART 5: DEALING WITH SPECIAL PROBLEMS

Not Enough Urine

Sometimes a donor cannot void or cannot provide at least 60 milliliters of urine. When this occurs, tell the donor that he or she must remain in the collection area until a specimen of sufficient quantity is obtained. The employee may be given 8 ounces of water, coffee, or a soft drink every 30 minutes. If the donor has not provided a specimen at the end of 2 hours, contact a higher level of supervision for guidance.

When a donor provides less than 60 milliliters of urine, have the donor cap the bottle and immediately apply a temperature patch. Note the temperature, make a color check, and record these findings in the Temperature section and the Remarks section of the Permanent Record and in Step 6 of the Urine Custody and Control Form.

Save this partial specimen and any other partial specimens from the same donor so that, if necessary, you can instruct the donor to combine them all into one bottle to obtain the needed 60 milliliters.

The donor may ask for permission to void elsewhere or to leave the collection area. Do not allow this to be done.

When the donor is ready to void, give him or her a new, unopened bag and pick up the process where you left off before.

Reasonable Suspicion

If you suspect a donor has deliberately contaminated his or her specimen or has substituted a bogus specimen, allow the collection to proceed as normal. After the processing for that donor has concluded, tell the donor to wait in the collection area and then immediately report your suspicions to a higher level supervisor. If the supervisor concurs, obtain without delay a second specimen under the direct observation of a same-gender collection site person.

Reasonable suspicion of contamination, adulteration, substitution, or dilution would exist in the following cases:

- A specimen's temperature falls outside the standard range.
- The color of the specimen is suspicious.
- The donor is discovered to have taken into the bathroom stall any equipment or devices that could be used to confound the test.

Direct observation also may be authorized by a higher level supervisor in the following cases:

- When the employee is being tested because his or her on-the-job conduct has indicated substance abuse
- When the employee is being tested on a follow-up basis because he or she has been previously identified as a substance abuser
- When the employee has previously tampered with a specimen

Conducting an Observed Collection

When an observed collection has been approved by a higher level supervisor, follow these procedures:

1. Act in a professional, discreet, and objective manner.
2. Make explanatory entries in the remarks sections of all forms pertaining to the individual and on extra sheets of paper if necessary.
3. Inform the donor that an observed collection will be conducted. Explain why and describe how an observed collection is conducted.
4. Make sure a collection site person of the same gender accompanies the donor into the bathroom. Only the donor and the collection site person will be in the bathroom at the same time.
5. Ask the donor to wash and dry his or her hands.
6. Hand the donor a factory-sealed plastic bag containing a specimen bottle.
7. Position yourself in a manner that will allow you to verify that the urine specimen passes directly from the donor's body into the specimen bottle.
8. Ask the donor to cap the bottle.
9. Continue the collection process in the usual manner.

Examples of Cheating

You should not be surprised if people try to fool you. Experience has shown that a donor is likely to do one or more of the following things:

- Add a foreign substance to the specimen, such as Drano, soap, iodine, sugar, salt, sweetener, bleach, tobacco, ashes, or soda pop
- Carry a concealed bottle of urine to the collection and try to switch it with the official bottle or try to pour the contents of the concealed bottle into the official bottle
- Try to con you into allowing the voiding to be done at home, in another bathroom, or someplace out of your control
- Try to switch his or her specimen with someone else's specimen
- Try to take the test for someone else
- Bring a urine-filled balloon or condom to the collection

  1. Men have been known to attach such items inside their pants and simulate voiding.
  2. Women have been known to conceal them in their undergarments.

Employee Fails to Report to the Collection Site

If an employee fails to report to the collection site, you should contact a higher level supervisor for guidance.

Employee Refuses to Provide a Specimen

If an employee refuses to provide a specimen, you should contact a higher level supervisor for guidance. Refusal could be in the nature of not signing the forms, not answering questions, or not cooperating in the collection process.

PART 6: A REVIEW OF THE MAJOR POINTS

Identify Each Donor

Make a positive identification of each donor by requiring presentation of a picture identification card or by obtaining verification from some other responsible person.

Obtain Medication Information

Get as much accurate information as you can concerning a donor's recent use of medication. Record that information on the Urine Custody and Control Form.

Fill Out the Forms Correctly

Take your time in filling out the forms completely and accurately and make sure they are signed in all the right places.

Seek Guidance from a Higher Supervisor

Do not hesitate to seek guidance from a higher level supervisor whenever in doubt about anything. Do not vary from the guidance in these procedures unless you have approval.

Do not take it upon yourself to collect a specimen under direct observation. You can and should recommend that action when it is needed, but the decision rests with a higher level supervisor.

Do Not Touch the Specimen Bottle

Make it a habit not to touch a specimen bottle. This is the best way to keep someone from later accusing you of rigging the test.

Get Specimens to the Lab Promptly

Specimens should be packaged and on the way to the lab on the same day they are collected.

Be Security Conscious

Prevent attempts at trickery by being alert and assuming a take-charge attitude.

Do not let the specimen bottles out of your control.

Remove from the bathroom any substances that can be slipped into a specimen.

Do not allow donors to go elsewhere to void.

Keep planned testing times and dates in strict confidence.

Limit the handling of specimens during the collection process to the donor and the collection site person processing that donor.

Do not rely on memory. Use this set of procedures and other preprinted guidance materials.

Do not be complacent. Concentrate on what you are doing when you are doing it.

Be Sensitive

Remember that many of the donors are giving urine specimens for the first time. They may be apprehensive and in need of assurance.

Conduct every collection with the full realization that the results of what you do can have a dramatic effect on someone else's life.

Appendix 7–B

Sample Consent Forms

GENERAL CONSENT TO DRUG TESTING

I have read and I understand the Company's drug-testing policy.

I understand that my employer reserves the right to conduct drug tests, such as tests that analyze urine, and that a positive finding of such a test may subject me to disciplinary action up to and including discharge.

I understand that I cannot be compelled to give a specimen of my urine for the purpose of determining the presence of drugs in my body system. I also understand that if I refuse to provide such a specimen or fail to cooperate with such tests, I may be subject to disciplinary action up to and including discharge.

I hereby agree to provide urine specimens when requested to do so by the Company and further authorize the testing agency to disclose to my employer the results of tests made of my urine specimens.

_____   _____
(Signature of witness)   (Signature of employee)

_____   _____
(Date)   (Printed name of employee)

These forms are provided courtesy of Forward Edge, Inc., Houston, Texas.

CONSENT TO A PREEMPLOYMENT DRUG TEST

I understand it is the policy of the Company to conduct urine tests of job applicants for the purpose of detecting drug abuse. I further understand that one of the requirements for consideration of employment with the Company is the satisfactory passing of the Company's urine drug test.

I agree to take a urine test as part of the regular preemployment screening conducted by the Company and understand that a favorable test result does not necessarily guarantee that I will be employed by the Company.

If I am accepted for employment, I agree to take urine tests whenever requested by the Company, and I understand that the taking of said tests is a condition of my continued employment.

I also give consent to the drug-testing agency to release to the Company the results of any drug tests made of my urine specimens so that I may qualify for employment.

At this time, I hereby consent to a drug test.

Signed _____

Printed name _____

Date _____

Witness _____

EMPLOYEE'S CONSENT TO A DRUG TEST

I have read and understand my employer's policy regarding drug abuse. I understand that it is the practice of my employer to conduct drug tests for the purpose of carrying out the policy.

I understand that I cannot be compelled to give a specimen of my urine. I understand that if I give a urine specimen, it will be tested for drugs. I understand that the giving of a urine specimen, when requested by my employer, is a condition of my continued employment.

I understand that if a test of my urine reveals an unexplained presence of a drug, my employer may take disciplinary action against me up to and including termination of my employment.

I authorize the officers, employees, and agents of the drug-testing agency and my employer to communicate among themselves for official purposes my drug test results, both orally and in writing, and to communicate such test results at any judicial or administrative proceeding. I also authorize the officers, employees, and agents of the drug-testing agency and my employer to have continued access to my urine specimen for the purpose of any further analysis or study that may be necessary.

At this time, I hereby agree to give a urine specimen.

Signed _____

Printed name _____

Date _____

Witness _____

TEST CONSENT FOR NONEMPLOYEES

Part 1: Notice to Specimen Donor

Company policy states that employees, contractors, subcontractors, vendors, and other nonemployees working on Company premises may be asked in certain situations to provide urine or blood specimens for drug-testing purposes. At this time, you are being asked to provide a urine or blood specimen relating to the situation checked below:

[ ] Accident   [ ] Cause based on reasonable belief

[ ] Random   [ ] Return to employment

[ ] Other _____

Part 2: Acknowledgment and Consent of Specimen Donor

In the past 30 days, I have taken medications that treat:

[ ] Pain   [ ] Muscle spasms   [ ] Allergies   [ ] Nervousness

[ ] Nausea, vomiting, and diarrhea   [ ] Asthma and wheezing

[ ] Coughing, sneezing, and congestion   [ ] Heart problems

[ ] Weight problems   [ ] Sleeping problems   [ ] Depression

[ ] Other _____

My employment status is: [ ] Contractor   [ ] Subcontractor

[ ] Vendor   [ ] Other _____

I am employed by _____

I understand the Company is now asking me to provide a specimen of my urine or blood for drug testing. I hereby agree and also authorize the specimen collecting and testing agencies to furnish the results of the test to the Company and to my employer.

_____   _____
(Signature of specimen donor)   (Signature of witness)

_____   _____
(Printed name of donor)   (Date)

CONSENT TO AN UNANNOUNCED TEST

I have read and understand the Company's policy regarding drug abuse.

I understand that the purpose of the policy is to provide a safe working environment for myself and fellow employees.

I understand that the Company may periodically conduct unannounced urine tests; that I may be asked to provide a specimen of my urine; and that if I give a specimen, it will be analyzed for the presence of drugs.

I understand that if a urine test reveals an unexplained presence of a drug in my body system, the Company may take disciplinary action against me, up to and including termination of employment, even for a first offense.

I understand that if I am asked to provide a urine specimen, I am not compelled to do so. However, I also understand that the giving of a urine specimen when requested by the Company is a condition of my continued employment and that I may be terminated for a failure to do so.

I acknowledge that the Company is at this time asking me to provide a specimen of my urine so that it may be analyzed for the presence of drugs. I hereby agree to give the specimen and consent to testing of it.

Signed _____

Printed name _____

Date _____

Witness _____

TEST CONSENT IN A REASONABLE CAUSE SITUATION

The Company's drug abuse policy provides that an employee may be required to submit to a urine drug and/or blood plasma test when the employee's performance or behavior on the job would cause a reasonable person to believe that the employee is under the influence of a chemical substance such as a drug or alcohol.

Reasonable cause has been shown to the effect that you may be under the influence of a chemical substance.

Employee

I am aware of the Company's drug abuse policy referred to above. I understand that I cannot be compelled to submit to a urine or blood plasma test but that if I refuse, I may be subject to disciplinary action, including discharge. I understand that if the results of such tests reveal an unexplained presence of a chemical substance in my body, I may be subject to disciplinary action, including discharge.

I hereby consent to a urine and/or blood plasma test, and I give consent to the Company and its agents, including the collecting and testing agencies, to disclose and discuss the results of such tests as they relate to me. I further agree to hold the Company and its agents harmless from any and all liability in connection with such tests.

To assist in the analysis of my urine and/or blood, please be informed that I have used, on the dates indicated, the following named chemical substances, legal or illegal drugs, prescription or nonprescription medicines, synthetic or look-alike drugs, or alcohol.

Name of Substance Taken   Date Last Used

_____   _____

_____   _____

_____   _____

_____   _____
(Date)   (Signature of employee)

_____   _____
(Signature of witness)   (Printed name of employee)

TEST CONSENT IN A RETURN-TO-DUTY SITUATION

Company policy provides that an employee suspended for having in his or her body system an unexplained presence of a prohibited substance such as a drug or alcohol may be required as a condition of reinstatement to enter the Employee Self-Help Program.

An element of the Employee Self-Help Program may require the suspended employee to undergo, cooperate with, and successfully complete an approved course of therapy as a condition of reinstatement. Further, if reinstated, the employee may be required to remain enrolled in the Employee Self-Help Program for the purpose of receiving follow-up, reinforcing, or maintenance therapy.

If you are reinstated, you will be expected to remain free of those substances prohibited by the Company's drug abuse policy and you may from time to time be asked on an unannounced basis to provide specimens of your urine and/or blood plasma for laboratory analysis. If you refuse to provide such specimens when requested to do so or if such specimens reveal an unexplained presence of the prohibited substances, you may be subject to disciplinary action, including discharge.

Response

I have read and understand the provisions regarding reinstatement following a violation of the Company's policy on drug abuse. I agree to comply with those provisions.

I specifically consent at this time to give a specimen of my urine and/or blood plasma for drug-testing purposes. I also give consent to the Company and its agents, including the collecting and testing agencies, to disclose and discuss the results of such testing. I further agree to hold the Company and its agents harmless from any and all liability in connection with such testing.

_____   _____

(Date)   (Signature of consenting person)

_____   _____

(Signature of witness)   (Printed name of consenter)

CONSENT TO RELEASE OF TEST RESULTS

I authorize the officers, employees, and agents of the drug-testing laboratory, specimen-collecting agency, and my employer to communicate among themselves for official purposes my drug test results, both orally and in writing, and to communicate such test results at any judicial or administrative proceeding. I also authorize the officers, employees, and agents of the drug-testing laboratory, specimen-collecting agency, and my employer to have continued access to my urine specimen for the purpose of any further analyses or studies that may be necessary.

_____   _____
(Date)   (Signature of consenting person)

_____   _____
(Signature of witness)   (Printed name of consenter)

Appendix 7–C

Disclosure of Medication and Ingested Substances

I understand that the drug test results pertaining to the analysis of a urine specimen I am about to give voluntarily can be affected by prescription medication, nonprescription medication, and some chemical and food substances such as poppy seeds.

I now wish to take this opportunity to identify any substances that could affect the proper analysis of my urine specimen.

In the past 30 days, I have taken the following named prescription or nonprescription medications:

_____

_____

The above medications were taken in order to treat:

[ ] Pain   [ ] Muscle spasms   [ ] Allergies   [ ] Nervousness

[ ] Nausea, vomiting, and diarrhea   [ ] Asthma and wheezing

[ ] Coughing, sneezing, and congestion   [ ] Heart problems

[ ] Weight problems   [ ] Sleeping problems   [ ] Depression

[ ] Other _____

In the past five days, I have ingested the following chemical or food substances:

_____

_____

This form is provided courtesy of Forward Edge, Inc., Houston, Texas.

At this time, I am not aware of any medications or other substances that may be in my body system that would affect the drug test I am about to take.

—————————   ——————————————————————
(Date)   (Signature)

Appendix 7–D

Consent and Waiver

Place _____   Date _____

I voluntarily agree to provide a specimen of my urine so that it may be analyzed for the presence of drugs.

I understand that collection of the urine specimen may be witnessed.

I hereby authorize the officers, employees, and agents of the collecting and testing agencies to disclose, both orally and in writing, the test results to the designated representatives of the Company.

For myself and successors, assigns, heirs, and executors and administrators, I hereby release, absolve, remise, agree to save harmless, forever discharge and hold free from all harm, liability, or damage to me the officers, employees, and agents of the collecting and testing agencies and the Company from any and all suits, actions, or causes of action at law, claim, demand, or liability that have now or may ever have resulted directly, indirectly, or remotely from my providing the said urine specimen so that it may be analyzed for the presence of drugs.

_____   _____
(Printed name)   (Signature)

_____   _____
(Date)   (Signature of witness)

_____

This form is provided courtesy of Forward Edge, Inc., Houston, Texas.

Identification of the Person Granting the Waiver

Type of picture ID card presented _____

Serial number of ID card _____

If no ID, name of person who vouched _____

[ ]   Identity could not be verified.

Chapter 8

Understanding the Drug-Testing Program

The evaluation of prospective employees to determine their fitness for work is not new. Physical examinations have long been used to ensure that selected applicants are free of medical conditions that might interfere with productivity and safety requirements. With the long-standing existence of alcohol abuse and the relatively recent rise of drug abuse in the United States, many companies have developed preemployment and in-service drug-testing programs. These programs are designed to protect the health and safety of all employees and are proving to be an effective way of managing substance abuse problems in industry.

URINALYSIS

Urinalysis is now part of the preemployment screening processes of many of the nation's largest employers, including major corporations, manufacturers, public utilities, and transportation companies. In general, these companies state they will not hire individuals who present positive urine specimens indicating current use of illicit substances.

The possible impact of a positive test result on an individual's livelihood or rights, together with the possibility of a legal challenge of the result, sets this type of test apart from most clinical laboratory testing. In fact, urine drug testing should be considered a special application of analytical forensic toxicology because the specimen must be treated as evidence, and all aspects of the testing procedure must be documented and available for possible court testimony.

Laboratories engaged in urine drug testing should require the services and advice of a qualified forensic toxicologist or an individual with equivalent qualifications (both training and experience) to address the specific needs of an employer's drug-testing program, including the demands of chain of custody, security, proper documentation, storage of positive specimens for later or independent testing, presentation of evidence in court, and expert witness testimony.

Although urine-testing technology is extremely effective in determining previous drug use, the positive results of a test cannot be used to prove intoxication or impaired performance. The evidence of drug use may appear in urine for several days or even weeks without related impairment. Positive urine tests do, however, show relatively recent drug use.

Several testing methods are available. Most of these are suitable for determining the presence or absence of a drug in a urine sample. The accuracy and reliability of these methods are assessed in the context of the total laboratory system. If the laboratory uses well-trained personnel who follow acceptable procedures, the accuracy of the results can be very high.

What Do Urine Tests Seek to Identify?

Urine tests are designed to identify drugs or drug metabolites. Some drug classes, such as opiates, can be identified directly, while other classes, such as cannabinoids and cocaine, are identified indirectly through the presence of metabolites.

For example, if a screening test finds a urine specimen positive for opiates, the sample is believed to contain an opioid. A confirmatory test of the specimen will identify which opioid is present—for instance, morphine, codeine, or heroin. Alternatively, a urine specimen that tests positive for cannabinoids (marijuana substances) will contain cannabinoid metabolites. There are more than 60 cannabinoid metabolites, and more than 30 of them are readily identifiable by a standard screening test. A confirmatory test will examine the specimen for one or more of the major metabolites.

How Does Urine Testing Work?

Urine testing follows a two-step process consisting of a screening test and a confirmatory test. When a specimen shows negative in the screen, testing stops for that specimen. When the specimen shows positive, it is subject to a confirmatory test. These two types of tests are discussed in the following sections.

Screening or Preliminary Tests

The purpose of screening or preliminary tests is to identify negative specimens so that they can be removed from further consideration. The immunoassay techniques are by far the most frequently used screening tests. They are specifically designed to detect small quantities of a drug or its metabolites. They lend themselves well to automation and can offer greater than 95 percent accuracy. Thin-layer chromatography (TLC), although still used and suitable for many other testing purposes, is losing favor as a technique for detecting drugs in urine. Its chief advantages are low operating costs, it can be performed with less training, and it detects many classes of drugs.

The main disadvantage is its dependence on human interpretation of test results.

Immunoassays

An immunoassay is an analysis of a body fluid for the purpose of detecting the presence of a drug or drug metabolite. It is based on the principle of competition between labeled and unlabeled antigens for binding sites on a specific antibody. An antibody is a protein substance to which a specific drug or drug metabolite will bind.

Enzyme Immunoassays. In the enzyme immunoassay (EIA) technique, the label on the antigen is an enzyme that produces a chemical reaction that allows for the detection of a drug or its metabolite. Urine is mixed with a reagent containing antibodies. The antibodies search for a compound or a group of closely related compounds characteristic of the drug. The drug in the urine competes for the limited number of antibody binding sites and in so doing increases the enzyme activity. The concentration of the drug present in the urine is determined by the extent of enzymatic activity.

The most widely used EIA method is EMIT (enzyme multiplied immunoassay technique), manufactured by Syva Company of Palo Alto, California. Syva markets two types of EMIT system. The first, called the EMIT st System, uses a portable testing unit and is often used in nonlaboratory situations. It is marketed to organizations that wish to conduct testing on their own. The EMIT st test does not measure the amount of a drug, only that a drug is present. The second type, called the EMIT dau System, is used in laboratories and large testing programs. It gives positive and negative test results and can estimate the concentrations of drugs and their metabolites.

In EMIT, a reagent that is specific for a particular drug or metabolite is combined with the urine. The reagent/urine is referred to a spectrophotometer, which reads the enzyme activity present, as indicated by the absorption of light waves. A numerical value is generated that represents the presence or absence of the drug or its metabolite.

The EMIT immunoassay tests have been shown to be among the most consistently accurate drug-testing methods in current use. The manufacturer reports that 96 to 99 percent of the results obtained with EMIT tests were confirmed as correct.

Radioimmunoassays. The radioimmunoassay (RIA) method of screening seeks to determine the concentration of a protein in a specimen by monitoring the reaction produced by the injection of a radioactive-labeled substance known to react in a particular way with the protein being studied. Known amounts of a radioactive-labeled drug are added to a urine sample with known amounts of antibodies. The mixture is then allowed to incubate, during which time the labeled drug and the unlabeled drug compete for binding sites on the antibody.

After precipitation and centrifugation of antigen-antibody complexes, either the supernatant fluid or the precipitated antibody is transferred to a gamma counter, an instrument that determines the radioactivity level of the sample. The presence or absence of the drug being looked for is indicated by the amount of radioactivity found.

RIA can detect drug concentrations on the order of 1 to 5 ng/ml. The required sample volume is small, and sample preparation is minimal. The use of automated pipetting and counting equipment allows for large-volume, multiple testing. Some of the disadvantages of this technique are associated with the use of radioactive substances and the high cost of reagents and instrumentation. The most frequently used RIA test is Abuscreen, manufactured by Roche Diagnostics of Nutley, New Jersey.

EMIT versus Abuscreen.   According to most scientists, EMIT and Abuscreen are roughly equivalent in value. Any comparison of their efficiency and accuracy must be done carefully, however, as they have different cutoff levels and there are different opinions about what constitutes a negative or a positive response. An EMIT test for marijuana, for example, will give a positive response only when the concentration of THC metabolites is above 20 ng/ml, whereas the cutoff level for Abuscreen is 100 ng/ml.

The important thing to remember about EMIT and Abuscreen is that they are screening tests. Although they are highly accurate when used by trained persons in a proper laboratory environment, they are not designed to be the final answer. Their main purpose is to separate the positive and the negative samples.

Thin-Layer Chromatography

Thin-layer chromatography (TLC) is a traditional analytical technique that can be used for both screening and confirming. It consists of a thin layer of silica on a plastic or glass plate having known standards spotted along the bottom. An extract of urine is prepared using an organic solvent. The urine extract is applied to the plate, and a developing solvent is added. The extract migrates (moves) up the plate by capillary action, and the developing solvent separates out any drugs present in the extract. A human interpretation is made based on a visual comparison between the known standards and the developed extract. The criteria for interpretation are the characteristics of the migration and color changes.

When the interpreting analyst has a doubt concerning the identification of a drug, a photograph may be made of the plate in question to allow for a second opinion. Alternatively, a questioned identification may be referred to a more sensitive technique, such as gas chromatography/mass spectrometry (GC/MS).

TLC can produce good results and for some classes of drugs is the only screening technique that will separate closely related compounds. The method, however, requires interpretation by a trained individual. The risk of legal challenges to TLC test results has caused this technique to lose favor in employee drug-testing programs.

Confirmatory Tests

If an initial screening test shows that a sample is positive, a second test is used to confirm the result. A confirmatory test is usually more specific (or selective) and reliable than a screening test and at least as sensitive as the testing method used in the initial screen. Examples of commonly used confirmation methods include high-performance liquid chromatography (HPLC), gas chromatography (GC), and gas chromatography/mass spectrometry (GC/MS). These are sophisticated instrumental methods requiring highly trained technicians who are capable of providing highly selective analyses for a variety of drugs. Confirmatory tests are more costly to conduct than screening tests, but when the two types are used together, much greater certainty is obtained.

High-Performance Liquid Chromatography

In the HPLC technique, the sample passes through a column while undergoing equilibration between two liquid phases. The technique measures the time it takes for the specimen to traverse the column at a given solvent flow rate. The speed of movement provides accurate indications as to the drug molecule in the sample.

Gas Chromatography

In the GC technique, the sample is converted to a gaseous state and injected into the gas chromatograph instrument, where it passes through a column of absorbent material. The gas is fractionated into compounds according to their chemical and physical properties. The compounds are portrayed as a pattern on a graph, which allows comparison with graphs of known drugs.

Gas Chromatography/Mass Spectrometry

The GC/MS technique combines the separating power of gas chromatography with the high sensitivity and specificity of spectrometric detection. GC/MS is generally considered to be the most conclusive method of confirming the presence of a drug in urine.

There are many different modes of operating a GC/MS system. It can be operated in a full-scan mode, which provides a complete mass spectrum for each component of the urine extract that passes through the GC component. Since a complete mass spectrum represents a unique pattern for each drug, this mode of operation will give the most conclusive identification of a sufficiently high concentration of a drug.

Alternatively, the GC/MS can be operated in the selected ion monitoring mode in which the MS component monitors the ion currents at only a few masses that are characteristic of a specific drug. This mode affords far greater sensitivity but provides a less specific pattern for identification. Other modes of operation include electron ionization (EI) and chemical ionization (CI). The mode selected depends on which drugs are to be detected, the cutoff level that constitutes a positive identification, and whether or not the concentration of the drug is to be quantitatively determined.

The reliability of a GC/MS test result depends on the skill and experience of the operator. In spite of the remarkable potential capabilities of GC/MS, it should not be assumed that the results of all tests performed with this technique are indisputably conclusive.

HAIR ANALYSIS

The biological basis for hair analysis is the contact between the blood supply and the hair follicles. Drugs circulating in the bloodstream are transferred to and embedded in the cortex of growing hair fibers. These deposits remain in the cortex and move away from the follicle as the hair strand grows. An individual's pattern of drug consumption is thus recorded. Hair analysis is a process of releasing the embedded drugs through chemical destruction of the hair fiber and then examining the resulting extract using RIA and GC/MS techniques.

The hair analyzed is typically taken from the head. Head hair grows at a rate of approximately 1.0 to 1.3 centimeters per month. Hair that is 12 centimeters long will provide a drug history of 9 to 12 months. Slower-growing body hair can extend the history to several years.

The collection method consists of taking strands of hair from the scalp and then cutting the strands into sections that correspond to the periods of interest. For example, if very recent drug use is of interest, a 2-centimeter section is cut from the follicle end of the strands. An analysis of this section will uncover drug use that occurred up to approximately two months prior to the test. Analyses of other sections can provide similar information about earlier time periods. This makes it possible to discover a person's history of drug use. It is not possible to isolate such use to a particular day or small group of days or to attribute a positive finding to very recent use, such as in the two or three days prior to collection of the hair specimen.

In contrast to urinalysis, which does not reveal much about the pattern of drug use, hair analysis can determine a time frame in which a particular drug was used and make general distinctions between heavy, medium, and light use.

The analytical techniques for evaluating hair are essentially the same as those used in urinalysis. RIA is used as a preliminary test, with gas GC/MS as the confirmatory test. Because hair analysis involves additional steps, however, it is more time-consuming and costly.

There are some obvious advantages of hair analysis. Hair specimens can be readily obtained from either sex in public without violating privacy and without the inherent intrusiveness related to the collection of urine specimens. In addition, a drug abuser cannot avoid detection by staying clean for a few days prior to a test or by flushing the body system with large quantities of fluids.

Hair analysis also offers an opportunity to obtain an additional specimen for further testing to verify or refute original test findings. Because urine is the product of a short-term metabolic process, a second specimen obtained even a few hours after the first is apt to be different. Hair, which is the product of a long-term organic process and contains its own record of growth, is ideally suited for comparison testing.

SOME TESTING CONCEPTS

The following concepts form a foundation for understanding how drug testing works.

Quality Assurance

A quality-assurance program is a documented set of procedures followed by a drug-testing laboratory to ensure the highest possible accuracy and reliability of its tests. These procedures control the way samples are handled and instruments are checked to be sure they are functioning correctly. The procedures focus strongly on the minimization of human error.

A quality-assurance program will include the analysis of known samples, blank samples, and spiked samples. Known samples are urine specimens having a precise purity or concentration that is known to the laboratory. They are also called quality-control samples because they are used to calibrate equipment.

A laboratory also must be able to analyze blank and spiked samples correctly. These are included with the regular specimens routinely sent to the laboratory and are used to check the laboratory's accuracy. A blank specimen contains no drugs, and a spiked specimen contains a known drug in a concentration above the cutoff level. The drug in a spiked specimen must be correctly identified and quantified within acceptable limits of error. The ability to measure the drug level accurately is an important indicator of a laboratory's quality-assurance program.

Quality assurance covers all aspects of the testing process, including chain of custody, personnel certification and recertification, instrument calibration and maintenance, and other processes that ensure an accurate test result.

Nanograms and Micrograms

Test results are frequently reported quantitatively. The actual concentration of the drug is expressed as a certain amount per volume of urine. Depending on the drug or the drug metabolite that is being analyzed, urine concentrations may be expressed either as nanograms per milliliter (ng/ml) or as micrograms per milliliter (μg/ml). There are 28 million micrograms in an ounce and 1,000 nanograms in a microgram.

Cocaine metabolites may be detected in amounts as high as several micrograms in a heavy user, but the level of metabolites from marijuana use rarely reaches 1 μg/ml and are usually expressed in ng/ml.

The Sensitivity Limit and Cutoff Level

The sensitivity limit of a test is the lowest concentration at which the test can detect the presence of a drug in a urine sample. The cutoff level is an administrative mechanism that distinguishes a positive specimen from a negative one. That is, a drug concentration at or above that level yields a positive result, whereas one below that level yields a negative result.

Manufacturers of commercial urine-screening systems set the cutoff level above the sensitivity limit. For example, although EMIT and Abuscreen are sufficiently sensitive to detect marijuana metabolites at levels below 20 ng/ml, the assays are usually used at cutoff levels of 20 and 100 ng/ml, respectively. This not only decreases the possibility of a false positive resulting from operating the assay too close to its sensitivity limit but also significantly decreases the possibility of a positive test resulting from passive inhalation.

False Positives

A false positive occurs when a drug or drug metabolite is reported in a sample but is not actually present. A false positive can be categorized in the following ways:

- A chemical false positive. This may occur if another substance in the sample is mistakenly identified as the drug being analyzed. A chemical false positive also may occur if the sample is contaminated or adulterated during handling or analysis.
- An administrative false positive. This may occur if the wrong sample is tested. It can result from improper labeling or recording or transcription errors.

- Operator error. This may occur during an analytical procedure, particularly if normal precautions are not followed for specimen handling, assay procedure, and operator qualification.

Although a few foods and medications may produce positive results, this occurs only with certain tests that seek to identify particular drugs. These interfering substances are well known to laboratories that specialize in drug testing and are easily resolved by using an alternate analytical technique. This circumstance alone is sufficient reason for all positive tests to be confirmed.

Probably the two most important reasons for the occurrence of false positives are poor quality-assurance procedures in the laboratory and the failure to conduct confirmation tests. A good laboratory will have a stringent and well-documented quality-assurance program and will perform confirmatory tests on all samples that test positive in a screen.

False Negatives

A false negative occurs when a test fails to identify a drug that was present in the specimen analyzed. In some cases, the screening test may be positive but the confirmatory test negative. EMIT, for example, is an extremely sensitive screening test. When a specimen shows positive with EMIT at a low or borderline level, the confirming test may not be sufficiently sensitive to find the drug or metabolite. This can be the case when the confirming test method is RIA, TLC, GC, or HPLC, but it is not generally true when GC/MS is used.

Another reason why a second test may not confirm the presence of a drug is that it seeks to detect different or fewer metabolites. For example, the screening test may identify a drug class, such as the opiates. A positive screening result means that the specimen contains an opiate, which could be any one of many. A false negative could occur if the confirmatory test is limited to a search for only one or a few of the opioids.

This also causes a problem in urine testing for cannabinoids. The EMIT system, which is widely used in screening programs, will detect more than 30 cannabinoid metabolites. This is a valuable characteristic because it increases the chances of detecting many cannabinoids. But if the second test uses a methodology that focuses on only one cannabinoid metabolite, such as delta-9-THC, a negative finding may ensue. This does not mean that the first test was a false positive but that the second test lacked the ability to confirm the presence of that drug metabolite. A better term for these conflicting results is *unconfirmed positive*, which more accurately reflects the possibility that the initial screening result may be correct.

Delta-9-THC comprises 20 to 33 percent of the total metabolites present in a urine specimen that tests positive for marijuana. If the nanograms reported in a positive screen just happened to be 100, about 20 to 33 of those nanograms would relate to delta-9-THC. If the confirmation test was done with a GC/MS technique that seeks to identify only the delta-9-THC metabolites, the total number of nanograms reported in this test would probably be 20 to 33 rather than 100, as in the screen. This explains why the nanogram concentration reported in a GC/MS test result is likely to be less than the concentration identified in the screen. A rule of thumb is to multiply the nanogram level in a GC/MS test result by 3 to obtain a rough estimate of the total marijuana metabolites that are present in a specimen. It is important to remember that a positive test result in a GC/MS test is regarded as a positive finding even though the nanogram level may be lower than the nanogram level measured in the initial screen.

Finally, test results are almost always reported by the laboratory simply as positive or negative. If a sample is reported as positive, the laboratory is saying that it detected the drug in an amount exceeding the cutoff level it has set for that drug. Different laboratories using different procedures and methods may have different cutoff levels. For this reason, one laboratory could determine a sample to be positive and another determine it to be negative.

Presumed, Confirmed, and Verified Positives

A laboratory test finding that has not been confirmed by an alternate and at least equally sensitive test is called a *presumed positive*. For example, a specimen that has been screened by an immunoassay test and found to be positive is considered to be presumptively positive until a second test confirms or refutes the initial finding. A positive finding with the second test is called a *confirmed positive*. When the second test is a repeat of the first test or uses a less sensitive or essentially similar methodology, the test finding is called a *verified positive*. In terms of being certain about accuracy, there is a vast difference between verification and confirmation.

The term *verified* has another connotation as well. In the federal drug-testing programs, an MRO is required to evaluate all confirmed positives. When an MRO concludes that a confirmed positive is in fact related to illegal drug use, the finding is considered to have been verified.

Administrative Error versus Analytical Error

There are no circumstances under which human error can be eliminated entirely. The major assurance of accuracy is the series of checks designed to detect and correct mistakes. An administrative error or clerical error is human error. Among these errors are incorrect transcription of test results, incorrect recording of donor identity, failure to obtain a signature, and so forth. These are not errors related to the accuracy of the analysis of specimens.

Precision of analysis, calibration of equipment, and interpretation of test results are examples of analytical errors.

An administrative error should not require that a batch of specimens be automatically retested. The decision of whether to retest will hinge on the type and extent of the error. If one employee's test result was incorrectly recorded, nothing would be gained by retesting all the specimens. Retesting would, however, be appropriate if it was not clear whose specimen was tested and which results belonged to which specimens.

An analytical error suggests that more than one test result may be faulty. For example, should a false positive occur and the error is determined to be technical or methodological, there is a possibility of error with other specimens in the batch. The corrective action would be to retest all the specimens that tested positive for that drug or metabolite from the time of final resolution of the error back to the time of the last satisfactory test cycle.

Cross-Reactivity

The immunoassays sometimes result in cross-reactivity. Because immunoassays rely on immune reactions, a certain degree of interference occurs among the various drug metabolites and structurally similar compounds of a particular drug. The manufacturer of an immunoassay wants to develop a test that will be fairly specific for the target drug, but if the test is too specific, it will tend to miss some related metabolites or compounds that are valid identifiers. For example, amphetamine and methamphetamine are so similar in chemical structure that a test for one might incorrectly identify the other. This can be a problem because methamphetamine has a cross-reactivity with some over-the-counter medications, such as diet pills and decongestants that contain ephedrine and phenylpropanolamine. The problem can be solved by confirming any positive screen with GC/MS.

Poppy seeds, which contain traces of opium/morphine, can cause some interferences in testing. If a person consumes enough poppy seeds within a few days prior to giving a urine specimen, a positive result can show up in screening and confirmatory tests. The tests in such a case cannot differentiate between oral ingestion of poppy seeds and intravenous injection of morphine. The tests can, however, differentiate between heroin and poppy seeds.

Not long ago, certain nonsteroidal antiinflammatory drugs caused false positives in the EMIT screen for marijuana. The pain killer ibuprofen, which is available over the counter in Advil and other products, reacted like marijuana in the test. This problem was eliminated by changing the enzyme.

Retesting a Challenged Specimen

When retesting a challenged specimen, the laboratory need only confirm the presence of the substance. It does not have to confirm a concentration above the cutoff level. This is because the amount of a drug may deteriorate over time, causing the detectable concentration to drop below the cutoff level.

Liquid Intake

The concentration of a drug in urine can change considerably depending on liquid intake. The more an individual drinks, the more the drug is diluted. A negative result in a sample taken a few hours after drinking a large amount of liquid is possible, even though a clearly positive sample might have been evident before the liquid intake. For this reason, a negative result does not mean that the person has not used the drug recently. As the excretion of marijuana metabolites reaches the approximate limit of detection by a given assay, repeated samples collected over several days may alternate between positive and negative before all becoming negative.

Patterns of Abuse

Impairment, intoxication, or time of last use cannot be predicted from a single urine test. In the case of Cannabis use, a true-positive urine test indicates only that the person used Cannabis (such as marijuana or hashish) in the recent past, which could be hours, days, or weeks depending on the specific use pattern. Repeated analyses over time would, however, allow a better understanding of the past and current use patterns. An infrequent user should be completely negative in a few days. Repeated positive analyses over a period of more than two weeks suggest either continuing use or previous heavy chronic use.

The principal psychoactive ingredient in Cannabis and its various substances is THC. The strength and duration of Cannabis effects is a direct function of how much THC is absorbed into the body. The amount of THC absorbed depends on the THC content of the substance ingested and the manner of ingestion.

Metabolites

Metabolites are the biochemical products of the process by which the body, using enzymes and other internal biochemicals, breaks down ingested substances such as foods and drugs so they may be consumed and eliminated.

When marijuana is ingested by smoking, the THC passes through the lungs and into the bloodstream, where it is bound to blood proteins and carried throughout the body. Because THC is extremely fat-soluble (meaning that it will not dissolve in water and will easily collect in the fatty tissues), it is quickly absorbed into almost all body tissues that contain fat.

Within about one-half hour after ingestion of marijuana by smoking, the THC absorbed in the body tissues begins to release slowly back into the blood, which eventually carries it to the liver, where it is metabolized and excreted. This process continues until all the THC is eliminated. If more marijuana is ingested before the previous amount is voided, the new THC is added to the THC already stored in the body tissues. Depending on rate of use, method of administration, and strength of the THC ingested, marijuana metabolites can remain in the body system at a detectable level for 30 days or longer.

For cocaine, the major metabolite is benzoylecgonine, and the urine test analyzes for that metabolite exclusively. Unlike marijuana, the metabolite for cocaine is quickly eliminated, and the urine test for it is effective for one to three days after the last use.

Detection Time

Detection time depends on the drug and the sensitivity of the assay. The more sensitive the assay, the longer the drug can be detected. Drug concentrations are initially highest hours after drug use and decrease to undetectable levels over time. The time it takes to reach the point of undetectability depends on the particular drug and other factors such as an individual's metabolism. The sensitivity of the urine assay methods generally available today allows detection of cocaine use for a period of one to three days and heroin or phencyclidine (PCP) use for two to four days. These detection times would be somewhat lengthened in cases of previous chronic drug use, but they would probably be no more than double these times. Methaqualone and phenobarbital can be detected for as long as two to three weeks, but some amphetamines and secobarbital pass through the body so quickly that a negative result is likely even after very recent use.

With regard to Cannabis, several studies show that, due to highly individualized excretory patterns, it is possible to see positive results for four weeks or more. Also, the manner in which the body stores Cannabis metabolites and releases them by excretion can be erratic over a period of days or weeks. The metabolites may vary in quantity each day depending on whether fat tissue is being broken down at a high rate, as with heavy exercise, or at a low rate. A person could test negative one day after smoking marijuana and positive the next day.

The metabolism of marijuana is extremely complex and is not fully understood. Marijuana contains well over 20 compounds labeled as cannabinoids, and since it can be taken by mouth or smoked, with variable absorption from either route, its metabolism is difficult to study. Literally hundreds of marijuana metabolites are produced in variable amounts according to the user's habit and personal pattern of metabolism. For most marijuana users, absorption of the drug varies with the route of administration. Oral ingestion (eating) results in about 2 to 4 percent of the drug being absorbed, while inhalation from smoking results in 15 to 20 percent absorption. Under efficient smoking conditions, absorption may go as high as 50 percent.

It also is difficult to determine a particular time of use. Urine specimens that test positive for cannabinoids indicate that a person has consumed marijuana or Cannabis derivatives from within one hour to four weeks or more before the specimen was collected. Generally, a single smoking session by a casual user of marijuana will result in subsequently collected urine samples being positive for two to five days, depending on the screening method used and on physiological factors that cause drug concentration to vary. Detection time increases significantly following a period of chronic use. The same issues apply to other drugs, although the time after use during which a positive analysis would be expected might be reduced to a few days rather than a week or more.

Metabolites of the active ingredients of marijuana may be detectable in urine for up to ten days after a single smoking session. Metabolites can sometimes be detected several weeks after a heavy chronic smoker (several joints a day) has ceased smoking.

THC can be accurately detected in blood as well as urine. RIA is the method commonly used to detect THC in blood serum. The lower limit of detection is approximately 10 nanograms of THC per 1 milliliter of serum. The rapid disappearance of THC from the blood limits the time of detection. For the smoking of a single marijuana cigarette of standard street strength, the detection time is three to four hours following last use. The analysis of blood in general drug testing is not feasible because of the time restriction, but it can be very valuable in situations where recent Cannabis use is suspected. Although behavioral impairment and THC in the blood have not been scientifically correlated, it can be assumed that a person whose blood is found to contain more than 10 ng/ml of THC has ingested Cannabis very recently. This is presumptive evidence that the person was intoxicated at the time the blood was drawn.

The Steady-State Level

Recent scientific studies have shown that THC is eliminated from the body at a relatively constant rate. This rate is defined in terms of the amount of time it takes for one-half of the drug to be eliminated from the body. The best estimate for this THC half-life is 18 to 24 hours. This means that 50 percent of the THC taken will be gone after one day, 75 percent will be gone after two days, and 87.5 percent will be gone after three days. This also means that an individual who smokes one or more marijuana cigarettes per day will excrete the same amount of THC taken in by smoking. Therefore, the level of THC and its metabolites in the body will remain constant at what is called the steady-state level.

Because the body of a chronic user is taking in much larger amounts of THC, more time is required to eliminate all the THC after use is discontinued. This explains why positive test findings can result after four weeks or longer.

An issue of practical concern is how long a chronic user will test positive. Because the half-life of THC is about 24 hours, the concentration of THC in the blood and the total amount of metabolite excreted in the urine will reach the steady-state level within five to six days. When the steady-state level has been reached, the detection time after cessation of smoking will be the same in any individual smoking the same amount daily, whether it is for a week, a month, or several years.

In cases where THC metabolites are detected for several weeks following discontinuation of use, the test applied is usually capable of detecting cannabinoids at the 20 ng/ml level, which is the lowest level of concentration that can be routinely detected. Some laboratories use a cutoff level of 100 ng/ml or higher in both the initial screening test and the confirmation test. Tests with higher cutoff levels are only able to detect drug use that has occurred within a short period of time.

Several studies bear this out. If the cutoff level is 100 ng/ml, it is highly unlikely that a person would test positive for more than three days after using a moderate amount of marijuana. If large amounts of the drug are consumed daily for more than a week, there is a small possibility that the user could test positive at that level for as long as a month after use has ended.

It also has been documented that after a person smokes one standard strength marijuana cigarette (that is, one that contains about 20 mg of THC) it is possible to detect THC metabolites at the 100 ng/ml level for one to three days and at the 20 ng/ml level for two to seven days. If more than one marijuana cigarette is smoked, the detection time can increase by one or two days at both the 100 and 20 ng/ml levels. Variations have been found among individuals, which can be attributed to variations in smoking efficiency and absorption of THC through the lungs.

DEFENSES AGAINST A POSITIVE RESULT

A number of defenses have been put forward to explain positive test results.

Passive Inhalation

Passive inhalation or inadvertent exposure to marijuana is frequently cited as the basis for a positive urine test. Clinical studies have shown, however, that it is highly unlikely that a nonsmoking individual could inhale sufficient smoke by passive inhalation to result in a high enough drug concentration to be detected at the cutoff level of currently used urinalysis methods.

One of the most important passive inhalation studies examined the effects of two different experimental conditions: exposure in a midsize automobile and exposure in an 8- by 8- by 10-foot room. The levels of exposure varied from two to four marijuana cigarettes per session, and one trial was conducted over three consecutive days to measure the possible cumulative effects. Only 2 of 75 urine specimens from six subjects tested positive at the 20 ng/ml level. Significantly, the two positive specimens were obtained from the first urine voidings, which were taken approximately five hours after exposure. The researcher concluded that given the severe conditions of exposure to marijuana smoke imposed by the experiment and the relatively short period of time between exposure and collection of urine specimens, it would be unreasonable to believe that any positive findings would have been made in real-life situations using standard testing techniques.

In other words, it is extremely improbable that a person who was not smoking would be exposed to the level of smoke and for the length of time required to produce a positive test. It is also improbable that a person would be called upon to give a urine specimen within the interval of time required to obtain a positive result. Even 24 hours is too long for passively inhaled THC to remain in the body at a detectable level. Consequently, this defense is rapidly losing favor.

Accidental Oral Ingestion

Although it is possible for an innocent person to test positive after eating food that contains marijuana, there are two limiting factors. The first is that marijuana contains THC as an inactive component that must be activated in order for it to be absorbed into the body and produce an effect. Heat, such as by smoking, is the quickest and most direct means of activating the THC. The only forms of Cannabis that generally have significant amounts of active THC are hashish and its extract, hashish oil.

Baking at high temperatures, such as those used to bake brownies and cookies, can activate the THC in marijuana, but the amount of marijuana and/or the strength of the THC must be substantially greater than those in marijuana cigarettes for the consumer to attain a definite high. Also, the effects of oral ingestion appear more slowly and last longer.

Marijuana that is boiled, as in the preparation of a tea, will almost certainly not release THC into the liquid. It is even less likely that THC can be made active in a cold drink, due to the extreme insolubility of THC in water.

The second limiting factor is the interval between the time of consumption and the time a urine specimen is taken. Generally, oral ingestion of THC at the standard dose (20 mg) can be detected at the 100 ng/ml level for one day and at the 20 ng/ml level for five days. Concentrations above these levels probably indicate that the person did not ingest the THC orally.

To ensure a fair and impartial interpretation of a test result in which the subject cites unknowing oral ingestion of Cannabis as a defense, it is important to determine the nature and quantity of Cannabis eaten and when it was ingested.

Melanin

In some cases, blacks and hispanics have held that their increased level of the skin pigment melanin led to a false-positive result. This is a scientifically absurd proposition because melanin is completely unlike the THC metabolites. Cross-reactivity of melanin with any illicit drug, including marijuana, does not occur in testing by EMIT, RIA, or any chromatographic procedure.

LABORATORY CERTIFICATION

The problem of choosing a qualified drug-testing laboratory was solved in April 1988 when the U.S. Department of Health and Human Services (DHHS) issued its Mandatory Guidelines for Federal Workplace Drug Testing Programs (see Appendix D). Subpart C of the guidelines is titled "Certification of Laboratories Engaged in Urine Drug Testing for Federal Agencies" and was developed in response to President Reagan's directive to establish standards and procedures for periodic reviews of laboratories and criteria for certification of laboratories to perform drug testing pursuant to Executive Order 12564 (see Appendix A).

For several years prior to 1988, standards for drug-testing laboratories were a thorny issue for the DHHS and the drug-testing industry. Executive Order 12564 and the attendant need to formulate a uniform approach to drug testing helped bring to a close a long-standing debate over standards and certification. The guidelines, which are really directives, apply to laboratories engaged in urine drug testing for federal agencies and private employers in certain regulated industries. The DHHS program of certification is by far the most stringent of the various certification programs for urine drug-testing laboratories and has come to be regarded by the courts as a standard for judging the accuracy and reliability of employer drug-testing activities.

Although most employers in the private sector are not required to use DHHS-certified laboratories, many have elected to do so because they were clients before certification or they recognized the advantage of being serviced by a laboratory that can meet the highest standards of competence. These guidelines have made it easier for many employers to select a competent laboratory. Employers still must make sure, however, that a laboratory's services are delivered as specified in the agreement or contract.

As of this writing, the fees charged by DHHS-certified laboratories have not increased appreciably despite the initial cost connected with obtaining certification and the ongoing cost of meeting higher standards relative to laboratory staff, equipment, and quality-control procedures. Two factors appear to have kept costs down: (1) competition among the growing number of companies that have entered the drug-testing field and (2) each competitor's desire to capture as much of the market as possible while the demand for drug testing is expanding.

Laboratory Staff

The laboratory staff requirements in the guidelines are designed to ensure that any individual responsible for test review or result reporting is qualified to perform the function and could, if necessary, appear as an expert witness to defend against a challenge of test results. This requires a wide range of knowledge related to test selection, quality assurance, interferences with various tests, maintenance of chain of custody, documentation of test findings, interpretation of test data, and validation and verification of test results.

Oversight and control of laboratory functions must be carried out by professionals who are directly responsible for day-to-day operations and are accountable for test results. These people must be available to consult with clients and to help them explain and defend drug testing at any legal or administrative proceeding. The objective of this requirement is to eliminate the practice of using consultants to intermittently or periodically oversee the technicians who perform the assays.

A certified laboratory must be managed by responsible individuals who select and monitor properly credentialed employees, who in turn perform well-defined functions that are constantly evaluated by objective techniques. At least one full-time manager is responsible for overall general management and for the scientific and technical performance of the laboratory. At least one full-time supervisor is responsible for directing laboratory operations and for supervising the analysts. One or both of these individuals must be able to attest to the validity of test results.

Testing Capability

To be certified, a laboratory must be capable of testing for at least five classes of drugs: marijuana, cocaine, opiates, amphetamines, and PCP. A laboratory seeking certification is surveyed and performance-tested regarding its ability to test for these drugs using an immunoassay technique for initial testing and quantitative GC/MS as the confirmatory test.

A certified laboratory must be able to perform both initial immunoassays and confirmatory GC/MS tests at the same site. The DHHS believes that this is the best approach to maintaining strict chain-of-custody control. Testing at more than one laboratory creates problems in filling out and maintaining multiple sets of chain-of-custody and laboratory forms, controlling and accounting for specimens moving between laboratories, and ensuring timely reporting of test results.

Quality Assurance and Quality Control

Perhaps the most important qualification for certification is to have a quality-assurance program that encompasses all aspects of the testing process, including specimen acquisition, chain of custody, security and reporting of results, initial and confirmatory testing, and validation of analytical procedures. Quality-control procedures must be designed and implemented to monitor the conduct of each step of the drug-testing process.

Security and Chain of Custody

A certified laboratory must be secure at all times and have in place security measures to control access. Controlled access must be such that unauthorized personnel will be prevented from entering the laboratory operations areas, handling specimens, or gaining entry to the areas where records or specimens are stored. Authorized individuals must have documented authorization, and all authorized visitors and maintenance and service personnel must be escorted at all times. Documentation of individuals accessing these areas, as well as the date, time, and purpose of entry, must be maintained.

A certified laboratory must use chain-of-custody procedures to maintain control and accountability of specimens from receipt through completion of testing, reporting of results, storage, and final disposition. The date and purpose of custody must be documented on a chain-of-custody form each time a specimen is handled or transferred, and every individual in the chain must be identified. The practical effect of these procedures is that the testing technicians are held responsible for each urine specimen in their possession and must fill out the chain-of-custody forms as the specimens are received for testing.

Storage for Confirmed Positives

All confirmed positive specimens are required to be retained in long-term frozen storage (− 20°C or colder) to ensure that positive urine specimens will be available for any necessary retest during administrative or disciplinary proceedings for at least one year. Within this one-year period, an employer can ask the laboratory to retain the specimen for an additional period of time, but if no such request is received, the laboratory is free to discard the specimen at the end of one year. Specimens that are the subject of legal challenge can be held for an indefinite period.

Documentation

A certified laboratory is expected to maintain and make available for at least two years documentation of all aspects of the testing process. The required documentation includes personnel files on all individuals authorized to have access to specimens, chain-of-custody documents, quality-assurance/quality-control records, procedure manuals, all test data (including calibration curves and any calculations used in determining test results), reports, performance records on certification inspections, and hard copies of computer-generated data.

Test Reports

In federal drug-testing programs, the laboratory's main contact concerning test results is an MRO employed or contracted by the employer. The laboratory reports test results to the MRO within an average of five working days after receipt of the specimen by the laboratory. The report identifies the drugs and/or metabolites tested for, whether the test was positive or negative, the cutoff level for each drug or metabolite, the specimen number assigned by the employer, and the drug-testing laboratory's specimen identification number.

All specimens that are negative on the initial or the confirmatory test are reported to the MRO as negative. Only specimens confirmed positive are reported as positive for a specific drug. The MRO may ask the laboratory to provide quantitation of test results, but the MRO will not disclose quantitation to the employer—only that the test was positive or negative.

A laboratory's reporting mode is typically by some electronic means, such as a teleprinter or facsimile machine. The manner of communication is designed to ensure confidentiality of the information. The reporting system expressly forbids reporting of results by telephone.

The laboratory also sends to the MRO a certified copy of the original chain-of-custody form. This will help the MRO determine whether a positive test finding could have resulted from a defect in the chain of custody.

In addition to reports relating to individual test specimens, the laboratory must provide the employer with a monthly statistical summary of urinalysis testing. This summary does not include any personal identifying information that would link an employee to a particular test result.

Performance Test Requirements

The performance testing program is part of the initial evaluation of a laboratory seeking certification and of the continuing assessment of laboratory performance necessary to maintain certification. Successful participation in three cycles of testing are required before a laboratory is eligible to be considered for inspection and certification. These initial three cycles can be compressed into a three-month period, one per month. After certification, laboratories are challenged every other month with one set of at least ten specimens, or a total of six cycles per year. To the greatest extent possible, the procedures associated with the handling and testing of the performance test specimens by the laboratory are carried out in a manner identical to that applied to routine laboratory specimens.

A certified laboratory is subject to blind performance testing. During the initial 90-day period of any new drug-testing program, an employer is expected to submit blind performance test specimens to the laboratory in the amount of at least 50 percent of the total number of samples submitted (up to a maximum of 500 samples) and thereafter a minimum of 10 percent of all samples (to a maximum of 250 samples) submitted per quarter. Approximately 80 percent of the blind performance test samples are blank (that is, certified to contain no drug), and the remaining samples are positive for one or more drugs per sample. The positive samples are spiked only with those drugs for which the employer is testing.

Should a false positive occur on a blind performance test specimen and it is determined to have resulted from an administrative error, the laboratory is required to take corrective action to minimize the occurrence of that particular error in the future. If there is reason to believe that the error could have been systematic, the laboratory may be compelled to reanalyze previously run specimens. If an error is determined to be technical or methodological, the laboratory is required to retest all specimens analyzed positive for that drug or metabolite from the time of final resolution of the error back to the time of the last satisfactory performance test cycle.

Performance Test Specimen Composition

Performance test specimens are spiked to contain those drugs and metabolites that the certified laboratory is prepared to assay. The laboratory is expected to detect the spiked drugs in concentration ranges that allow identification of the analyte by commonly used immunoassay screening techniques. These concentrations are generally in the range of what might be expected in the urine of recent drug users. For some drug analytes, the specimen composition will consist of the parent drug as well as major metabolites. In some cases, more than one drug class may be included in one specimen container, but generally no more than two drugs will be present in any one specimen. The idea is to imitate the type of specimen that a laboratory normally encounters. The composition of test kits going to different laboratories during a particular test cycle will vary, but within any one year, all laboratories will analyze the same total set of specimens.

In the federal drug-testing program, the performance test specimens are spiked for marijuana, cocaine, opiates, amphetamines, and PCP. The concentration levels are set at least 20 percent above the cutoff levels for either the initial assay or the confirmatory test.

Inspections

Prior to receiving laboratory certification and at least twice a year after certification, a DHHS team of three qualified inspectors, at least two of whom
have been trained as laboratory inspectors, conduct an on-site inspection of
the laboratory. They document the overall quality of the laboratory setting
and make recommendations for improvements.

CONCLUSION

At laboratories where urine drug testing is performed as a forensic specialty,
the urinalysis technology is at an extremely high level. In life, nothing is
ever absolutely certain, but drug-testing reliability can get as close to 100
percent as the laws of science permit.

Drug testing is not the total answer to an organization's drug problem,
but it can be the driving force in a larger process that includes employee
education, supervisor intervention, and medical rehabilitation. These major
components of abuse prevention can be greatly enhanced by a skillfully
applied program of drug testing.

Chapter 9

Drug Testing in the Federal Workplace

The rationale for drug testing in the federal workplace comes largely from the experience of the U.S. military forces. In 1980, 27 percent of military personnel surveyed said that they had used an illicit drug within the month preceding the survey. In 1985, only 9 percent reported similar use. What caused such a sharp decline? A program of urinalysis was instituted during that five-year period, and 64 percent of the military personnel asked said that they believed urinalysis was the main reason for reduced drug use. Three years later, drug use in the military dropped to 5.3 percent, a decline of more than 80 percent in eight years.

EXECUTIVE ORDER 12564

On September 15, 1986, President Reagan issued Executive Order 12564 (see Appendix A) mandating a drug-free federal workplace with the intent that the federal work force would serve as a model for all American business. The order requires that all federal employees refrain from using illegal drugs on or off the job. It directs federal agency heads to do the following:

- Develop policies regarding the use of illicit drugs and the consequences of policy violations
- Initiate EAPs
- Conduct supervisory training
- Provide for supervisory referrals and self-referrals of employees to treatment
- Use drug testing to identify employees who are in violation of policy

The order allows agency heads to require urine testing in the following cases:

- When candidates apply for federal employment
- When there is a reasonable suspicion that an employee uses drugs

- Following an accident or unsafe practice
- As a follow-up to drug counseling or rehabilitation
- On a random basis among employees who hold positions that are designated as sensitive or critical

In developing the order, President Reagan required that those employees who tested positive for drug use be referred to appropriate treatment or counseling. The order also contains provisions designed to protect the rights of employees.

SECTION 503 OF PUBLIC LAW 100-73

On July 11, 1987, Congress passed legislation effecting implementation of Executive Order 12564 under Section 503 of Public Law 100-73 (the Supplemental Appropriations Act of 1987) (see Appendix B). In addition to providing funds to carry out the executive order, Section 503 established uniformity among federal agency drug-testing plans, ensured confidentiality of drug test results, and centralized oversight of the government's drug-testing program.

MANDATORY GUIDELINES FOR
FEDERAL WORKPLACE DRUG TESTING PROGRAMS

Under the executive order and Section 503, the secretary of the Department of Health and Human Services (DHHS) was tasked with promulgating technical and scientific guidelines. On April 11, 1988, the DHHS published the Mandatory Guidelines for Federal Workplace Drug Testing Programs (see Appendix D), sometimes referred to as the NIDA (National Institute on Drug Abuse) guidelines, which play a critical part in ensuring that the requirements of the executive order are met. All federal agencies must follow the procedures outlined in these guidelines and may not deviate from them without written approval of the DHHS.

The guidelines require that all federal agency programs must, at a minimum, test for marijuana and cocaine. Agencies also may elect to test for opiates, amphetamines, and PCP without additional authorization. No other substances may be tested for without written authorization from the DHHS.

The apparent rationale for this testing scheme is that marijuana and cocaine are by far the drugs most frequently abused, with opiates, amphetamines, and PCP the next most common drugs of abuse. Although there is little doubt that federal employees, like employees in other sectors, suffer a heavy burden of illness and death from alcohol, this drug is excluded from the testing portion of the drug-free workplace program.

AGENCY PLANS

Each agency head is required to develop a plan for carrying out the requirements of the executive order. Although each plan will contain language specific to its mission and work environment, all plans must contain the following:

- A clear policy statement that describes the impact of illegal drug use on the agency's mission and specifies the agency's expectations regarding drug use and the actions to be anticipated in response to identified drug use
- A commitment to employee assistance through development of a program emphasizing education, counseling, referral to rehabilitation, and coordination with available community resources
- An assurance to employees that personal dignity and privacy will be respected in reaching the goal of a drug-free workplace
- A commitment that management will seek ways in which recognized bargaining unit representatives might assist in program implementation
- Provisions for self-referrals as well as supervisory referrals to treatment, with maximum respect for individual confidentiality consistent with safety and security priorities
- A commitment to develop an employee education component that may, for example, use videotapes, lunchtime forums, drug awareness days, and distribution of written materials to educate employees about drug abuse
- Review by a licensed physician of any positive test result before such result is made known to agency officials
- A requirement that any employee with a confirmed positive test result will be referred to the EAP
- The opportunity for an employee to seek administrative relief if he or she believes that his or her position has been wrongly selected as a testing-designated position
- Compliance with all applicable provisions of law, the executive order, and the mandatory guidelines
- A recommendation for "safe harbor" provisions that protect an employee from disciplinary action if he or she voluntarily admits to illegal drug use, obtains counseling or rehabilitation through the EAP, and thereafter refrains from illegal drug use
- A recommendation for extension of EAP services to the spouses and dependents of employees

The agency's plan also will provide training to assist supervisors and managers in identifying and responding to illegal drug use. Training courses must include information on the following:

- Policies relevant to work performance problems, drug use, and the EAP
- How to recognize employees with possible drug problems
- The agency's procedures for referring employees to the EAP
- The roles and responsibilities of key personnel charged with carrying out the plan
- The agency's procedures for reintegrating employees into the work force

Each federal agency must certify to Congress that its drug-free workplace program plan meets all requirements of the executive order and the mandatory guidelines.

CUTOFF LEVELS

In the federal drug-testing programs, the following initial cutoff levels are used when screening specimens to determine whether they are negative for these five drugs or classes of drugs:

Marijuana metabolites	100 ng/ml
Cocaine metabolites	300 ng/ml
Opiate metabolites	300 ng/ml*
PCP	25 ng/ml
Amphetamines	1,000 ng/ml

*25 ng/ml if the immunoassay is specific for free morphine.

All specimens identified as positive on the initial test are confirmed using GC/MS techniques at the cutoff values listed below:

Marijuana metabolite*	15 ng/ml
Cocaine metabolite**	150 ng/ml
Opiates	
Morphine	300 ng/ml
Codeine	300 ng/ml
PCP	25 ng/ml
Amphetamines	
Amphetamine	500 ng/ml
Methamphetamine	500 ng/ml

*Delta-9-tetrahydrocannabinol-9-carboxylic acid
**Benzoylecgonine

All test levels are subject to change by the DHHS as advances in technology or other considerations warrant identification of these substances at other concentrations.

REPORTING OF TEST RESULTS

A laboratory is expected to report test results to the agency's MRO within an average of five working days of receipt of the specimen. Before any test result is reported, it is reviewed and certified as accurate by the responsible individual. The report identifies the drugs or drug metabolites tested for, whether the result was positive or negative, the cutoff level for each substance, the specimen number assigned by the agency, and the drug-testing laboratory's specimen identification number. The results (positive or negative) for all specimens submitted at the same time to the laboratory are reported back to the MRO at the same time.

The laboratory will report as negative all specimens that are negative on the initial or the confirmatory test. Only specimens confirmed positive are reported as positive for a specific drug.

The MRO may request from the laboratory quantitation of test results. He or she will not disclose quantitation to the agency but will report only whether the test was positive or negative.

In most cases, the laboratory will transmit results to the MRO by various electronic means (for example, a teleprinter, facsimile machine, or computer). Results may not be provided verbally by telephone. The laboratory must ensure the security of the data transmission and limit access to any data transmission, storage, or retrieval system.

The laboratory will send to the MRO a certified copy of the original chain-of-custody form signed by the individual responsible for day-to-day management of the drug-testing laboratory or the individual responsible for attesting to the validity of test reports. Unless otherwise instructed by the agency in writing, the laboratory will retain all records pertaining to a given urine specimen for a minimum of two years.

CONFIDENTIALITY

The procedures for protecting the confidentiality of drug test results must comply with the Privacy Act, 5 USC 552a, and the patient access and confidentiality provisions of Section 503 of Public Law 100-73. This is done by setting up a Privacy Act System of Records, modifying an existing system, or using any applicable government-wide system of records to cover both the agency's and the laboratory's records of employee urinalysis results. The contract procedures must specifically require that employee records be maintained and used with the highest regard for employee privacy.

In accordance with Section 503, any federal employee who is the subject of a drug test shall, upon written request, have access to any records relating to his or her drug test and any records relating to the results of any relevant certification, review, or revocation-of-certification proceedings.

EMPLOYEE ASSISTANCE PROGRAMS

Federal EAPs are designed to assist employees and their families with problems that may affect their well-being and their ability to perform their jobs. These worksite-based programs offer both counseling activities (such as assessment and referral services) and work-related activities (such as supervisory and union representative training). The EAP also may provide services such as prevention, education, and health promotion activities. The primary goal of an EAP is to maintain the ability of employees to be fully productive by offering a wide range of services, including early intervention and prevention. The objectives of a federal EAP are as follows:

- To effectively and efficiently provide services for ameliorating the mental health and alcohol- and other drug-related problems of the work force
- To identify employees with job performance problems and to respond to those seeking assistance; to direct employees toward the best assistance possible; and to provide continuing support and guidance throughout the problem-solving period
- To serve as a resource for management and labor in intervening with employees whose personal problems affect their job performance
- To benefit both the organization and the employees and their families

Each agency designs its own EAP based on the agency's unique mission, operation, and culture. An effective program will be broad enough to respond to a wide range of employee problems. The focus is on individuals and families seeking or requiring assistance for personal and/or job performance problems. These problems may fall into several categories: alcohol and drugs, marital, family/child, emotional, medical, AIDS, legal, financial, career vocational, or organizational. Since EAPs offer assessment and referral services, they should be able to match employee needs with the appropriate services. Short-term counseling may be provided during the assessment process.

A variety of EAPs can be provided internally or purchased from external service providers, or the agency may use some combination of the two. Smaller organizations often provide EAPs through participation in consortiums. Regardless of the exact structure used to provide EAP services, ethical factors are considered in every aspect of the design, implementation, and delivery of the program.

A key component of a federal EAP is the provision of training and consultation to management and union leaders concerning the particular and changing needs of the agency. These needs will be greatest during the early implementation of a drug-testing program. The following areas are included in training and consultation efforts:

- The impact of mental well-being on job performance
- Use of the EAP

- Identification of employees in need of assistance
- Methods for referral
- Management of employees with problems
- Positive return-to-work experience
- Confidentiality
- Relationship of the EAP to personnel actions

Active efforts by EAP administrators to incorporate such information into ongoing supervisor and manager training help ensure that the work force is kept informed about the services available.

In summary, three important points need to be made concerning EAPs in the federal workplace:

1. Each agency will have its own EAP, but all EAPs will contain the core components discussed previously.
2. Although a major focus of the EAP will be drug use, many other employee problems will be covered.
3. An agency's drug-testing program will be inextricably linked to its EAP.

THE MEDICAL REVIEW OFFICER

The MRO is a physician knowledgeable in the medical use of prescription drugs and the pharmacology and toxicology of illicit drugs. The MRO's primary responsibility is to review and interpret positive test results obtained through the agency's drug-testing program. It is important to remember that a positive test result does not automatically identify an employee or applicant as an illegal drug user. The MRO must assess and determine whether alternate medical explanations could account for the positive test result.

Responsibilities

The DHHS's mandatory guidelines specify these MRO responsibilities:

- Receive and evaluate all confirmed positive test results from the drug-testing laboratory
- Obtain as required a quantitative description of test results
- Examine a certified copy of the original chain of custody related to each confirmed positive test result
- Review and interpret positive test results
- Inform the tested individual of positive test results and provide those results
- Conduct a medical interview with an individual who has tested positive
- Review the medical history or any other relevant biomedical factors related to an individual who has tested positive

- Allow a discussion (although not necessarily face-to-face) of positive test results related to an individual who has tested positive
- Order a reanalysis of the original specimen if necessary
- Consult with others if a question of accuracy arises
- Consult with laboratory officials
- Refuse to accept test results that do not comply with the mandatory guidelines
- Not declare as positive an opiate-positive urine without clinical evidence
- Determine whether a test result is scientifically insufficient
- Determine whether a test result is consistent with legal drug use
- Forward results of verified positive tests to the EAP and management officials empowered to recommend or take administrative action

These are perhaps the most critical points regarding the function of the MRO. Essentially, the MRO determines whether some reason other than illegal drug use explains a drug-positive urine. If the MRO verifies illegal drug use, the case is referred to the agency's EAP representative and to the appropriate management official. If drug use is not verified by the MRO, the test result is deemed negative, the employee is so informed, and no further action is taken.

Giving the Employee an Opportunity for an Interview

The mandatory guidelines require that the MRO must provide the opportunity for an interview if the individual requests it, and the MRO must review all medical records that the tested individual submits when a confirmed positive test could have resulted from legally prescribed medication. For example, a cocaine-positive urine may result from the proper medical use of cocaine as a local vasoconstrictive anesthetic in bronchoscopy and dentistry.

If any question arises as to the accuracy or validity of a positive test result, the MRO should, in collaboration with the drug-testing laboratory director and consultants, review the laboratory records to determine whether the required procedures were followed. The MRO then makes a determination as to whether the result is scientifically sufficient to take further action. Moreover, if records from collection sites or laboratories raise doubts about the handling of samples, the MRO may deem the urinary evidence insufficient, and no further actions relative to individual employees would occur. In such situations, the MRO should note indications of possible errors in laboratory analysis or chain-of-custody procedures and bring these to the attention of the appropriate program officials. Each DHHS-certified laboratory must have a scientific director or a consultant forensic toxicologist available to consult with the MRO on interpretations of laboratory reports.

Special consideration is given in the case of a positive assay for opiates.

Because the ingestion of a variable quantity of poppy seeds, which contain a small amount of morphine, can produce a confirmed positive test for opiates, the mandatory guidelines require that the MRO must determine whether there is clinical evidence of illegal opiate use. The term *clinical evidence* means the signs and symptoms of use, such as needle tracks on the body.

While there may be wide agreement that there should be an opportunity for some type of medical interview between the MRO and the employee prior to the MRO's final decision concerning a positive test result, a face-to-face interview may not always be feasible or possible. The employee and the MRO may be far apart, in which case the practical solution is to confer by telephone. An employee who does not make himself or herself available for an interview, either in person or by telephone, has in effect rejected the opportunity for an interview. The course of action in this event would be for the MRO to document the attempt to conduct the interview and allow a reasonable period (ten days is recommended) for the employee to make contact. In the absence of contact and after having made a good-faith attempt, the MRO would report the positive test result to the employer.

The role of the MRO may be broader in some agencies. He or she may advise and assist management in the planning and oversight of the overall substance abuse control program, including specimen collection, chain-of-custody procedures, laboratory quality control, and treatment. The MRO may offer advice when suspected substance abusers are thought to be avoiding detection by various manipulative maneuvers or claims of medical illness.

The MRO also may assist management in determining the degree of impairment as it affects occupationally related performance and safety. This service may naturally extend to providing guidance to management regarding the rehabilitation of impaired employees.

It is important to note that the MRO does not adjudicate, punish, or otherwise arrange consequences for employees whose drug-positive urines apparently do not result from medical treatment or from problems in handling or analyzing samples.

Interaction with the Employee Assistance Program

When the MRO verifies an employee's illegal drug use, the agency is required to follow its plan concerning counseling, rehabilitative care, and random testing to confirm successful therapy. In general, these matters fall within the scope of the EAP. The rules of an agency's EAP will determine the extent and nature of assistance and treatment, if and when an employee may safely return to work, and the circumstances that dictate termination. The MRO may be asked to consult with EAP officials but usually does not play a directing role in that program.

An agency's plan will provide for written notice to employees, in advance of specimen collection, describing policy and the actions that will be taken if laboratory findings are positive. When, and under what conditions, such positive results and any related information will be shared with management and other sources also must be specified in writing.

Summary

These points summarize an MRO's role in the drug-testing program:

- The MRO's major function is to determine whether the laboratory evidence indicating the use of illegal drugs is justified.
- If there is no reasonable medical explanation (such as a legitimate prescription) or other explanation (such as a breakdown in the chain of custody or a laboratory error) for a positive test result, the result is disclosed to management and EAP officials as required by the agency's plan. Any medical information disclosed during testing or by the MRO's investigation that is not related to the use of illegal drugs (such as pregnancy) is treated as confidential and not disclosed.
- If it is determined with reasonable certainty that there is a legitimate medical or other explanation for the positive finding, no information identifying the specific employee is disclosed. Any medical information is treated as confidential.
- Although the MRO may assist in employee rehabilitation efforts related to substance abuse, any such assistance is made within the framework of the agency's plan, policy, and procedures.

DRUG-TESTING PROGRAMS OF THE DEPARTMENT OF TRANSPORTATION

On November 21, 1988, the Department of Transportation (DOT) issued antidrug program rules through its six operating administrations. The DOT program requires a DOT employee to be removed from federal service under several circumstances:

- Refusal to enter or to successfully complete a drug rehabilitation or abatement program
- Repeated use of drugs
- Refusal to provide a urine specimen for drug testing
- Adulteration or substitution of a urine specimen
- On-duty use of illegal drugs
- A determination that the employee has engaged in illegal drug trafficking

Following are highlights and summaries of the rules.

Federal Highway Administration

Motor carrier safety has been delegated to the Federal Highway Administration (FHWA) by a number of authorities. Under 49 USC, the FHWA may prescribe requirements for the qualifications and maximum hours of service of employees and the safety of operation and equipment of motor carriers. Under the Motor Carrier Safety Act of 1984, the FHWA established safety standards ensuring that, among other things, the physical condition of operators of commercial motor vehicles is adequate to allow them to drive safely.

The FHWA rules issued on November 21, 1988, require motor carriers that operate commercial vehicles in interstate commerce to have an antidrug program, including testing of drivers for the use of controlled substances. Testing is a responsibility of the motor carrier and must be conducted prior to employment, periodically (biannually), based on reasonable cause, and randomly. Postaccident testing also must be performed; however, because most accidents occur on highways away from the effective control of the motor carrier, the driver is made responsible for providing the specimens necessary for testing. The rules cover drivers of commercial motor vehicles with a gross vehicle weight rating (GVWR) over 26,000 pounds and vehicles transporting hazardous materials that must be placarded.

A driver may not use controlled substances on or off duty, and if controlled substance use is detected, an individual is disqualified from driving a commercial motor vehicle involved in interstate commerce. A driver cannot be hired or used if he or she has a confirmed positive drug test and continues to be disqualified until such time as he or she is medically recertified on the basis of a negative drug test.

The primary goal of the FHWA testing program is to reduce accidents and casualties in motor carrier operations. A secondary goal is to reduce absenteeism, health care costs, and other drug-related problems.

These antidrug program rules supplement earlier rules pertaining to the use of drugs by drivers of commercial motor vehicles. Under the Commercial Motor Vehicle Safety Act of 1986, the FHWA established a regulation that disqualifies motor vehicle drivers who operate while under the influence. The regulation disqualifies a driver for one year from driving in intrastate or interstate commerce upon his or her first violation of driving a commercial motor vehicle while under the influence of alcohol or a controlled substance. The disqualification period is extended to three years if the cargo includes hazardous materials. A second offense results in a lifetime ban from driving a commercial motor vehicle.

The Anti–Drug Abuse Act of 1986 makes it a federal crime for the operator of a common carrier (that is, a rail carrier, sleeping car carrier, bus transporting passengers in interstate commerce, water common carrier, or air common carrier) to operate under the influence. The maximum penalty is five years imprisonment and a $10,000 fine.

Under its regulatory authority, the FHWA has adopted regulations that prohibit driver use of a Schedule I drug or other substance, an amphetamine, a narcotic, or any other habit-forming drug. A driver who uses such a drug is not qualified to operate a commercial motor vehicle in interstate commerce and is subject to civil and criminal penalties.

The prohibition of alcohol use by drivers is covered in a rule stemming from the Commercial Motor Vehicle Safety Act. The rule establishes 0.04 percent as the blood alcohol concentration (BAC) level at or above which a driver can be disqualified. Enforcement of the BAC level through state laws is linked to federal-aid highway funds.

In summary, alcohol and drug use by commercial motor vehicle drivers has been an issue of long-standing concern with the FHWA. The earlier rules generally address impairment and disqualification. The rules extending from Executive Order 12564 are complementary and focus on drug testing as a means for identifying drivers whose drug or alcohol use makes them medically unqualified to drive.

Federal Railroad Administration

The Federal Railroad Administration (FRA) antidrug program rules build on an extensive history of efforts by the FRA, the railroads, and the rail unions to curb alcohol and drug abuse within the industry. Rule G, one of the earliest standard operating rules of the railroads, prohibits employees from going or remaining on duty while using, possessing, or being under the influence of alcohol. In recent years, mind-altering drugs have been included in the rule. Unions formed within the past century have included sobriety and mutual assistance in their organizational goals.

The FRA has actively promoted peer prevention programs led by employees and supported by rail management. These efforts provide a means for rank-and-file workers to protect their own safety while assisting fellow employees with substance abuse problems. In these programs, workers who come to work impaired may be confronted by fellow workers. In some situations, railroad management will withhold discipline for first-offense violations uncovered by active employee involvement.

Drug testing is not new to the railroad industry. Of the seven large rail systems that provide roughly 85 percent of the United States' rail service, five conduct drug screening in conjunction with physical examinations that are part of company medical qualifications programs. The examinations are typically done on a regularly scheduled basis, and when an employee returns to work after an extended absence, or when an employee is transferred to a safety-sensitive job. Most of these programs have been challenged in litigation under the Railway Labor Act, even though it is a uniform practice of the railroads to return drug-afflicted employees to service upon successful completion of substance abuse treatment.

For several years, all the major rail systems have had programs for making employees aware of the consequences of abuse and for teaching supervisors how to intervene. The unions also have been active in prevention and control activities.

Historically, considerable attempts have been made by the FRA, the employers, and the unions to eliminate alcohol and drug abuse from the railroad industry workplace. Some progress has been made, but the problem persists and railroad employees and the public they serve remain at risk.

The rules issued by the FRA in November 1988 prohibit use of controlled substances without medical authorization by certain safety-sensitive railroad employees. They also require random drug testing and amend prior regulations with respect to drug testing.

U.S. Coast Guard

Rules of the U.S. Coast Guard (USCG) antidrug program target drug abuse by crew members on commercial vessels. The program includes chemical testing in preemployment, periodic, random, postaccident, and reasonable cause situations. The postaccident provision also includes testing for alcohol use.

The USCG has explicit statutory authority to deny a license, certificate of registry, or merchant mariner's document to any individual who has been convicted of a dangerous drug law violation in the ten years preceding application. The USCG also must revoke such documents when it discovers individuals who have been convicted of drug law violations within ten years preceding the initiation of revocation proceedings. Further, the USCG has the authority to deny issuance of and to revoke such documents for any individual who has ever been a user of, or addicted to, a dangerous drug.

The methods for gathering evidence to support remedial or punitive steps include examining criminal conviction records of license and document applicants and holders. Denial and revocation actions are usually carried out only after an incident occurs.

Federal Aviation Administration

Domestic and supplemental air carriers, commercial operators of large aircraft, air taxi and commuter operators, certain commercial operators, certain contractors to these operators, and air traffic control facilities not operated by the Federal Aviation Administration (FAA) or the U.S. military are required to have an antidrug program for employees who perform sensitive safety or security functions. Testing is conducted by the employer prior to employment, periodically, randomly, after an accident, based on reasonable cause, and after an employee returns to duty.

Like the trucking, railroad, and maritime industries, aviation has a long history of regulatory actions to curb the use of drugs and alcohol. The main focus has been on pilots, navigators, flight engineers, and flight attendants. Laws that go back more than 30 years, for example, prohibit crew members from working within eight hours after drinking an alcoholic beverage, working with 0.04 percent or more of alcohol in their blood, or working while using any drug that affects their faculties in any way. Crew members may be tested for drugs and alcohol while receiving medical care immediately after an accident.

The FAA has had broad authority to deny, suspend, and revoke flight certificates and ratings for reasons related to drugs and alcohol, including drug trafficking. These new FAA drug-testing rules are complementary to and consistent with preexisting laws and previous actions taken by the FAA to combat drug and alcohol use in the aviation industry.

Urban Mass Transportation Administration

Recipients of federal financial assistance from the Urban Mass Transportation Administration (UMTA), and operators for such recipients, are required by UMTA drug-testing rules to have an antidrug program for employees who perform safety-sensitive functions. The required program includes testing for drugs prior to employment, for reasonable cause, randomly, and before returning to duty after a positive drug test.

The UMTA rules apply to recipients of financial assistance under the Urban Mass Transit Act of 1964 and to recipients of interstate transfer transit funds under 23 USC. A recipient also must apply the rules to any public or private operator that provides transportation services to the recipient. Interestingly, some recipients also are subject to the related rules of the FRA, FHWA, and USCG. For instance, several UMTA recipients provide commuter rail service or operate ferryboats.

Under the UMTA's federal financial assistance program, a recipient is a state. A state receives funds directly from the UMTA and then generally makes the funds available to users (subrecipients). The state certifies to UMTA that it and the subrecipients are complying with UMTA's drug testing rules. Administration of the rules can be done by the state government directly or by the state's requiring each subrecipient to abide by the rules as a condition of qualifying for funds.

The UMTA recognizes that because the anti-drug program does not preempt state law, conflicts may occur. In such cases, a recipient is permitted to seek a temporary waiver from the part of the program it believes it cannot follow. The temporary waiver is intended to provide time for the conflicting law to be changed. In the meantime, the recipient must comply with all other parts of the program to continue receiving federal financial aid.

Research and Special Programs Administration

The Research and Special Programs Administration (RSPA) is the DOT's operating administration for matters related to natural gas, liquefied natural gas, and hazardous liquid pipeline operations. Its drug-testing rules require operators of pipeline facilities, other than master meter systems, that are used for the transportation of natural gas or hazardous liquids and operators of liquefied natural gas facilities to have an antidrug program for employees who perform safety-sensitive functions. Testing is conducted prior to employment, after an accident, randomly, and for reasonable cause. The rules also require that an operator provide an EAP to conduct education and training sessions concerning the effects and consequences of drug use.

Procedures for DOT Workplace
Drug-Testing Programs

In addition to the six sets of rules outlined in the previous sections, the DOT published a modified version of the DHHS's Mandatory Guidelines for Federal Workplace Drug Testing Programs. The DOT version is called the Procedures for Transportation Workplace Drug Testing Programs and is codified in 49 CFR Part 40.

The DHHS procedures apply to the physical and organizational circumstances of federal agencies. In contrast, the DOT testing procedures apply specifically to drug-testing programs in industries regulated by the DOT's operating administrations. These procedures were meant to clear up any confusion regarding application of the DHHS procedures in the industrial context. The revisions removed much of the potentially confusing terminology and left intact the safeguards for accuracy and privacy in drug testing.

The major thrust of the DOT procedures is to require employers subject to regulation to conduct drug testing in a specific and uniform manner. They include provisions for collecting urine specimens, establishing and maintaining chain of custody, transmitting specimens to testing laboratories, analyzing the specimens, applying quality-control measures, evaluating test results, ensuring confidentiality of test results, keeping detailed records, and engaging DHHS-certified laboratories.

An employer may test a specimen only for the five major classes of drugs listed in the rules of each DOT operating administration. An operating administration may, however, authorize (with DHHS approval) testing for another drug class. For example, the USCG has authorized and instructed employers to include alcohol testing in postaccident situations.

This restriction applies only to specimens collected under the DOT testing rules. Nothing prevents an employer from testing for other drug classes, provided the testing is done on a separate specimen. The employer needs to keep in mind that the authority or justification for additional testing cannot be founded on the DOT rules.

In the matter of specimen collection, the DOT rules reflect a balance between the practical experience the agency has gained in the administration of drug-testing programs for its own employees in the federal sector and a concern for employee privacy. On the one hand, practical experience has shown that some employees will cheat. On the other hand, the DOT does not wish to require witnessed collections. The result is a compromise in which a witnessed collection could be ordered in the following situations:

- When there is a discrepancy in the temperature of the collected specimen
- When there is a record of an employee's having previously given a specimen that had a suspect measurement of specific gravity or creatinine concentration
- When the collection site person observed that the employee attempted to tamper with a specimen

A specimen collection also can be witnessed when the drug test is part of a rehabilitation program or when an employee is being tested as a follow-up to a previous positive test. The rationale is that employees in these situations may have a greater incentive to cheat.

The DOT procedures require employers with 2,000 or more employees subject to drug testing to send blind specimens to the laboratory periodically as a means of assessing the laboratory's accuracy. Employers with fewer than 2,000 employees are relieved of this requirement on the assumption that most, if not all, DHHS-certified laboratories will have contracts with one or more federal agencies or large employers and will therefore be subject to assessment by blind specimen testing.

The use of a consortium is mentioned in the procedures as a means for two or more employers to jointly achieve compliance with the requirement for 50 percent random testing per year of an employer's covered work force. Participation in a consortium does not relieve an employer of complying with any of the rules or procedures; it simply allows an employer's covered work force to be included in the total population of the consortium, which is subject to the 50 percent rule. For example, a member of a consortium might not meet the 50 percent rule within its own work force, but the member company would be in compliance if the consortium met the rule. A consortium or joint enterprise also offers economic benefits to participants through the savings derived from volume testing.

Objections to the DOT Drug-Testing Programs

Many objections have been registered in response to the rules proposed by the DOT's operating administrations.

Accuracy of Testing

Some objections were based on the perceived inaccuracy of analysis and test results. Issues were raised with respect to false-positive results, cross-reactivity, passive inhalation of marijuana smoke, misidentification of legal drugs, accidental or unknowing ingestion of illegal substances, and ingestion of poppy seeds.

The government's answer was that the rules require GC/MS confirmatory tests, which are extremely accurate when conducted by DHHS-certified drug-testing laboratories. Also, the rules require a medical review process designed to preclude false-positive results.

Insufficient Evidence of Drug Problems

Spokespersons from the maritime and pipeline industries expressed the belief that there is insufficient evidence of drug problems in their industries to warrant mandated drug testing. They further noted that in most cases where drug use can be linked to accidents, the involved persons are third-party employees over which the maritime or pipeline operators have little control.

The DOT made no attempt to document the existence of drug problems in the maritime and pipeline industries but pointed out that employees in those occupations are not immune to the drug problems that exist in society. Further, some employers in these industries have reported significant decreases in lost-time accidents after having instituted drug interdiction programs.

Aviation industry representatives also raised the issue of lack of evidence of a drug problem in commercial aviation. In this case, however, the government was able to offer evidence of illegal drug use by airline flight crew members and expressed a strong belief that any such drug use warrants preventive and proactive intervention.

Interestingly, spokespersons from the railroad and trucking industries were in agreement that drug use is a pervasive problem in their work forces.

Overly Broad Regulations

Some people argued that the definitions of persons subject to testing were vague and overly broad. Persons who did not need to be tested would be included, and the use of fuzzy terms such as *sensitive safety* would lead to varying interpretations by different employers. For a variety of reasons, practically all commenters objected to including employees of contractors.

The DOT revised many of its definitions of affected employees by naming the types of safety- or security-related duties that would be covered by the regulations and made requirements for contractors to implement their own drug-testing programs subject to monitoring by the operator.

Cost

Some objectors believed that testing would lead to unbearable and unnecessary implementation costs. Small- to medium-size businesses were especially distressed by a random sampling rate that went as high as 125 percent. Businesses with many employees were concerned about the costs of going from no testing to full testing. The final rules accommodated most objectors by providing for a 50 percent random testing rate and phased-in testing.

A cost objection also was raised in relation to the requirement that employers engage an MRO to evaluate positive test results. The DOT felt that the evaluation and review functions of an MRO are irreducible employee safeguards. The final rule does make it possible for small entities to associate with larger companies or to participate in a consortium in order to obtain the services of an MRO at a reasonable cost.

The high level of personal and institutional development necessary to create and administer antidrug programs was frequently mentioned as an added cost, as was the time and effort needed to negotiate labor contracts and other agreements affected by the DOT rules. The potential exposure to legal challenge and the costs associated with litigation and damages also were put forth as objections.

A Resulting Shortage of Employees

There was a concern that mandatory testing would result in a shortage of employees, who would opt to work elsewhere. The maritime industry believed that requiring tests of seasonal workers, who are mostly high school and college students, would cause many to seek jobs in other industries. The DOT countered with the observation that safety concerns are not lessened because employees are used seasonally and that the documented incidence of drug use in high school and college populations is further reason for testing.

Forced Abandonment of Existing Programs

A common complaint was that the DOT testing programs would force employers with existing programs to abandon these programs and implement the DOT programs. Many felt that it would be costly and administratively difficult to combine or to operate separately two different antidrug programs. Further, some critics believed that their own company programs were more stringent than the DOT programs, pointing out that the DOT forbade witnessed collection of specimens and testing for more than five classes of drugs.

The DOT did not argue whether or not employers would be compelled to abandon their existing programs but did point out that an employer who wished to collect specimens in another manner or wished to test for additional classes of drugs could do so—but not in the context of, or with any authority flowing from, the DOT regulations.

Constitutional Issues

The notices of proposed rule making that preceded implementation of the DOT testing programs provoked spirited discussions of the constitutionality of mandatory drug testing. Many commenters urged the DOT not to proceed with the regulations until the Supreme Court could resolve the constitutional issues.

The Fourth Amendment Argument

The issue most frequently debated was the relevance of the Fourth Amendment to drug testing. The Fourth Amendment applies to searches conducted by the government and protects individuals against unreasonable searches and seizures. The action of a private party does not constitute government action unless a close connection exists between the government and the action in question.

The DOT's position was that it remains to be decided whether the testing regulations implicate the government, but assuming that they do, there is a question about whether a drug test is a search within the meaning of the Fourth Amendment. The DOT went on to say that even if it is established that a drug test falls under the Fourth Amendment, the government may not be required to obtain warrants whenever testing is conducted. The Supreme Court has already ruled that although a search is ordinarily conducted pursuant to a warrant issued on probable cause grounds, such a requirement is not always necessary. Further, the Court has held that a warrant is not required by the Fourth Amendment when obtaining the warrant is likely to frustrate the purpose behind the search.

The fundamental thrust of the Fourth Amendment is that searches and seizures must be reasonable. To support a claim that a search is reasonable, the government must demonstrate that the public's interest in conducting the search outweighs the individual's expectation of privacy. The DOT asserts that when drug testing is viewed in this light, it does not violate the Fourth Amendment.

The Invasion of Privacy Argument

The related issue of invasion of privacy was put forth as an argument against the DOT testing rules. The DOT acknowledged that when searches are undertaken in situations where individualized suspicion is lacking, other safeguards must ensure that the discretion of the searching party is properly defined and the scope of the search is limited. Accordingly, the DOT rules place constraints on an employer's discretion with respect to the procedures for selecting employees for random testing (for example, computer-based random selection), collecting the specimens (for example, nonwitnessed testing and strict chain of custody), analyzing the specimens (for instance, state-of-the-art methodologies by certified laboratories), maintaining the confidentiality of test results (for instance, restricted access), and allowing for review and appeal of positive results (such as evaluation by an MRO).

Another significant consideration is the context of the employment relationship. As the Supreme Court has noted, the operational realities of the workplace may make some employees' expectations of privacy unreasonable. This is particularly applicable in industries in which employee activities are subject to extensive regulation. Persons who choose to work in such industries in effect consent to the regulation placed on them. The DOT's bottom-line stance is that the privacy interest of employees who perform safety- or security-related functions in DOT-regulated industries is outweighed by a greater public need.

CONCLUSION

The federal government has moved to require antidrug programs by federal employers and private employers in industries regulated by the DOT. These programs provide for drug testing of employees who perform sensitive safety and security functions and are aimed at the enhancement of safety and the protection of physical and information assets through the maintenance of drug-free work forces.

Appendix A

Executive Order 12564: A Drug-Free Federal Workplace

September 15, 1986

I, Ronald Reagan, President of the United States of America, find that:

Drug use is having serious adverse effects upon a significant proportion of the national work force and results in billions of dollars of lost productivity each year;

The Federal government, as an employer, is concerned with the well-being of its employees, the successful accomplishment of agency missions, and the need to maintain employee productivity;

The Federal government, as the largest employer in the Nation, can and should show the way towards achieving drug-free workplaces through a program designed to offer drug users a helping hand and, at the same time, demonstrating to drug users and potential drug users that drugs will not be tolerated in the Federal workplace;

The profits from illegal drugs provide the single greatest source of income for organized crime, fuel violent street crime, and otherwise contribute to the breakdown of our society;

The use of illegal drugs, on or off duty, by Federal employees is inconsistent not only with the law-abiding behavior expected of all citizens, but also with the special trust placed in such employees as servants of the public;

Federal employees who use illegal drugs, on or off duty, tend to be less productive, less reliable, and prone to greater absenteeism than their fellow employees who do not use illegal drugs;

The use of illegal drugs, on or off duty, by Federal employees impairs the efficiency of Federal departments and agencies, undermines public confidence in them, and makes it more difficult for other employees who do not use illegal drugs to perform their jobs effectively. The use of illegal drugs, on or off duty, by Federal employees also can pose a serious health and safety threat to members of the public and to other Federal employees;

The use of illegal drugs, on or off duty, by Federal employees in certain positions evidences less than the complete reliability, stability, and good judgment that is consistent with access to sensitive information and creates the possibility of coercion, influence and irresponsible action under pressure that may pose a serious risk to national security, the public safety, and the effective enforcement of the law; and

Federal employees who use illegal drugs must themselves be primarily responsible for changing their behavior and, if necessary, begin the process of rehabilitating themselves.

By the authority vested in me as President by the Constitution and laws of the United States of America, including section 3301(2) of Title 5 of the United States Code, section 7301 of Title 5 of the United States Code, section 290ee-1 of Title 42 of the United States Code, deeming such action in the best interests of national security, public health and safety, law enforcement and the efficiency of the Federal service, and in order to establish standards and procedures to ensure fairness in achieving a drug-free Federal workplace and to protect the privacy of Federal employees, it is hereby ordered as follows:

Section 1.   Drug-Free Workplace.

(a) Federal employees are required to refrain from the use of illegal drugs.

(b) The use of illegal drugs by Federal employees, whether on duty or off duty, is contrary to the efficiency of the service.

(c) Persons who use illegal drugs are not suitable for Federal employment.

Section 2.   Agency Responsibilities.

(a) The head of each executive agency shall develop a plan for achieving the objective of a drug free workplace with due consideration of the rights of the government, the employee, and the general public.

(b) Each agency plan shall include:

(1) A statement of policy setting forth the agency's expectations regarding drug use and the action to be anticipated in response to identified drug use;

(2) Employee Assistance Programs emphasizing high level direction, education, counseling, referral to rehabilitation, and coordination with available community resources;

(3) Supervisory training to assist in identifying and addressing illegal drug use by agency employees;

(4) Provision for self-referrals as well as supervisory referrals to treatment with maximum respect for individual confidentiality consistent with safety and security issues; and

(5) Provision for identifying illegal drug users, including testing on a controlled and carefully monitored basis in accordance with this Order.

Section 3.   Drug Testing Programs.

(a) The head of each Executive agency shall establish a program to test for the use of illegal drugs by employees in sensitive positions. The extent to which such employees are tested and the criteria for testing shall be determined by the head of each agency, based upon the nature of the agency's mission and its employees' duties, the efficient use of agency resources, and the danger to the public health and safety or national security that could result from the failure of an employee adequately to discharge his or her position.

(b) The head of each Executive agency shall establish a program for voluntary employee drug testing.

(c) In addition to the testing authorized in subsections (a) and (b) of this section, the head of each Executive agency is authorized to test an employee for illegal drug use under the following circumstances:

(1) When there is a reasonable suspicion that any employee uses illegal drugs;

(2) In an examination authorized by the agency regarding an accident or unsafe practice; or

(3) As part of or as a follow-up to counseling or rehabilitation for illegal drug use through an Employee Assistance Program.

(d) The head of each Executive agency is authorized to test any applicant for illegal drug use.

Section 4.   Drug Testing Procedures.

(a) Sixty days prior to the implementation of a drug testing program pursuant to this Order, agencies shall notify employees that testing for the use of illegal drugs is to be conducted and they may seek counseling and rehabilitation and inform them of the procedures for obtaining such assistance through the agency's Employee Assistance Program. Agency drug testing programs already ongoing are exempted from the 60-day notice requirement. Agencies may take action under section 3(c) of this Order without reference to the 60-day notice period.

(b) Before conducting a drug test, the agency shall inform the employee to be tested of the opportunity to submit medical documentation that may support a legitimate use for a specific drug.

(c) Drug testing programs shall contain procedures for timely submission of requests for retention of records and specimens; procedures for retesting; and procedures, consistent with applicable law, to protect the confidentiality of test results and related medical and rehabilitation records. Procedures for providing urine specimens must allow individual privacy, unless the agency has reason to believe that a particular individual may alter or substitute the specimen to be provided.

(d) The Secretary of Health and Human Services is authorized to promulgate scientific and technical guidelines for drug testing programs, and agencies shall conduct their drug testing programs in accordance with these guidelines once promulgated.

Section 5.   Personnel Actions.

(a) Agencies shall, in addition to any appropriate personnel actions, refer any employee who is found to use illegal drugs to an Employee Assistance Program for assessment, counseling, and referral for treatment or rehabilitation as appropriate.

(b) Agencies shall initiate action to discipline any employee who is found to use illegal drugs, provided that such action is not required for an employee who:

(1) Voluntarily identifies himself as a user of illegal drugs or who volunteers for drug testing pursuant to section 3(b) of this Order, prior to being identified through other means;

(2) Obtains counseling or rehabilitation through an Employee Assistance Program; and

(3) Thereafter refrains from using illegal drugs.

(c) Agencies shall not allow any employee to remain on duty in a sensitive position who is found to use illegal drugs, prior to successful completion of rehabilitation through an Employee Assistance Program. However, as part of a rehabilitation or counseling program, the head of an Executive agency may, in his or her discretion, allow an employee to return to duty in a sensitive position if it is determined that this action would not pose a danger to public health or safety or the national security.

(d) Agencies shall initiate action to remove from the service any employee who is found to use illegal drugs and:

(1) Refuses to obtain counseling or rehabilitation through an Employee Assistance Program; or

(2) Does not thereafter refrain from using illegal drugs.

(e) The results of a drug test and information developed by the agency in the course of drug testing of the employee may be considered in processing any adverse action against the employee or for other administrative purposes. Preliminary test results may not be used in an administrative proceeding unless they are confirmed by a second analysis of the same sample or unless the employee confirms the accuracy of the initial test by admitting the use of illegal drugs.

(f) The determination of an agency that any employee uses illegal drugs can be made on the basis of any appropriate evidence, including direct observation, a criminal conviction, administrative inquiry, or the results of an authorized testing program. Positive drug results may be rebutted by other evidence that an employee has not used illegal drugs.

(g) Any action to discipline an employee who is using illegal drugs (including removal from the service, if appropriate) shall be taken in compliance with otherwise applicable procedures, including the Civil Service Reform Act.

(h) Drug testing shall not be conducted pursuant to this Order for the purpose of gathering evidence for use in criminal proceedings. Agencies are not required to report to the Attorney General for investigation or prosecution any information, allegation, or evidence relating to violations of Title 21 of the United States Code received as a result of the operation of drug testing programs established pursuant to this Order.

Section 6.   Coordination of Agency Programs.

(a) The Director of the Office of Personnel Management shall:

(1) Issue government-wide guidance to agencies on the implementation of the terms of this Order;

(2) Ensure that appropriate coverage for drug abuse is maintained for employees and their families under the Federal Employees Health Benefits Program;

(3) Develop a model Employee Assistance Program for Federal agencies and assist the agencies in putting programs in place;

(4) In consultation with the Secretary of Health and Human Services, develop and improve training programs for Federal supervisors and managers on illegal drug use; and

(5) In cooperation with the Secretary of Health and Human Services and heads of Executive agencies, mount an intensive drug awareness campaign through the Federal work force.

(b) The Attorney General shall render legal advice regarding the implementation of this Order and shall be consulted with regard to all guidelines, regulations, and policies proposed to be adopted pursuant to this Order.

(c) Nothing in this Order shall be deemed to limit the authorities of the Director of Central Intelligence under the National Security Act of 1947, as amended, or the statutory authorities of the National Security Agency or the Defense Intelligence Agency. Implementation of this Order within the Intelligence Community, as defined in Executive Order 12333, shall be subject to the approval of the head of the affected agency.

Section 7. Definitions.

(a) This Order applies to all agencies of the Executive Branch.

(b) For purposes of this Order, the term "agency" means an Executive agency, as defined in 5 U.S.C. 105; the Uniformed Services, as defined in 5 U.S.C. 2101(3) (but excluding the armed forces as defined by 5 U.S.C. 2101(2)); or any other employing unit or authority of the Federal government, except the United States Postal Service, the Postal Rate Commission, and employing units or authorities in the Judicial and Legislative Branches.

(c) For purposes of this Order, the term "illegal drugs" means a controlled substance included in Schedule I or II, as defined by section 802(6) of Title 21 of the United States Code, the possession of which is unlawful under chapter 13 of that Title. The term "illegal drugs" does not mean the use of a controlled substance pursuant to a valid prescription or other uses authorized by law.

(d) For purposes of this Order, the term "employee in a sensitive position" refers to:

(1) An employee in a position that an agency head designates Special Sensitive, Critical-Sensitive, or Noncritical Sensitive under Chapter 731 of the Federal Personnel Manual or an employee in a position that an agency head designates as sensitive in accordance with Executive Order 10450, as amended;

(2) An employee who has been granted access to classified information or may be granted access to classified information pursuant to a determination of trustworthiness by an agency head under Section 4 of Executive Order 12356;

(3) Individuals serving under Presidential appointments;

(4) Law enforcement officers as defined in 5 U.S.C. 8331(20);

(5) Other positions that the agency head determines involve law enforcement, national security, the protection of life and property, public health or safety, or other functions requiring a high degree of trust and confidence.

(e) For purposes of this Order, the term "employee" means all persons appointed in the Civil Service as described in 5 U.S.C. 2105 (but excluding persons appointed in the armed services as defined in 5 U.S.C. 2102(2)).

(f) For purposes of this Order, the term "Employee Assistance Program" means agency-based counseling programs that offer assessment, short-term counseling, and referral services to employees for a wide range of drug, alcohol, and mental health programs that affect employee job performance. Employee Assistance Programs are responsible for referring drug-using employees for rehabilitation and for monitoring employees' progress while in treatment.

Section 8.   Effective Date.

This Order is effective immediately.

RONALD REAGAN

THE WHITE HOUSE
September 15, 1986

Appendix B

Section 503, Public Law 100-73

CHAPTER 73. SUITABILITY, SECURITY, AND CONDUCT

7301. Presidential regulations.

History; Ancillary Laws and Directives

Other provisions:

Availability of funds for drug testing pursuant to Executive Order No. 12564. Act July 11, 1987, PL 100-71, Title V, 503, 101 Stat 468 provides:

(a)(1) Except as provided in subsection (b) or (c), none of the funds appropriated or made available by this Act, or any other Act, with respect to any fiscal year, shall be available to administer or implement any drug testing pursuant to Executive Order Numbered 12564 (dated September 15, 1986), or any subsequent order, unless and until—

"(A) the Secretary of Health and Human Services certifies in writing to the Committees on Appropriations of the House of Representatives and the Senate, and other appropriate committees of the Congress, that—

"(i) each agency has developed a plan for achieving a drug-free workplace in accordance with Executive Order Numbered 12564 and applicable provisions of law (including applicable provisions of this section);

"(ii) the Department of Health and Human Services, in addition to the scientific and technical guidelines dated February 13, 1987, and any subsequent amendments thereto, has, in accordance with paragraph (3), published mandatory guidelines which—

"(I) establish comprehensive standards for all aspects of laboratory testing and laboratory procedures to be applied in carrying out Executive Order Numbered 12564, including standards which require the use of the best available technology for ensuring the full reliability and accuracy of drug tests and strict procedures governing the chain of custody of specimens collected for drug testing;

"(II) specify the drugs for which Federal employees may be tested; and

"(III) establish appropriate standards and procedures for periodic review of laboratories and criteria for certification and revocation of certification of laboratories to perform drug testing in carrying out Executive Order Numbered 12564; and

"(B) the Secretary of Health and Human Services has submitted to the Congress, in writing, a detailed, agency-by-agency analysis relating to—

"(i) the criteria and procedures to be applied in designating employees or positions for drug testing, including the justification for such criteria and procedures;

"(ii) the position titles designated for random drug testing;

"(iii) the nature, frequency, and type of drug testing proposed to be instituted; and

"(C) the Director of the Office of Management and Budget has submitted in writing to the Committees on Appropriations of the House of Representatives and the Senate a detailed, agency-by-agency analysis (as of the time of certification under subparagraph (A)) of the anticipated annual costs associated with carrying out Executive Order Numbered 12564 and all other requirements under this section during the 5-year period beginning on the date of the enactment of this Act (enacted July 11, 1987).

"(2) Notwithstanding subsection (g), for purposes of this subsection, the term 'agency' means—

"(A) the Executive Office of the President;

"(B) an Executive department under section 101 of Title 5, United States Code;

"(C) the Environmental Protection Agency;

"(D) the General Services Administration;

"(E) the National Aeronautics and Space Administration;

"(F) the Office of Personnel Management;

"(G) the Small Business Administration;

"(H) the United States Information Agency; and

"(I) the Veterans Administration;

except that such term does not include the Department of Transportation or any other entity (or component thereof) covered by subsection (b).

"(3) Notwithstanding any provision of chapter 5 of title 5, United States Code (5 USC 500 et seq), the mandatory guidelines to be published pursuant to subsection (a)(1)(A)(ii) shall be published and made effective exclusively according to the provisions of this paragraph. Notice of the mandatory guidelines proposed by the Secretary of Health and Human Services shall be published in the Federal Register, and interested persons shall be given not less than 60 days to submit written comments on the proposed mandatory guidelines. Following review and consideration of written comments, final mandatory guidelines shall be published in the Federal Register and shall become effective upon publication.

"(b)(1) Nothing in subsection (a) shall limit or otherwise affect the availability of funds for drug testing by—

"(A) the Department of Transportation;

"(B) the Department of Energy, for employees specifically involved in the handling of nuclear weapons or nuclear materials;

"(C) any agency with an agency-wide drug-testing program in existence as of September 15, 1986; or

"(D) any component of an agency if such component had a drug-testing program in existence as of September 15, 1986.

"(2) The Departments of Transportation and Energy and any agency or component thereof with a drug-testing program in existence as of September 15, 1986—

"(A) shall be brought into full compliance with Executive Order Numbered 12564 no later than the end of the 6-month period beginning on the date of the enactment of this Act (enacted July 11, 1987).

"(B) shall take such actions as may be necessary to ensure that their respective drug-testing programs or plans are brought into full compliance with the mandatory guidelines published under subsection (a)(1)(A)(ii) no later than 90 days after such mandatory guidelines take effect, except that any judicial challenge that affects such guidelines should not affect drug-testing programs or plans subject to this paragraph.

"(c) In the case of an agency (or component thereof) other than an agency as defined by subsection (a)(2) or an agency (or component thereof) covered under subsection (b), none of the funds appropriated or made available by this Act, or any other Act, with respect to any fiscal year, shall be available to administer or implement any drug testing pursuant to Executive Order Numbered 12564, or any subsequent order, unless and until—

"(1) the Secretary of Health and Human Services provides written certification with respect to that agency (or component) in accordance with clauses (i) and (iii) of subsection (a)(1)(A);

"(2) the Secretary of Health and Human Services has submitted a written, detailed analysis with respect to that agency (or component) in accordance with subsection (a)(1)(B); and

"(3) the Director of the Office of Management and Budget has submitted a written, detailed analysis with respect to that agency (or component) in accordance with (a)(1)(C).

"(d) Any Federal employee who is the subject of a drug test under any program or plan shall, upon written request, have access to—

"(1) any records relating to such employee's drug test; and

"(2) any records relating to the results of any relevant certification, review, or revocation-of-certification proceedings, as referred to in subsection (a)(1)(A)(ii)(III).

"(e) The results of a drug test of a Federal employee may not be disclosed without the prior written consent of such employee, unless the disclosure would be—

"(1) to the employee's medical review official (as defined in the scientific and technical guidelines referred to in subsection (a)(1)(A)(ii));

"(2) to the administrator of any Employee Assistance Program in which the employee is receiving counseling or treatment or is otherwise participating;

"(3) to any supervisory or management official within the employee's agency having authority to take the adverse personnel action against such employee; or

"(4) pursuant to the order of a court of competent jurisdiction where required by the United States Government to defend against any challenge against any adverse personnel action.

"(f) Each agency covered by Executive Order Numbered 12564 shall submit to the Committees on Appropriations of the House of Representatives and the Senate, and other appropriate committees of the Congress, an annual report relating to drug-testing activities conducted by such agency pursuant to such executive order. Each such annual report shall be submitted at the time of the President's budget submission to the Congress under section 11045(a) of title 31, United States Code.

"(g) For purposes of this section, the terms 'agency' and 'Employee Assistance Program' each has the meaning given such term under section 7(b) of Executive Order Numbered 12564, as in effect on September 15, 1986."

Appendix C

Drug-Free Workplace Act of 1988

Section 5152. Drug-Free Workplace Requirements for Federal Contractors

(a) Drug-Free Workplace Requirement.

(1) Requirement for persons other than individuals. No person, other than an individual, shall be considered a responsible source, under the meaning of such term as defined in section 4(8) of the Office of Federal Procurement Policy Act (41 USC 403(8)), for the purposes of being awarded a contract for the procurement of any property or services of a value of $25,000 or more from any Federal agency unless such person has certified to the contracting agency that it will provide a drug-free workplace by—

(A) publishing a statement notifying employees that the unlawful manufacture, distribution, dispensation, possession, or use of a controlled substance is prohibited in the person's workplace and specifying the actions that will be taken against employees for violations of such prohibition;

(B) establishing a drug-free awareness program to inform employees about—

(i) the dangers of drug abuse in the workplace;

(ii) the person's policy of maintaining a drug-free workplace;

(iii) any available drug counseling, rehabilitation, and employee assistance programs; and

(iv) the penalties that may be imposed upon employees for drug abuse violations;

(C) making it a requirement that each employee to be engaged in the performance of such contract be given a copy of the statement required by subparagraph (A);

(D) notifying the employee in the statement required by subparagraph (A), that as a condition of employment on such contract, the employee will—

(i) abide by the terms of the statement; and

(ii) notify the employer of any criminal drug statute conviction for a violation occurring in the workplace no later than 5 days after such conviction;

(E) notifying the contracting agency within 10 days after receiving notice under subparagraph (D)(ii) from an employee or otherwise receiving actual notice of such conviction;

(F) imposing a sanction on, or requiring the satisfactory participation in a drug abuse assistance or rehabilitation program by any employee who is so convicted, as required by section 5154; and

(G) making a good faith effort to continue to maintain a drug-free workplace through implementation of subparagraphs (A), (B), (C), (D), (E), and (F).

(2) Requirement for individuals. No Federal agency shall enter into a contract with an individual unless such contract includes a certification by the individual that the individual will not engage in the unlawful manufacture, distribution, dispensation, possession, or use of a controlled substance in the performance of the contract.

(b) Suspension, Termination, or Debarment of the Contractor.

(1) Grounds for Suspension, Termination, or Debarment. Each contract awarded by a Federal agency shall be subject to suspension of payments under the contract or termination of the contract, or both, and the contractor thereunder or the individual who entered the contract with the Federal agency, as applicable, shall be subject to suspension or debarment in accordance with the requirements of this section if the head of the agency determines that—

(A) the contractor or individual has made a false certification under subsection (a);

(B) the contractor violates such certification by failing to carry out the requirements of subparagraph (A), (B), (C), (D), (E), or (F) of subsection (a)(1); or

(C) such a number of employees of such contractor have been convicted of violations of criminal drug statutes for violations occurring in the workplace as to indicate that the contractor has failed to make a good faith effort to provide a drug-free workplace as required by subsection (a).

(2) Conduct of Suspension, Termination, and Debarment Proceedings.

(A) If a contracting officer determines, in writing, that cause for suspension of payments, termination, or suspension or debarment exists, an appropriate action shall be initiated by the contracting officer of the agency, to be conducted by the agency concerned in accordance with the Federal Acquisition Regulation and applicable agency procedures.

(B) The Federal Acquisition Regulation shall be revised to include rules for conducting suspension and debarment proceedings under this subsection, including rules providing notice, opportunity to respond in writing or in person, and such other procedures as may be necessary to provide a full and fair proceeding to a contractor or individual in such proceeding.

(3) Effect of debarment. Upon issuance of any final decision under this subsection requiring debarment of a contractor or individual, such contractor or individual shall be ineligible for award of any contract by any Federal agency, and for participation in any future procurement by any Federal agency, for a period specified in the decision, not to exceed 5 years.

Section 5153. Drug-Free Workplace Requirements for Federal Grant Recipients

(a) Drug-Free Workplace Requirement.

(1) Persons other than individuals. No person, other than an individual, shall receive a grant from any Federal agency unless such person has certified to the granting agency that it will provide a drug-free workplace by—

(A) publishing a statement notifying employees that the unlawful manufacture, distribution, dispensation, possession, or use of a controlled substance is prohibited in the grantee's workplace and specifying the actions that will be taken against employees for violations of such prohibition;

(B) establishing a drug-free awareness program to inform employees about—

(i) the dangers of drug abuse in the workplace;

(ii) the grantee's policy of maintaining a drug-free workplace;

(iii) any available drug counseling, rehabilitation, and employee assistance programs; and

(iv) the penalties that may be imposed upon employees for drug abuse violations;

(C) making it a requirement that each employee to be engaged in the performance of such grant be given a copy of the statement required by subparagraph (A);

(D) notifying the employee in the statement required by subparagraph (A), that as a condition of employment on such grant, the employee will—

(i) abide by the terms of the statement; and

(ii) notify the employer of any criminal drug statute conviction for a violation occurring in the workplace no later than 5 days after such conviction;

(E) notifying the granting agency within 10 days after receiving notice under subparagraph (D)(ii) from an employee or otherwise receiving actual notice of such conviction;

(F) imposing a sanction on, or requiring the satisfactory participation in a drug abuse assistance or rehabilitation program by any employee who is so convicted, as required by section 5154; and

(G) making a good faith effort to continue to maintain a drug-free workplace through implementation of subparagraphs (A), (B), (C), (D), (E), and (F).

(2) Individuals. No Federal agency shall make a grant to any individual unless such individual certifies to the agency as a condition of such grant that the individual will not engage in the unlawful manufacture, distribution, dispensation, possession, or use of a controlled substance in conducting any activity with such grant.

(b) Suspension, Termination, or Debarment of the Grantee.

(1) Grounds for Suspension, Termination, or Debarment. Each grant awarded by a Federal agency shall be subject to suspension of payments under the grant or termination of the grant, or both, and the grantee thereunder shall be subject to suspension or debarment in accordance with the requirements of this section if the agency of the granting agency determines, in writing, that—

(A) the grantee has made a false certification under subsection (a);

(B) the grantee violates such certification by failing to carry out the requirements of subparagraph (A), (B), (C), (D), (E), or (F) of subsection (a)(1); or

(C) such a number of employees of such grantee have been convicted of violations of criminal drug statutes for violations occurring in the workplace as to indicate that the grantee has failed to make a good faith effort to provide a drug-free workplace as required by subsection (a)(1).

(2) Conduct of Suspension, Termination, and Debarment Proceedings. A suspension of payments, termination, or suspension or debarment proceeding subject to this subsection shall be conducted in accordance with applicable law, including Executive Order 12549 or any superseding Executive order and regulations promulgated to implement such law or Executive order.

(3) Effect of debarment. Upon issuance of any final decision under this subsection requiring debarment of a grantee, such grantee shall be ineligible for award of any grant by any Federal agency, and for participation in any future grant from any Federal agency for a period specified in the decision, not to exceed 5 years.

Section 5154. Employee Sanctions and Remedies

A grantee or contractor shall, within 30 days after receiving notice from an employee of a conviction pursuant to section 5152(a)(1)(D)(ii) or 5153(a)(1)(D)(ii)—

(1) take appropriate personnel action against such employee up to and including termination; or

(2) require such employee to satisfactorily participate in a drug abuse assistance or rehabilitation program approved for such purposes by a Federal, State, or local health, law enforcement, or other appropriate agency.

Section 5155. Waiver

(a) In general. A termination, suspension of payments, or suspension or debarment under this subtitle may be waived by the head of an agency with respect to a particular contract or grant if—

(1) in the case of a waiver with respect to a contract, the head of the agency determines under section 5152(b)(1), after the issuance of a final determination under such section, that suspension of payments, or termination of the contract, or suspension or debarment of the contractor, or refusal to permit a person to be treated as a responsible source for a contract, as the case may be, would severely disrupt the operation of such agency to the detriment of the Federal Government or the general public; or

(2) in the case of a waiver with respect to a grant, the head of the agency determines that suspension of payments, termination of the grant, or suspension or debarment of the grantee would not be in the public interest.

(b) Exclusive authority. The authority of the head of an agency under this section to waive a termination, suspension or debarment shall not be delegated.

Section 5156. Regulations

Not later than 90 days after the date of enactment of this subtitle, the government-wide regulations governing actions under this subtitle shall be issued pursuant to the Office of Federal Procurement Policy Act (41 USC 401 et seq.).

Section 5157. Definitions

For the purpose of this subtitle—

(1) the term "drug-free workplace" means a site for the performance of work done in connection with a specific grant or contract described in section 5152 or 5153 or an entity at which employees of such entity are prohibited from engaging in the unlawful manufacture, distribution, dispensation, possession, or use of a controlled substance in accordance with the requirements of this Act;

(2) the term "employee" means the employee of a grantee or contractor directly engaged in the performance of work pursuant to the provisions of the grant or contract described in section 5152 or 5153;

(3) the term "controlled substance" means a controlled substance in schedules I through V of section 202 of the Controlled Substances Act (21 USC 812);

(4) the term "conviction" means a finding of guilt (including a plea of nolo contendere) or imposition of sentence, or both, by any judicial body charged with the responsibility to determine violations of the Federal or State criminal drug statutes;

(5) the term "criminal drug statute" means a criminal statute involving manufacture, distribution, dispensation, use or possession of any controlled substance;

(6) the term "grantee" means the department, division, or other unit of a person responsible for the performance under the grant;

(7) the term "contractor" means the department, division, or other unit of a person responsible for the performance under the contract; and

(8) the term "Federal agency" means an agency as that term is defined in section 552(f) of title 5, United States Code.

Section 5158. Construction of Subtitle

Nothing in this subtitle shall be construed to require law enforcement agencies, if the head of the agency determines it would be inappropriate in connection with the agency's undercover operations, to comply with the provisions of this subtitle.

Section 5159. Repeal of Limitation on Use of Funds

Section 628 of Public Law 100-440 (relating to restrictions on the use of certain appropriated amounts) is amended—

(1) by striking "(a)" after "Sec 628."; and

(2) by striking subsection (b).

Section 5160. Effective Date

Sections 5152 and 5153 shall be effective 120 days after the date of the enactment of this subtitle.

EMPLOYEE'S ACKNOWLEDGMENT OF AWARENESS
OF THE DRUG-FREE WORKPLACE ACT OF 1988

I, _____, acknowledge that I have attended a drug awareness program as required by the Drug-Free Workplace Act of 1988.

In this drug awareness program:

I have been given information on the company's policy on a drug-free workplace and had it explained to me.

I have been given information on the company's policy on illegal drug activity in the workplace. I understand that penalties up to and including termination can be imposed for conviction of a drug related offense that occurs in the workplace.

I have been made aware that illegal drug use is dangerous.

I have been given information about resources for drug counseling and rehabilitation.

I have been informed that the company intends to have a drug-free workplace and wants to provide assistance to any employee who has a drug related problem.

I have been informed that I must report any conviction of a drug related offense committed on the job to my supervisor within five days.

_____

SIGNED

_____

DATE

Appendix D

Mandatory Guidelines for Federal Workplace Drug Testing Programs

3.16 Recertification

3.17 Performance Test Requirement for Certification

3.18 Performance Test Specimen Composition

3.19 Evaluation of Performance Testing

3.20 Inspections

3.21 Results of Inadequate Performance

Subpart A—General

1.1 Applicability

(a) These mandatory guidelines apply to:

(1) Executive Agencies as defined in 5 USC 105;

(2) The Uniformed Services, as defined in 5 USC 2101(3) (but excluding the Armed Forces as defined in 5 USC 2101(2));

(3) And any other employing unit or authority of the Federal Government except the United States Postal Service, the Postal Rate Commission, and employing units or authorities in the Judicial and Legislative Branches.

(b) Any agency or component of an agency with a drug testing program in existence as of September 15, 1986, and the Departments of Transportation and Energy shall take such action as may be necessary to ensure that the agency is brought into compliance with these Guidelines no later than 90 days after they take effect, except that any judicial challenge that affects these Guidelines shall not affect drug testing programs subject to this paragraph.

(c) Except as provided in 2.6, Subpart C of these Guidelines (which establishes laboratory certification standards) applies to any laboratory which has or seeks certification to perform urine drug testing for Federal agencies under a drug testing program conducted under Executive Order No. 12564. Only laboratories certified under these standards are authorized to perform urine drug testing for Federal agencies.

(d) The Intelligence Community, as defined by Executive Order No. 12333, shall be subject to these Guidelines only to the extent agreed to by the head of the affected agency.

(e) These Guidelines do not apply to drug testing conducted under legal authority other than E.O. 12564, including testing of persons in the criminal justice system, such as arrestees, detainees, probationers, incarcerated persons, or parolees.

(f) Agencies may not deviate from the provisions of these Guidelines without the written approval of the Secretary. In requesting approval for a deviation, an agency must petition the Secretary in writing and describe the specific provision or provisions for which a deviation is sought and the rationale therefor. The Secretary may approve the request upon a finding of good cause as determined by the Secretary.

1.2 Definitions

For purposes of these Guidelines the following definitions are adopted:

Aliquot. A portion of a specimen used for testing.

Chain of Custody. Procedures to account for the integrity of each urine specimen by tracking its handling and storage from point of specimen collection to final disposition of the specimen. These procedures shall require that an approved agency chain of custody form be used from time of collection to receipt by the laboratory and that upon receipt of the laboratory an appropriate laboratory chain of custody form(s) account for the sample or sample aliquots within the laboratory. Chain of custody forms shall, at a minimum, include an entry documenting date and purpose each time a specimen or aliquot is handled or transferred and identifying every individual in the chain of custody.

Collection Site. A place designated by the agency where individuals present themselves for the purpose of providing a specimen of their urine to be analyzed for the presence of drugs.

Collection Site Person. A person who instructs and assists individuals at a collection site and who receives and makes an initial examination of the urine specimen provided by those individuals. A collection site person shall have successfully completed training to carry out this function.

Confirmatory Test. A second analytical procedure to identify the presence of a specific drug or metabolite which is independent of the initial test and which uses a different technique and chemical principle from that of the initial test in order to ensure reliability and accuracy. (At this time gas chromatography/mass spectrometry (GC/MS) is the only authorized confirmation method for cocaine, marijuana, opiates, amphetamines, and phencyclidine.)

Initial Test (also known as Screening Test). An immunoassay screen to eliminate "negative" urine specimens from further consideration.

Medical Review Officer. A licensed physician responsible for receiving laboratory results generated by an agency's drug testing program who has knowledge of substance abuse disorders and has appropriate medical training to interpret and evaluate an individual's positive test result together with his or her medical history and any other relevant biomedical information.

Permanent Record Book. A permanently bound book in which identifying data on each specimen collected at a collection site are permanently recorded in the sequence of collection.

Reason to Believe. Reason to believe that a particular individual may alter or substitute the urine specimen as provided in section 4(c) of E.O. 12564.

Secretary. The Secretary of Health and Human Services or the Secretary's designee. The Secretary's designee may be a contractor or other recognized organization which acts on behalf of the Secretary in implementing these Guidelines.

1.3 Future Revisions

In order to ensure the full reliability and accuracy of drug assays, the accurate reporting of test results, and the integrity and efficacy of Federal drug testing programs, the Secretary may make changes to these Guidelines to reflect improvements in the available science and technology. These changes will be published in final as a notice in the Federal Register.

Subpart B—Scientific and Technical Requirements

2.1   The Drugs

(a) The President's Executive Order 12564 defines "illegal drugs" as those included in Schedule I or II of the Controlled Substances Act (CSA), but not when used pursuant to a valid prescription or when used as otherwise authorized by law. Hundreds of drugs are covered under Schedule I and II and while it is not feasible to test routinely for all of them, Federal drug testing programs shall test for drugs as follows:

(1) Federal agency applicant and random drug testing programs shall at a minimum test for marijuana and cocaine;

(2) Federal agency applicant and random drug testing programs are also authorized to test for opiates, amphetamines, and phencyclidine; and

(3) When conducting reasonable suspicion, accident, or unsafe practice testing, a Federal agency may test for any drug listed in Schedule I or II of the CSA.

(b) Any agency covered by these Guidelines shall petition the Secretary in writing for approval to include in its testing protocols any drugs (or classes of drugs) not listed for Federal agency testing in paragraph (a) of this section. Such approval shall be limited to the use of the appropriate science and technology and shall not otherwise limit agency discretion to test for any drugs covered under Schedule I and II of the CSA.

(c) Urine specimens collected pursuant to Executive Order 12564, Pub L 100-71, and these Guidelines shall be used only to test for those drugs included in agency drug-free workplace plans and may not be used to conduct any other analysis or test unless otherwise authorized by law.

(d) These Guidelines are not intended to limit any agency which is specifically authorized by law to include additional categories of drugs in the drug testing or its own employees or employees in its regulated industries.

2.2   Specimen Collection Procedures

(a) Designation of Collection Site. Each agency drug testing program shall have one or more designated collection sites which have all necessary personnel, materials, equipment, facilities, and supervision to provide for the collection, security, temporary storage, and shipping or transportation of urine specimens to a certified drug testing laboratory.

(b) Security. Procedures shall provide for the designated collection site to be secure. If a collection site facility is dedicated solely to urine collection, it shall be secure at all times. If a facility cannot be dedicated solely to drug testing, the portion of the facility used for testing shall be secured during drug testing.

(c) Chain of Custody. Chain of custody standardized forms shall be properly executed by the authorized collection site personnel upon receipt of specimens. Handling and transportation of urine specimens from one authorized individual or place to another shall always be accomplished through chain of custody procedures. Every effort shall be made to minimize the number of persons handling specimens.

(d) Access to Authorized Personnel Only. No unauthorized personnel shall be permitted in any part of the designated collection site when urine specimens are collected or stored.

(e) Privacy. Procedures for collecting urine specimens shall allow the individual privacy unless there is reason to believe that a particular individual may alter or substitute the specimen to be provided.

(f) Integrity and Identity of Specimen. Agencies shall take precautions to ensure that a urine specimen not be adulterated or diluted during the collection procedure and that information on the urine bottle and in the record book can identify the individual from whom the specimen was collected. The following minimum precautions shall be taken to ensure that unadulterated specimens are obtained and correctly identified:

(1) To deter the dilution of specimens at the collection site, toilet bluing agents shall be placed in toilet tanks wherever possible, so the reservoir of water in the toilet bowl remains blue. There shall be no other source of water (e.g., no shower or sink) in the enclosure where urination occurs.

(2) When an individual arrives at the collection site, the collection site person shall request the individual to present photo identification. If the individual does not have proper photo identification, the collection site person shall contact the supervisor of the individual, the coordinator of the drug testing program, or any other agency official who can positively identify the individual. If the individual's identity cannot be established, the collection site person shall not proceed with the collection.

(3) If the individual fails to arrive at the assigned time, the collection site person shall contact the appropriate authority to obtain guidance on the action to be taken.

(4) The collection site person shall ask the individual to remove any unnecessary outer garments such as a coat or jacket that might conceal items or substances that could be used to tamper with or adulterate the individual's urine specimen. The collection site person shall ensure that all personal belongings such as a purse or briefcase remain with the outer garments. The individual may retain his or her wallet.

(5) The individual shall be instructed to wash and dry his or her hands prior to urination.

(6) After washing hands, the individual shall remain in the presence of the collection site person and shall not have access to any water fountain, faucet, soap dispenser, cleaning agent or any other materials which could be used to adulterate the specimen.

(7) The individual may provide his/her specimen in the privacy of a stall or otherwise partitioned area that allows for individual privacy.

(8) The collection site person shall note any unusual behavior or appearance in the permanent record book.

(9) In the exceptional event that an agency-designated collection site is not accessible and there is an immediate requirement for specimen collection (e.g., an accident investigation), a public rest room may be used according to the following procedures: A collection site person of the same gender as the individual shall

accompany the individual into the public rest room which shall be made secure during the collection procedure. If possible, a toilet bluing agent shall be placed in the bowl and any accessible toilet tank. The collection site person shall remain in the rest room, but outside the stall, until the specimen is collected. If no bluing agent is available to deter specimen dilution, the collection site person shall instruct the individual not to flush the toilet until the specimen is delivered to the collection site person. After the collection site person has possession of the specimen, the individual will be instructed to flush the toilet and to participate with the collection site person in completing the chain of custody procedures.

(10) Upon receiving the specimen from the individual, the collection site person shall determine that it contains at least 60 milliliters of urine. If there is less than 60 milliliters of urine in the container, additional urine shall be collected in a separate container to reach a total of 60 milliliters. (The temperature of the partial specimen in each separate container shall be measured in accordance with paragraph (f)(12) of this section, and the partial specimens shall be combined in one container.) The individual may be given a reasonable amount of liquid to drink for this purpose (e.g., a glass of water). If the individual fails for any reason to provide 60 milliliters of urine, the collection site person shall contact the appropriate authority to obtain guidance on the action to be taken.

(11) After the specimen has been provided and submitted to the collection site person, the individual shall be allowed to wash his or her hands.

(12) Immediately after the specimen is collected, the collection site person shall measure the temperature of the specimen. The temperature measuring device used must accurately reflect the temperature of the specimen and not contaminate the specimen. The time from urination to temperature measurement is critical and in no case shall exceed 4 minutes.

(13) If the temperature of a specimen is outside the range of 32.5 to 37.7 degrees Centigrade or 90.5 to 99.8 degrees Fahrenheit, that is reason to believe that the individual may have altered or substituted the specimen, and another specimen shall be collected under direct observation of a same gender collection site person and both specimens shall be forwarded to the laboratory for testing. An individual may volunteer to have his or her oral temperature taken to provide evidence to counter the reason to believe the individual may have altered or substituted the specimen caused by the specimen's temperature falling outside the prescribed range.

(14) Immediately after the specimen is collected, the collection site person shall also inspect the specimen to determine its color and look for any signs of contaminants. Any unusual findings shall be noted in the permanent record book.

(15) All specimens suspected of being adulterated shall be forwarded to the laboratory for testing.

(16) Whenever there is reason to believe that a particular individual may alter or substitute the specimen to be provided, a second specimen shall be obtained as soon as possible under the direct observation of a same gender collection site person.

(17) Both the individual being tested and the collection site person shall keep the specimen in view at all times prior to its being sealed and labeled. If the specimen is transferred to a second bottle, the collection site person shall request the individual

to observe the transfer of the specimen and the placement of the tamperproof seal over the bottle cap and down the sides of the bottle.

(18) The collection site person and individual shall be present at the same time during procedures outlined in paragraphs (f)(19)–(f)(22) of this section.

(19) The collection site person shall place securely on the bottle an identification label which contains the date, the individual's specimen number, and any other identifying information provided or required by the agency.

(20) The individual shall initial the identification label on the specimen bottle for the purpose of certifying that it is the specimen collected from him or her.

(21) The collection site person shall enter in the permanent record book all information identifying the specimen. The collection site person shall sign the permanent record book next to the identifying information.

(22) The individual shall be asked to read and sign a statement in the permanent record book certifying that the specimen identified as having been collected from him or her is in fact that specimen he or she provided.

(23) A higher level supervisor shall review and concur in advance with any decision by a collection site person to obtain a specimen under the direct observation of a same gender collection site person based on a reason to believe that the individual may alter or substitute the specimen to be provided.

(24) The collection site person shall complete the chain of custody form.

(25) The urine specimen and chain of custody form are now ready for shipment. If the specimen is not immediately prepared for shipment, it shall be appropriately safeguarded during temporary storage.

(26) While any part of the above chain of custody procedures is being performed, it is essential that the urine specimen and custody documents be under the control of the involved collection site person. If the involved collection site person leaves his or her work station momentarily, the specimen and custody form shall be taken with him or her or shall be secured. After the collection site person returns to the work station, the custody process will continue. If the collection site person is leaving for an extended period of time, the specimen shall be packaged for mailing before he or she leaves the site.

(g) Collection Control. To the maximum extent possible, collection site personnel shall keep the individual's specimen bottle within sight both before and after the individual has urinated. After the specimen is collected, it shall be properly sealed and labeled. An approved chain of custody form shall be used for maintaining control and accountability of each specimen from the point of collection to final disposition of the specimen. The date and purpose shall be documented on an approved chain of custody form each time a specimen is handled or transferred and every individual in the chain shall be identified. Every effort shall be made to minimize the number of persons handling specimens.

(h) Transportation to Laboratory. Collection site personnel shall arrange to ship the collected specimens to the drug testing laboratory. The specimens shall be placed in containers designed to minimize the possibility of damage during shipment, for example, specimen boxes or padded mailers; and those containers shall be sealed to eliminate the possibility of undetected tampering. On the tape sealing the container, the collection site supervisor shall sign and enter the date specimens were sealed in the containers for shipment. The collection site personnel shall ensure that the chain of custody documentation is attached to each container sealed for shipment to the drug testing laboratory.

2.3   Laboratory Personnel

(a) Day-to-Day Management.

(1) The laboratory shall have a qualified individual to assume professional, organizational, educational, and administrative responsibility for the laboratory's urine drug testing facility.

(2) This individual shall have documented scientific qualifications in analytical forensic toxicology. Minimum qualifications are:

(i) Certification as a laboratory director by the State in forensic or clinical laboratory toxicology; or

(ii) A Ph.D. in one of the natural sciences with an adequate undergraduate and graduate education in biology, chemistry, and pharmacology or toxicology; or

(iii) Training and experience comparable to a Ph.D. in one of the natural sciences, such as a medical or scientific degree with additional training and laboratory/research experience in biology, chemistry, and pharmacology or toxicology; and

(iv) In addition to the requirements in (i), (ii), and (iii) above, minimum qualifications also require:

(A) Appropriate experience in analytical forensic toxicology including experience with the analysis of biological material for drugs of abuse, and

(B) Appropriate training and/or experience in forensic applications of analytical toxicology, e.g., publications, court testimony, research concerning analytical toxicology of drugs of abuse, or other factors which qualify the individual as an expert witness in forensic toxicology.

(3) This individual shall be engaged in and responsible for the day-to-day management of the drug testing laboratory even where another individual has overall responsibility for an entire multispecialty laboratory.

(4) This individual shall be responsible for ensuring that there are enough personnel with adequate training and experience to supervise and conduct the work of the drug testing laboratory. He or she shall assure the continued competency of laboratory personnel by documenting their inservice training, reviewing their work performance, and verifying their skills.

(5) This individual shall be responsible for the laboratory's having a procedure manual which is complete, up-to-date, available for personnel performing tests, and followed by those personnel. The procedure manual shall be reviewed, signed, and dated by this responsible individual whenever procedures are first placed into use or changed or when a new individual assumes responsibility for management of the

drug testing laboratory. Copies of all procedures and dates on which they are in effect shall be maintained. (Specific contents of the procedure manual are described in 2.4(n)(1)).

(6) This individual shall be responsible for maintaining a quality assurance program to assure the proper performance and reporting of all test results; for maintaining acceptable analytical performance for all controls and standards; for maintaining quality control testing; and for assuring and documenting the validity, reliability, accuracy, precision, and performance characteristics of each test and test system.

(7) This individual shall be responsible for taking all remedial actions necessary to maintain satisfactory operation and performance of the laboratory in response to quality control systems not being within performance specifications, errors in result reporting or in analysis of performance testing results. This individual shall ensure that sample results are not reported until all corrective actions have been taken and he or she can assure that the test results provided are accurate and reliable.

(b) Test Validation. The laboratory's urine drug testing facility shall have a qualified individual(s) who reviews all pertinent data and quality control results in order to attest to the validity of the laboratory's test reports. A laboratory may designate more than one person to perform this function. This individual(s) may be any employee who is qualified to be responsible for day-to-day management or operation of the drug testing laboratory.

(c) Day-to-Day Operations and Supervision of Analysis. The laboratory's urine drug testing facility shall have an individual to be responsible for day-to-day operations and to supervise the technical analysts. This individual(s) shall have at least a bachelor's degree in the chemical or biological sciences or medical technology or equivalent. He or she shall have training and experience in the theory and practice of the procedures used in the laboratory, resulting in his or her thorough understanding of quality control practices and procedures; the review, interpretation, and reporting of test results; maintenance of chain of custody; and proper remedial actions to be taken in response to test systems being out of control limits or detecting aberrant test or quality control results.

(d) Other Personnel. Other technicians or nontechnical staff shall have the necessary training and skills for the tasks assigned.

(e) Training. The laboratory's urine drug testing program shall make available continuing education programs to meet the needs of laboratory personnel.

(f) Files. Laboratory personnel files shall include: resume of training and experience; certification or license, if any; references; job descriptions; records of performance evaluation and advancement; incident reports; and results of tests which establish employee competency for the position he or she holds, such as a test for color blindness, if appropriate.

2.4 Laboratory Analysis Procedures

(a) Security and Chain of Custody.

(1) Drug testing laboratories shall be secure at all times. They shall have in place sufficient security measures to control access to the premises to ensure that no

unauthorized personnel handle specimens or gain access to the laboratory processes or to areas where records are stored. Access to these secured area shall be limited to specifically authorized individuals whose authorization is documented. With the exception of personnel authorized to conduct inspections on behalf of Federal agencies for which the laboratory is engaged in urine testing or on behalf of the Secretary, all authorized visitors and maintenance and service personnel shall be escorted at all times. Documentation of individuals accessing these areas, dates, and time of entry and purpose of entry must be maintained.

(2) Laboratories shall use chain of custody procedures to maintain control and accountability of specimens from receipt through completion of testing, reporting of results, during storage, and continuing until final disposition of specimens. The date and purpose shall be documented on an appropriate chain of custody form each time a specimen is handled or transferred, and every individual in the chain shall be identified. Accordingly, authorized technicians shall be responsible for each urine specimen or aliquot in their possession and shall sign and complete chain of custody forms for those specimens or aliquots as they are received.

(b) Receiving.

(1) When a shipment of specimens is received, laboratory personnel shall inspect each package for evidence of possible tampering and compare information on specimen bottles within each package to the information on the accompanying chain of custody forms. Any direct evidence of tampering or discrepancies in the information on specimen bottles and the agency's chain of custody forms attached to the shipment shall be reported to the agency and shall be noted on the laboratory's chain of custody form which shall accompany the specimens while they are in the laboratory's possession.

(2) Specimen bottles will normally be retained within the laboratory's accession area until all analyses have been completed. Aliquots and the laboratory's chain of custody forms shall be used by laboratory personnel for conducting initial and confirmatory tests.

(c) Short-Term Refrigerated Storage. Specimens that do not receive an initial test within 7 days of arrival at the laboratory shall be placed in secure refrigeration units. Temperatures shall not exceed 6 degrees Celsius. Emergency power equipment shall be available in case of prolonged power failure.

(d) Specimen Processing. Laboratory facilities for urine drug testing will normally process specimens by grouping them into batches. The number of specimens in each batch may vary significantly depending on the size of the laboratory and its workload. When conducting either initial or confirmatory tests, every batch shall contain an appropriate number of standards for calibrating the instrumentation and a minimum of 10 percent controls. Both quality control and blind performance test samples shall appear as ordinary samples to laboratory analysts.

(e) Initial Test.

(1) The initial test shall use an immunoassay which meets the requirements of the Food and Drug Administration for commercial distribution. The following initial cutoff levels shall be used when screening specimens to determine whether they are negative for these five drugs or classes of drugs:

	Initial test level (ng/ml)
Marijuana metabolites	100
Cocaine metabolites	300
Opiate metabolites	300*
Phencyclidine	25
Amphetamines	1000

*25 ng/ml if immunoassay specific for free morphine.

(2) These test levels are subject to change by the Department of Health and Human Services as advances in technology or other considerations warrant identification of these substances at other concentrations. Initial test methods and testing levels for other drugs shall be submitted in writing by the agency for the written approval of the Secretary.

(f) Confirmatory Test.

(1) All specimens identified as positive on the initial test shall be confirmed using gas chromatography/mass spectrometry (GC/MS) techniques at the cutoff values listed in this paragraph for each drug. All confirmations shall be by quantitative analysis. Concentrations which exceed the linear region of the standard curve shall be documented in the laboratory record as "greater than highest standard curve value."

	Confirmatory test level (ng/ml)
Marijuana metabolite*	15
Cocaine metabolite**	150
Opiates	
Morphine	300
Codeine	300
Phencyclidine	25
Amphetamines	
Amphetamine	500
Methamphetamine	500

*Delta-9-tetrahydrocannabinol-9-carboxylic acid.
**Benzoylecgonine.

(2) These test levels are subject to change by the Department of Health and Human Services as advances in technology or other considerations warrant identification of these substances at other concentrations. Confirmatory test methods and testing levels for other drugs shall be submitted in writing by the agency for the written approval of the Secretary.

(g) Reporting Results.

(1) The laboratory shall report test results to the agency's Medical Review Officer within an average of 5 working days after receipt of the specimen by the laboratory. Before any test result is reported (the results of initial tests, confirmatory tests, or

quality control data), it shall be reviewed and the test certified as an accurate report by the responsible individual. The report shall identify the drugs/metabolites tested for, whether positive or negative, and the cutoff for each, the specimen number assigned by the agency, and the drug testing laboratory specimen identification number. The results (positive or negative) for all specimens submitted at the same time to the laboratory shall be reported back to the Medical Review Officer at the same time.

(2) The laboratory shall report as negative all specimens which are negative on the initial test or negative on the confirmatory test. Only specimens confirmed positive shall be reported positive for a specific drug.

(3) The Medical Review Officer may request from the laboratory and the laboratory shall provide quantitation of test results. The Medical Review Officer may not disclose quantitation of test results to the agency but shall report only whether the test was positive or negative.

(4) The laboratory may transmit results to the Medical Review Officer by various electronic means (for example, teleprinters, facsimiles, or computer) in a manner designed to ensure confidentiality of the information. Results may not be provided verbally by telephone. The laboratory must ensure the security of the data transmission and limit access to any data transmission, storage, and retrieval system.

(5) The laboratory shall send only to the Medical Review Officer a certified copy of the original chain of custody form signed by the individual responsible for day-to-day management of the drug testing laboratory or the individual responsible for attesting to the validity of test reports.

(6) The laboratory shall provide to the agency official responsible for the coordination of the drug-free workplace program a monthly statistical summary of urinalysis testing of Federal employees and shall not include in the summary any personal identifying information. Initial and confirmation data shall be included from test results reported within that month. Normally this summary shall be forwarded by registered or certified mail not more than 14 calendar days after the end of the month covered by the summary. The summary shall contain the following information:

(i) Initial Testing:

(A) Number of specimens received;

(B) Number of specimens reported out; and

(C) Number of specimens screened positive for:

Marijuana metabolites
Cocaine metabolites
Opiate metabolites
Phencyclidine
Amphetamines

(ii) Confirmatory Testing:

(A) Number of specimens received for confirmation;

(B) Number of specimens confirmed positive for:

Marijuana metabolite
Cocaine metabolite
Morphine, codeine
Phencyclidine
Amphetamine
Methamphetamine

(7) The laboratory shall make available copies of all analytical results for Federal drug testing programs when requested by DHHS or any Federal agency for which the laboratory is performing drug testing services.

(8) Unless otherwise instructed by the agency in writing, all records pertaining to a given urine specimen shall be retained by the drug testing laboratory for a minimum of 2 years.

(h) Long-Term Storage. Long-term frozen storage (− 20 degrees Celsius or less) ensures that positive urine specimens will be available for any necessary retest during administrative or disciplinary proceedings. Unless otherwise authorized in writing by the agency, drug testing laboratories shall retain and place in properly secured long-term frozen storage for a minimum of 1 year all specimens confirmed positive. Within this 1-year period an agency may request the laboratory to retain the specimen for an additional period of time, but if no such request is received the laboratory may discard the specimen after the end of 1 year, except that the laboratory shall be required to maintain any specimens under legal challenge for an indefinite period.

(i) Retesting Specimens. Because some analytes deteriorate or are lost during freezing and/or storage, quantitation for a retest is not subject to a specific cutoff requirement but must provide data sufficient to confirm the presence of the drug or metabolite.

(j) Subcontracting. Drug testing laboratories shall not subcontract and shall perform all work with their own personnel and equipment unless otherwise authorized by the agency. The laboratory must be capable of performing testing for the five classes of drugs (marijuana, cocaine, opiates, phencyclidine, and amphetamines) using the initial immunoassay and confirmatory GC/MS methods specified in these Guidelines.

(k) Laboratory Facilities.

(1) Laboratory facilities shall comply with applicable provisions of any State licensure requirements.

(2) Laboratories certified in accordance with Subpart C of these Guidelines shall have the capability, at the same laboratory premises, of performing initial and confirmatory tests for each drug or metabolite for which service is offered.

(l) Inspections. The Secretary, any Federal agency utilizing the laboratory, or any organization performing laboratory certification on behalf of the Secretary shall reserve the right to inspect the laboratory at any time. Agency contracts with laboratories for drug testing, as well as contracts for collection site services, shall permit the agency to conduct unannounced inspection. In addition, prior to the award of a contract the agency shall carry out preaward inspections and evaluation of the procedural aspects of the laboratory's drug testing operation.

(m) Documentation. The drug testing laboratories shall maintain and make available for at least 2 years documentation of all aspects of the testing process. This 2-year period may be extended upon written notification by DHHS or by any Federal agency for which laboratory services are being provided. The required documentation shall include personnel files on all individuals authorized to have access to specimens; chain of custody documents; quality assurance/quality control records; procedure manuals; all test data (including calibration curves and any calculations used in determining test results); reports; performance records on certification inspections; and hard copies of computer-generated data. The laboratory shall be required to maintain documents for any specimen under legal challenge for an indefinite period.

(n) Additional Requirements for Certified Laboratories.

(1) Procedure Manual. Each laboratory shall have a procedure manual which includes the principles of each test, preparation of reagents, standards and controls, calibration procedures, derivation of results, linearity of methods, sensitivity of the methods, cutoff values, mechanisms for reporting results, controls, criteria for unacceptable specimens and results, remedial actions to be taken when the test systems are outside of acceptable limits, reagents and expiration dates, and references. Copies of all procedures and dates on which they are in effect shall be maintained as part of the manual.

(2) Standards and Controls. Laboratory standards shall be prepared with pure drug standards which are properly labeled as to content and concentration. The standards shall be labeled with the following dates: when received; when prepared or opened; when placed in services; and expiration date.

(3) Instruments and Equipment.

(i) Volumetric pipettes and measuring devices shall be certified for accuracy or be checked by gravimetric, colorimetric, or other verification procedure. Automatic pipettes and dilutors shall be checked for accuracy and reproducibility before being placed in service and checked periodically thereafter.

(ii) There shall be written procedures for instrument set-up and normal operation, a schedule for checking critical operating elements, tolerance limits for acceptable function checks and instructions for major trouble shooting and repair. Records shall be available on preventive maintenance.

(4) Remedial Actions. There shall be written procedures for the actions to be taken when systems are out of acceptable limits or errors are detected. There shall be documentation that these procedures are followed and that all necessary corrective actions are taken. There shall also be in place systems to verify all stages of testing and reporting and documentation that these procedures are followed.

(5) Personnel Available to Testify at Proceedings. A laboratory shall have qualified personnel available to testify in an administrative or disciplinary proceeding against a Federal employee when that proceeding is based on positive urinalysis results reported by the laboratory.

2.5   Quality Assurance and Quality Control

(a) General. Drug testing laboratories shall have a quality assurance program which encompasses all aspects of the testing process including but not limited to specimen acquisition, chain of custody, security and reporting of results, initial and confirmatory testing, and validation of analytical procedure. Quality assurance procedures shall be designed, implemented, and reviewed to monitor the conduct of each step of the process of testing for drugs.

(b) Laboratory Quality Control Requirements for Initial Tests. Each analytical run of specimens to be screened shall include:

   (1) Urine specimens certified to contain no drug;

   (2) Urine specimens fortified with known standards; and

   (3) Positive controls with the drug or metabolite at or near the threshold (cutoff).

In addition, with each batch of samples a sufficient number of standards shall be included to ensure and document the linearity of the assay method over time in the concentration area of the cutoff. After acceptable values are obtained for the known standards, those values will be used to calculate sample data. Implementation of procedures to ensure that carryover does not contaminate the testing of an individual's specimen shall be documented. A minimum of 10 percent of all test samples shall be quality control specimens. Laboratory quality control samples, prepared from spiked urine samples of determined concentration, shall be included in the run and should appear as normal samples to laboratory analysis. One percent of each run, with a minimum of at least one sample, shall be the laboratory's own quality control samples.

(c) Laboratory Quality Control Requirements for Confirmation Tests. Each analytical run of specimens to be confirmed shall include:

   (1) Urine specimens certified to contain no drug;

   (2) Urine specimens fortified with known standards; and

   (3) Positive controls with the drug or metabolite at or near the threshold (cutoff).

The linearity and precision of the method shall be periodically documented. Implementation of procedures to ensure that carryover does not contaminate the testing of an individual's specimen shall also be documented.

(d) Agency Blind Performance Test Procedures.

   (1) Agencies shall purchase drug testing services only from laboratories certified by DHHS or a DHHS-recognized certification program in accordance with these Guidelines. Laboratory participation is encouraged in other performance testing surveys by which the laboratory's performance is compared with peers and reference laboratories.

   (2) During the initial 90-day period of any new drug testing program, each agency shall submit blind performance test specimens to each laboratory it contracts with in the amount of at least 50 percent of the total number of samples submitted (up to a maximum of 500 samples) and thereafter a minimum of 10 percent of all samples (to a maximum of 250) submitted per quarter.

   (3) Approximately 80 percent of the blind performance test samples shall be blank (i.e., certified to contain no drug) and the remaining samples shall be positive for one or more drugs per sample in a distribution such that all the drugs to be tested

are included in approximately equal frequencies of challenge. The positive samples shall be spiked only with those drugs for which the agency is testing.

(4) The Secretary shall investigate any unsatisfactory performance testing result and, based on this investigation, the laboratory shall take action to correct the cause of the unsatisfactory performance test result. A record shall be made of the Secretary's investigative findings and the corrective action by the laboratory, and that record shall be dated and signed by the individuals responsible for the day-to-day management and operation of the drug testing laboratory. Then the Secretary shall send the document to the agency contracting officer as a report of the unsatisfactory performance testing incident. The Secretary shall ensure notification of the finding to all other Federal agencies for which the laboratory is engaged in urine drug testing and coordinate any necessary action.

(5) Should a false positive error occur on a blind performance test specimen and the error is determined to be an administrative error (clerical, sample mix-up, etc.), the Secretary shall require the laboratory to take corrective action to minimize the occurrence of the particular error in the future; and, if there is reason to believe the error could have been systematic, the Secretary may also require review and reanalysis of previously run specimens.

(6) Should a false positive occur on a blind performance test specimen and the error is determined to be a technical or methodological error, the laboratory shall submit all quality control data from the batch of specimens which included the false positive specimen. In addition, the laboratory shall retest all specimens analyzed positive for that drug or metabolite from the time of final resolution of the error back to the time of the last satisfactory performance test cycle. This retesting shall be documented by a statement signed by the individual responsible for day-to-day management of the laboratory's drug testing. The Secretary may require an on-site review of the laboratory which may be conducted unannounced during any hours of operations of the laboratory. The Secretary has the option of revoking (3.13) or suspending (3.14) the laboratory's certification or recommending that no further action be taken if the case is one of less serious error in which corrective action has already been taken, thus reasonably assuring that the error will not occur again.

2.6   Interim Certification Procedures.

During the interim certification period as determined under paragraph (c), agencies shall ensure laboratory competence by one of the following methods:

(a) Agencies may use agency or contract laboratories that have been certified for urinalysis testing by the Department of Defense; or

(b) Agencies may develop interim self-certification procedures by establishing pre-award inspections and performance testing plans approved by DHHS.

(c) The period during which these interim certification procedures will apply shall be determined by the Secretary. Upon notice by the Secretary that these interim certification procedures are no longer available, all Federal agencies subject to these Guidelines shall only use laboratories that have been certified in accordance with Subpart C of these Guidelines and all laboratories approved for interim certification under paragraphs (a) and (b) of the section shall become certified in accordance with Subpart C within 120 days of the date of this notice.

2.7   Reporting and Review of Results.

(a) Medical Review Officer Shall Review Results. An essential part of the drug testing program is the final review of results. A positive test result does not automatically identify an employee/applicant as an illegal drug user. An individual with a detailed knowledge of possible alternate medical explanations is essential to the review of results. This review shall be performed by the Medical Review Officer prior to the transmission of results to agency administrative officials.

(b) Medical Review Officer—Qualifications and Responsibilities. The Medical Review Officer shall be a licensed physician with knowledge of substance abuse disorders and may be an agency or contract employee. The role of the Medical Review Officer is to review and interpret positive test results obtained through the agency's testing program. In carrying out this responsibility, the Medical Review Officer shall examine alternate medical explanations for any positive test result. This action could include conducting a medical interview with the individual, review of the individual's medical history, or review of any other relevant biomedical factors. The Medical Review Officer shall review all medical records made available by the tested individual when a confirmed positive test could have resulted from legally prescribed medication. The Medical Review Officer shall not, however, consider the results of urine samples that are not obtained or processed in accordance with these Guidelines.

(c) Positive Test Result. Prior to making a final decision to verify a positive test result, the Medical Review Officer shall give the individual an opportunity to discuss the test result with him or her. Following verification of a positive test result, the Medical Review Officer shall refer the case to the agency Employee Assistance Program and to the management official empowered to recommend or take administrative action.

(d) Verification for Opiates; Review for Prescription Medication. Before the Medical Review Officer verifies a confirmed positive result for opiates, he or she shall determine that there is clinical evidence—in addition to the urine test—of illegal use of any opium, opiate or opium derivative (e.g., morphine/codeine) listed in Schedule I or II of the Controlled Substances Act. (This requirement does not apply if the agency's GC/MS confirmation testing for opiates confirms the presence of 6-monoacetylmorphine.)

(e) Reanalysis Authorized. Should any question arise as to the accuracy or validity of a positive test result, only the Medical Review Officer is authorized to order a reanalysis of the original sample and such retests are authorized only at laboratories certified under these Guidelines.

(f) Result Consistent with Legal Drug Use. If the Medical Review Officer determines there is a legitimate medical explanation for the positive test result, he or she shall determine that the result is consistent with legal drug use and take no further action.

(g) Result Scientifically Insufficient. Additionally, the Medical Review Officer, based on review of inspection reports, quality control data, multiple samples, and other pertinent results, may determine that the result is scientifically insufficient for further action and declare the test specimen negative. In this situation the Medical Review Officer may request reanalysis of the original sample before making this decision. (The Medical Review Officer may request that the reanalysis be performed by the same laboratory or, as provided in 2.7(e), that an aliquot of the original specimen be sent for reanalysis to an alternate laboratory which is certified in accordance with these Guidelines. The laboratory shall assist in this review process as requested by the Medical Review Officer by making available the individual responsible for day-to-day management of the urine drug testing laboratory or other employee who is a forensic toxicologist or who has equivalent forensic experience in urine drug testing, to provide specific consultation as required by the agency. The Medical Review Officer shall report to the Secretary all negative findings based on scientific insufficiency but shall not include any personal identifying information in such reports.

2.8   Protection of Employee Records.

Consistent with 5 U.S.C. 522a(m) and 48 CFR 24.101-24.104, all laboratory contracts shall require that the contractor comply with the Privacy Act, 5 U.S.C. 552a. In addition, laboratory contracts shall require compliance with the patient access and confidentiality provisions of section 503 of Pub. L. 100-71. The agency shall establish a Privacy Act System of Records or modify an existing system, or use any applicable Government-wide system of records to cover both the agency's and the laboratory's records of employee urinalysis results. The contract and the Privacy Act System shall specifically require that employee records be maintained and used with the highest regard for employee privacy.

2.9   Individual Access to Test and Laboratory Certification Results.

In accordance with section 503 of Pub. L. 100-71, any Federal employee who is the subject of a drug test shall, upon written request, have access to any records relating to his or her drug test and any records relating to the results of any relevant certification, review, or revocation-of-certification proceedings.

Subpart C—Certification of Laboratories Engaged in Urine Drug Testing for Federal Agencies

3.1   Introduction.

Urine drug testing is a critical component of efforts to combat drug abuse in our society. Many laboratories are familiar with good laboratory practices but may be unfamiliar with the special procedures required when drug test results are used in the employment context. Accordingly, the following are minimum standards to certify laboratories engaged in urine drug testing for Federal agencies. Therefore, results from laboratories certified under these Guidelines must be interpreted with a complete understanding of the total collection, analysis, and reporting process before a final conclusion is made.

3.2   Goals and Objectives of Certification.

(a) Uses of Urine Drug Testing. Urine drug testing is an important tool to identify drug users in a variety of settings. In the proper context, urine drug testing can be used to deter drug abuse in general. To be a useful tool, the testing procedure must be capable of detecting drugs or their metabolites at concentrations indicated in 2.4(e) and (f).

(b) Need to Set Standards; Inspections. Reliable discrimination between the presence, or absence, of specific drugs or their metabolites is critical, not only to achieve the goals of the testing program but to protect the rights of the Federal employees being tested. Thus, standards have been set which laboratories engaged in Federal employee urine drug testing must meet in order to achieve maximum accuracy of test results. These laboratories will be evaluated by the Secretary or the Secretary's designee as defined in 1.2 in accordance with these Guidelines. The qualifying evaluation will involve three rounds of performance testing plus on-site inspection. Maintenance of certification requires participation in an every-other-month performance testing program plus periodic, on-site inspections. One inspection following successful completion of a performance testing regimen is required for initial certification. This must be followed by a second inspection within 3 months, after which biannual inspections will be required to maintain certification.

(c) Urine Drug Testing Applies Analytical Forensic Toxicology. The possible impact of a positive test result on an individual's livelihood or rights, together with the possibility of a legal challenge of the result, sets this type of test apart from most clinical laboratory testing. In fact, urine drug testing should be considered a special application of analytical forensic toxicology. That is, in addition to the application of appropriate analytical methodology, the specimen must be treated as evidence, and all aspects of the testing procedure must be documented and available for possible court testimony. Laboratories engaged in urine drug testing for Federal agencies will require the services and advice of a qualified forensic toxicologist, or individual with equivalent qualifications (both training and experience) to address the specific needs of the Federal drug testing program, including the demands of chain of custody of specimens, security, property documentation of all records, storage of positive specimens for later or independent testing, presentation of evidence in court, and expert witness testimony.

3.3   General Certification Requirements.

A laboratory must meet all the pertinent provisions of these Guidelines in order to qualify for certification under these standards.

3.4   Capability to Test for Five Classes of Drugs.

To be certified, a laboratory must be capable of testing for at least the following five classes of drugs: marijuana, cocaine, opiates, amphetamines, and phencyclidine, using the initial immunoassay and quantitative confirmatory GC/MS methods specified in these Guidelines. The certification program will be limited to the five classes of drugs (2.1(a)(1) and (2)) and the methods (2.4(e) and (f)) specified in these Guidelines. The laboratory will be surveyed and performance tested only for these methods and drugs. Certification of a laboratory indicates that any test result reported by the laboratory for the Federal Government meets the standards in these Guidelines for the five classes of drugs using the methods specified. Certified laboratories must clearly inform non-Federal clients when procedures followed for those clients conform to the standards specified in these Guidelines.

3.5   Initial and Confirmatory Capability at Same Site.

Certified laboratories shall have the capability, at the same laboratory site, of performing both initial immunoassays and confirmatory GC/MS tests (2.4(e) and (f)) for marijuana, cocaine, opiates, amphetamines, and phencyclidine and for any other drug or metabolite for which agency drug testing is authorized (2.1(a)(1) and (2)). All positive initial test results shall be confirmed prior to reporting them.

3.6   Personnel.

Laboratory personnel shall meet the requirements specified in 2.3 of these Guidelines. These Guidelines establish the exclusive standards for qualifying or certifying those laboratory personnel involved in urinalysis testing whose functions are prescribed by these Guidelines. A certification of a laboratory under these Guidelines shall be a determination that these qualification requirements have been met.

3.7   Quality Assurance and Quality Control.

Drug testing laboratories shall have a quality assurance program which encompasses all aspects of the testing process, including but not limited to specimen acquisition, chain of custody, security and reporting of results, initial and confirmatory testing, and validation of analytical procedures. Quality control procedures shall be designed, implemented, and reviewed to monitor the conduct of each step of the process of testing for drugs as specified in 2.5 of these Guidelines.

3.8   Security and Chain of Custody.

Laboratories shall meet the security and chain of custody requirements provided in 2.4(a).

3.9   One-Year Storage for Confirmed Positives.

All confirmed positive specimens shall be retained in accordance with the provisions of 2.4(h) of these Guidelines.

3.10   Documentation.

The laboratory shall maintain and make available for at least 2 years documentation in accordance with specifications in 2.4(m).

3.11   Reports.

The laboratory shall report test results in accordance with the specifications in 2.4(g).

3.12   Certification.

(a) General. The Secretary may certify any laboratory that meets the standards in these Guidelines to conduct urine drug testing. In addition, the Secretary may consider to be certified any laboratory that is certified by a DHHS-recognized certification program in accordance with these Guidelines.

(b) Criteria. In determining whether to certify a laboratory or to accept the certification of a DHHS-recognized certification program in accordance with these Guidelines, the Secretary shall consider the following criteria:

(1) The adequacy of the laboratory facilities;

(2) The expertise and experience of the laboratory personnel;

(3) The excellence of the laboratory's quality assurance/quality control program;

(4) The performance of the laboratory on any performance tests;

(5) The laboratory's compliance with standards as reflected in any laboratory inspections; and

(6) Any other factors affecting the reliability and accuracy of drug tests and reporting done by the laboratory.

3.13   Revocation.

(a) General. The Secretary shall revoke certification of any laboratory certified under these provisions or accept revocation by a DHHS-recognized certification program in accordance with these Guidelines if the Secretary determines that revocation is necessary to ensure the full reliability and accuracy of drug tests and the accurate reporting of test results.

(b) Factors to Consider. The Secretary shall consider the following factors in determining whether revocation is necessary:

(1) Unsatisfactory performance in analyzing and reporting the results of drug tests; for example, a false positive error in reporting the results of an employee's drug test;

(2) Unsatisfactory participation in performance evaluations or laboratory inspections;

(3) A material violation of a certification standard or a contract term or other condition imposed on the laboratory by a Federal agency using the laboratory's services;

(4) Conviction for any criminal offense committed as an incident to operation of the laboratory; or

(5) Any other cause which materially affects the ability of the laboratory to ensure the full reliability and accuracy of drug tests and the accurate reporting of results.

(c) Period and Terms.

The period and terms of the revocation shall be determined by the Secretary and shall depend upon the facts and circumstances of the revocation and the need to ensure accurate and reliable drug testing of Federal employees.

3.14   Suspension.

(a) Criteria. Whenever the Secretary has reason to believe that revocation may be required and that immediate action is necessary in order to protect the interests of the United States and its employees, the Secretary may immediately suspend a laboratory's certification to conduct urine drug testing for Federal agencies. The Secretary may also accept suspension of certification by a DHHS-recognized certification program in accordance with these Guidelines.

(b) Period and Terms. The period and terms of suspension shall be determined by the Secretary and shall depend upon the facts and circumstances of the suspension and the need to ensure accurate and reliable drug testing of Federal employees.

3.15   Notice; Opportunity for Review.

(a) Written Notice. When a laboratory is suspended or the Secretary seeks to revoke certification, the Secretary shall immediately serve the laboratory with written notice of the suspension or proposed revocation by personal service or registered or certified mail, return receipt requested. This notice shall state the following:

(1) The reasons for the suspension or proposed revocation;

(2) The terms of the suspension or proposed revocation; and

(3) The period of suspension or proposed revocation.

(b) Opportunity for Informal Review. The written notice shall state the laboratory will be afforded an opportunity for an informal review of the suspension or proposed revocation if it so requests in writing within 30 days of the date of mailing or service of the notice. The review shall be by a person or persons designated by the Secretary and shall be based on written submissions by the laboratory and the Department of Health and Human Services and, at the Secretary's discretion, may include an opportunity for an oral presentation. Formal rules of evidence and procedures applicable to proceedings in a court of law shall not apply. The decision of the reviewing official shall be final.

(c) Effective Date. A suspension shall be effective immediately. A proposed revocation shall be effective 30 days after written notice is given or, if review is requested, upon the reviewing official's decision to uphold the proposed revocation. If the reviewing official decides not to uphold the suspension or proposed revocation, the suspension shall terminate immediately and any proposed revocation shall not take effect.

(d) DHHS-Recognized Certification Program. The Secretary's responsibility under this section may be carried out by a DHHS-recognized certification program in accordance with these Guidelines.

3.16   Recertification.

Following the termination of expiration of any suspension or revocation, a laboratory may apply for recertification. Upon the submission of evidence satisfactory to the Secretary that the laboratory is in compliance with these Guidelines or any DHHS-recognized certification program in accordance with these Guidelines, and any other conditions imposed as part of the suspension or revocation, the Secretary may recertify the laboratory or accept the recertification of the laboratory by a DHHS-recognized certification program.

3.17   Performance Test Requirement for Certification.

(a) An Initial and Continuing Requirement. The performance testing program is part of the initial evaluation of a laboratory seeking certification (both performance testing and laboratory inspection are required) and of the continuing assessment of laboratory performance necessary to maintain this certification.

(b) Three Initial Cycles Required. Successful participation in three cycles of testing shall be required before a laboratory is eligible to be considered for inspection and certification. These initial three cycles (and any required for recertification) can be compressed into a 3-month period (one per month).

(c) Six Challenges Per Year. After certification, laboratories shall be challenged every other month with one set of at least 10 specimens a total of six cycles per year.

(d) Laboratory Procedures Identical for Performance Test and Routine Employee Specimens. All procedures associated with the handling and testing of the performance test specimens by the laboratory shall to the greatest extent possible be carried out in a manner identical to that applied to routine laboratory specimens, unless otherwise specified.

(e) Blind Performance Test. Any certified laboratory shall be subject to blind performance testing (see 2.5(d)). Performance on blind test specimens shall be at the same level as for the open or non-blind performance testing.

(f) Reporting-Open Performance Test. The laboratory shall report results of open performance tests to the certifying organization in the same manner as specified in 2.4(g)(2) for routine laboratory specimens.

3.18   Performance Test Specimen Composition.

(a) Description of the Drugs. Performance test specimens shall contain those drugs and metabolites which each certified laboratory must be prepared to assay in concentration ranges that allow detection of the analyte by commonly used immunoassay screening techniques. These levels are generally in the range of concentrations which might be expected in the urine of recent drug users. For some drug analytes, the specimen composition will consist of the parent drug as well as major metabolites. In some cases, more than one drug class may be included in one specimen container, but generally no more than two drugs will be present in any one specimen in order to imitate the type of specimen which a laboratory normally encounters. For any particular performance testing cycle, the actual composition of kits going to different laboratories will vary but, within any annual period, all laboratories participating will have analyzed the same total set of specimens.

(b) Concentrations. Performance test specimens shall be spiked with the drug classes and their metabolites which are required for certification: marijuana, cocaine, opiates, amphetamines, and phencyclidine, with concentration levels set at least 20 percent above the cutoff limit for either the initial assay or confirmatory test, depending on which is to be evaluated. Some performance test specimens may be identified for GC/MS assay only. Blanks shall contain less than 2 ng/ml of any of the target drugs. These concentrations and drug types shall be changed periodically in response to factors such as changes in detection technology and patterns of drug use.

3.19   Evaluation of Performance Testing.

(a) Initial Certification. (1) An applicant laboratory shall not report any false positive test result during performance testing for initial certification. Any false positives will automatically disqualify a laboratory from further consideration.

(2) An applicant laboratory shall maintain an overall grade level of 90 percent for the three cycles of performance testing required for initial certification, i.e., it must correctly identify and confirm 90 percent of the total drug challenges for each shipment. Any laboratory which achieves a score on any one cycle of the initial certification such that it can no longer achieve a total grade of 90 percent over the three cycles will be immediately disqualified from further consideration.

(3) An applicant laboratory shall obtain quantitative values for at least 80 percent of the total drug challenges which are plus or minus 20 percent or plus or minus 2 standard deviations of the calculated reference group mean (whichever is larger). Failure to achieve 80 percent will result in disqualification.

(4) An applicant laboratory shall not obtain any quantitative values that differ by more than 50 percent from the calculated reference group mean. Any quantitative values that differ by more than 50 percent will result in disqualification.

(5) For any individual drug, an applicant laboratory shall successfully detect and quantitate in accordance with paragraphs (a)(2), (a)(3), and (a)(4) of this section at least 50 percent of the total drug challenges. Failure to successfully quantitate at least 50 percent of the challenges for any individual drug will result in disqualification.

(b) Ongoing Testing of Certified Laboratories. (1) False Positives and Procedures for Dealing with Them. No false drug identifications are acceptable for any drugs for which a laboratory offers service. Under some circumstances a false positive test may result in suspension or revocation of certification. The most serious false positives are by drug class, such as reporting THC in a blank specimen or reporting cocaine in a specimen known to contain only opiates. Misidentifications within a class (e.g., codeine for morphine) are also false positives which are unacceptable in an appropriately controlled laboratory, but they are clearly less serious errors than misidentification of a class. The following procedures shall be followed when dealing with a false positive:

(i) The agency detecting a false positive error shall immediately notify the laboratory and the Secretary of any such error.

(ii) The laboratory shall provide the Secretary with a written explanation of the reasons for the error within 5 working days. If required by paragraph (b)(1)(v) below, this explanation shall include the submission of all quality control data from the batch of specimens that included the false positive specimen.

(iii) The Secretary shall review the laboratory's explanation within 5 working days and decide what further action, if any, to take.

(iv) If the error is determined to be an administrative error (clerical, sample mixup, etc.), the Secretary may direct the laboratory to take corrective action to minimize the occurrence of the particular error in the future and, if there is reason to believe the error could have been systematic, may require the laboratory to review and reanalyze previously run specimens.

(v) If the error is determined to be a technical or methodological error, the laboratory shall submit to the Secretary all quality control data from the batch of specimens which included the false positive specimen. In addition, the laboratory shall retest all specimens analyzed positive by the laboratory from the time of the last satisfactory performance test cycle. This retesting shall be documented by a statement signed by the individual responsible for the day-to-day management of the laboratory's urine drug testing. Depending on the type of error which caused the false positive, this retesting may be limited to one analyte or may include any drugs a laboratory certified under these Guidelines must be prepared to assay. The laboratory shall immediately notify the agency if any result on a retest sample must be corrected because the criteria for a positive are not satisfied. The Secretary may suspend or revoke the laboratory's certification for all drugs or for only the drug or drug class in which the error occurred. However, if the case is one of a less serious error for which effective corrections have already been made, thus reasonably assuring that the error will not occur again, the Secretary may decide to take no further action.

(vi) During the time required to resolve the error, the laboratory shall remain certified but shall have a designation indicating that a false positive result is pending resolution. If the Secretary determines that the laboratory's certification must be suspended or revoked, the laboratory's official status will become "Suspended" or "Revoked" until the suspension or revocation is lifted or any recertification process is complete.

(2) Requirement to Identify and Confirm 90 Percent of Total Drug Challenges. In order to remain certified, laboratories must successfully complete six cycles of performance testing per year. Failure of a certified laboratory to maintain a grade of 90 percent on any required performance test cycle, i.e., to identify 90 percent of the total drug challenges and to correctly confirm 90 percent of the total drug challenges, may result in suspension or revocation of certification.

(3) Requirement to Quantitate 80 Percent of Total Drug Challenges at Plus or Minus 20 Percent or Plus or Minus 2 Standard Deviations. Quantitative values obtained by a certified laboratory for at least 80 percent of the total drug challenges must be plus or minus 20 percent or plus or minus 2 standard deviations of the calculated reference group mean (whichever is larger).

(4) Requirement to Quantitate Within 50 Percent of Calculated Reference Group Mean. No quantitative values obtained by a certified laboratory may differ by more than 50 percent from the calculated reference group mean.

(5) Requirement to Successfully Detect and Quantitate 50 Percent of the Total Drug Challenges for Any Individual Drug. For any individual drug, a certified laboratory must successfully detect and quantitate in accordance with paragraphs (b)(2), (b)(3), and (b)(4) of this section at least 50 percent of the total drug challenges.

(6) Procedures When Requirements in Paragraphs (b)(2)–(b)(5) of this Section Are Not Met. If a certified laboratory fails to maintain a grade of 90 percent per test cycle after initial certification as required by (b)(2) of this section or if it fails to successfully quantitate results as required by paragraphs (b)(3), (b)(4), or (b)(5) of this section, the laboratory shall be immediately informed that its performance fell under the 90 percent level or that it failed to successfully quantitate test results and how it failed to successfully quantitate. The laboratory shall be allowed 5 working days in which to provide any explanation for its unsuccessful performance, including administrative error or methodological error, and evidence that the source of the poor performance has been corrected. The Secretary may revoke or suspend the laboratory's certification or take no further action, depending on the seriousness of the errors and whether there is evidence that the source of the poor performance has been corrected and that current performance meets requirements for a certified laboratory under these Guidelines. The Secretary may require that additional performance tests be carried out to determine whether the source of the poor performance has been removed. If the Secretary determines to suspend or revoke the laboratory's certification, the laboratory's official status will become "Suspended" or "Revoked" until the suspension or revocation is lifted or until any recertification process is complete.

(c) 80 Percent of Participating Laboratories Must Detect Drug. A laboratory's performance shall be evaluated for all samples for which drugs were spiked at concentrations above the specified performance test level unless the overall response from participating laboratories indicates that less than 80 percent of them were unable to detect a drug.

(d) Participation Required. Failure to participate in a performance test or to participate satisfactorily may result in suspension or revocation of certification.

3.20   Inspections.

Prior to laboratory certification under these Guidelines and at least twice a year after certification, a team of three qualified inspectors, at least two of whom have been trained as laboratory inspectors, shall conduct an on-site inspection of laboratory premises. Inspections shall document the overall quality of the laboratory setting for the purposes of certification to conduct urine drug testing. Inspection reports may also contain recommendations to the laboratory to correct deficiencies noted during the inspection.

3.21   Results of Inadequate Performance.

Failure of a laboratory to comply with any aspect of these Guidelines may lead to revocation or suspension of certification as provided in 3.13 and 3.14 of these Guidelines.

Bibliography

Bensinger, Peter B. *A Practical Approach to Drugs in the Workplace.* Abbott Park, Ill.: Abbott Diagnostics Educational Services, 1988.

———. *Drugs and Crime in America.* Abbott Park, Ill.: Abbott Diagnostics Educational Services, 1988.

Broder, Joseph F., and Peyton B. Schur. *Investigation of Drug Abuse in the Workplace.* Stoneham, Mass.: Butterworth Publishers, 1990.

Burns Security Institute. *Report of a Panel Discussion on Drugs in Industry.* Briarcliff Manor, N.Y.: Burns Security Institute, 1975.

Cornish, Craig M. *Drugs and Alcohol in the Workplace.* Wilmette, Ill.: Callaghan and Company, 1988.

Cull, J.G., and R.E. Hardy. *Types of Drug Abusers and Their Abuse.* Springfield, Ill.: Charles C. Thomas, 1974.

Dogoloff, Lee I., and Robert R. Angarola. *Urine Testing in the Workplace.* New York: American Council for Drug Education, 1985.

Fay, Calvina L. "Lay Down the Law Carefully." *Security Management,* March 1987.

Fay, John. *Managing Drug Abuse in the Workplace.* Houston: Forward Edge, 1987.

———. *Alcohol/Drug Abuse Dictionary and Encyclopedia.* Springfield, Ill.: Charles C. Thomas, 1988.

———. "Let's Be Honest About Drug Testing." *Security Management,* December 1988.

———. *The Supervisor's Handbook for Preventing Drug Abuse in the Workplace.* Houston: Forward Edge, 1989.

Fedorko, Steve, and Mark E. McKinney. "Refreshing Our Memories." *Employee Assistance,* April 1989.

Francek, Jim. "Taking Our Pulse." *Employee Assistance,* July 1989.

Googins, Bradley K. "Looking in the Mirror." *Employee Assistance,* April 1989.

———. "Make Hay While the Sun Shines." *Employee Assistance,* July 1989.

Haynes, Richard A. "Drugs in the Workplace." *Security Management,* December 1983.

Hoffman-La Roche, Inc. *Fighting Drug Abuse in Corporate America: A Special Report of the National Conference on Corporate Initiatives for a Drug Free Workplace.* Nutley, N.J.: Hoffman-La Roche, 1988.

Kline, N.S., et al. *Psychotropic Drugs: A Manual for Emergency Management of Overdose.* Oradell, N.J.: Medical Economics Company, 1974.

Maurer, D.W., and V.H. Vogel. *Narcotics and Narcotic Addiction.* Springfield, Ill.: Charles C. Thomas, 1973.

Miller, Jeri. "Simple Eye Test Highly Effective in Quickly Determining Drug Influence." *Psychiatric Times,* December 1988.

Midwest Research Institute. *Drug Atlas.* Kansas City, Mo.: Midwest Research Institute, 1971.

National Institute on Alcohol Abuse and Alcoholism. *Alcohol Abuse in the Hard-to-Reach Work Force*. Rockville, Md.: NIAAA, 1982.

National Institute on Drug Abuse. *Developing an Occupational Drug Abuse Program*. Washington: GPO, 1985.

National Institute on Drug Abuse. *Employee Counseling Service Program: A Supervisor's Guide*. Washington: GPO, 1986.

National Institute on Drug Abuse. *Strategic Planning for Workplace Drug Abuse Programs*. Washington: GPO, 1987.

National Institute on Drug Abuse. *Guidelines for the Development and Assessment of a Comprehensive Federal Employee Assistance Program*. Washington: GPO, 1988.

National Institute on Drug Abuse. *Medical Review Officer Manual: A Guide to Evaluating Urine Drug Analysis*. Washington: GPO, 1988.

National Institute on Drug Abuse. *Urinalysis Collection Handbook for Federal Drug Testing Programs*. Washington: GPO, 1988.

Novitt, Mitchell S. *Employer Liability for Employee Misconduct*. New York: Amacom, 1982.

Patin, Harold C., and Raymond R. Egan. *Industrial Drug Abuse*. Metairie, La.: Drug Education Associates, 1981.

Pendleton, Charles S. *The Employee Handbook on Drug and Alcohol Awareness*. Austin, Tex.: Texas Safety Association, 1984.

Pradhan, S.N., and S.N. Dutta. *Drug Abuse: Clinical and Basic Aspects*. St. Louis: Mosby Books, 1977.

Swint, J. Michael, and David R. Lairson. "Employee Assistance Programs." *Alcohol Health and Research World*, Winter 1983/84.

U.S. Bureau of Justice Assistance. *Urinalysis as Part of a Treatment Alternative to Street Crime (TASC) Program*. Washington: GPO, 1988.

U.S. Bureau of Justice Statistics. *BJS Data Report, 1988*. Washington: GPO, 1989.

U.S. Department of the Army. *Drug Abuse: Clinical Recognition and Treatment*. Washington: GPO, 1973.

U.S. Department of Health and Human Services. *Drug Use in Industry*. Washington: GPO, 1979.

U.S. Department of Health and Human Services. *Guide to Drug Abuse Research Terminology*. Research Issue 26. Washington: GPO, 1982.

U.S. Department of Health and Human Services. *Preventing Drug Abuse in the Workplace*. Washington: GPO, 1982.

U.S. Department of Health and Human Services. *Employer's Guide to the Employment of Former Drug and Alcohol Abusers*. Washington: GPO, 1983.

U.S. Department of Health and Human Services. *Employee Drug Screening: Detection of Drug Use by Urinalysis*. Washington: GPO, 1986.

U.S. Department of Health and Human Services. *Urine Testing for Drugs of Abuse*. Research Issue 73. Washington: GPO, 1986.

U.S. Department of Health and Human Services. "Mandatory Guidelines for Federal Workplace Drug Testing Programs." *Federal Register* 53, no. 69 (1988).

U.S. Department of Justice. *List of Controlled Substances and Drug Code Numbers*. Washington: GPO, 1987.

U.S. Department of Justice. Office of Justice Programs. *Drug Recognition Program: A Monograph*. Washington: GPO, 1989.

U.S. Department of Labor. *What Works: Workplaces without Drugs*. Washington: GPO.

U.S. Department of Transportation. "Procedures for Transportation Workplace Drug Testing Programs." *Federal Register* 53, no. 224 (1988).

U.S. Department of Transportation. Coast Guard. "Programs for Chemical Drug and Alcohol Testing of Commercial Vessel Personnel." *Federal Register* 53, no. 224 (1988).

U.S. Department of Transportation. Coast Guard. "Programs for Chemical Drug and Alcohol Testing of Commercial Vessel Personnel." *Federal Register* 53, no. 230 (1989).

U.S. Department of Transportation. Federal Aviation Administration. "Anti-Drug Program for Personnel Engaged in Specified Aviation Activities." *Federal Register* 53, no. 224 (1988).

U.S. Department of Transportation. Federal Highway Administration. "Controlled Substances Testing." *Federal Register* 53, no. 224 (1988).

U.S. Department of Transportation. Federal Railroad Administration. "Random Drug Testing: Amendments to Alcohol/Drug Regulations." *Federal Register* 53, no. 224 (1988).

U.S. Department of Transportation. Research and Special Programs Administration. "Control of Drug Use in Natural Gas, Liquefied Natural Gas, and Hazardous Liquid Pipeline Operations." *Federal Register* 53, no. 224 (1988).

U.S. Department of Transportation. Research and Special Programs Administration. "Control of Drug Use in Natural Gas, Liquefied Natural Gas, and Hazardous Liquid Pipeline Operations." *Federal Register* 54, no. 70 (1989).

U.S. Department of Transportation. Urban Mass Transportation Administration. "Control of Drug Use in Mass Transportation Operations." *Federal Register* 53, no. 224 (1988).

U.S. Nuclear Regulatory Commission. *NRC Drug Testing Plan.* Washington: GPO, 1988.

Walsh, Timothy J., and Richard J. Healy. *The Protection of Assets Manual.* Santa Monica, Calif.: The Merritt Company, 1983.

White House. *National Strategy for Prevention of Drug Abuse and Drug Trafficking.* Washington: GPO, 1984.

White House Conference for a Drug Free America. Washington: GPO, 1988.

Selected Glossary

active ingredient   The alkaloid or chemical in a plant that produces mind-altering and toxic effects. Cocaine, for example, is the active ingredient of coca leaf.

aftercare   In drug abuse treatment, the services provided the client after successful discharge from the program; community interventions designed to permit a client's effective integration or reintegration into society. Aftercare activities would include involvement in self-help groups, supported work programs, and staff follow-up contacts and interventions.

Al-Anon   A group that helps family members and friends of alcoholic persons cope with related difficulties within and outside the home.

Alateen   A subgroup of Al-Anon that assists young people whose lives have been affected by the alcoholism of a family member or close friend.

Alcohol, Drug Abuse, and Mental Health Administration (ADAMHA)   An umbrella agency within the Public Health Service of the U.S. Department of Health and Human Services. In addition to its own administrative staff, ADAMHA consists of the National Institute on Alcoholism and Alcohol Abuse, the National Institute on Drug Abuse, and the National Institute of Mental Health.

alcoholic   A frequently used term with many shades of meaning about which there is little consensus. It is sometimes used narrowly as a synonym for addict and at other times to refer to an alcohol abuser generally. An alcoholic is sometimes viewed as a person with physical dependence characteristics and sometimes as one with psychological dependence characteristics. Other definitions include the following: (1) a person unable to correct the physiological and other bodily disturbances that have accumulated as the result of drinking; (2) a person with a chronic and usually progressive disease or a symptom of an underlying psychological or physical disorder, which is characterized by dependence on alcohol (manifested by loss of control over drinking) for relief from psychological or physical distress or for gratification from alcohol intoxication itself and by a consumption of alcoholic beverages sufficiently great and consistent to cause physical, mental, social, or economic disability; and (3) a person with a learned or conditioned dependence on alcohol that activates consumption whenever a critical internal or environmental stimulus occurs.

alcoholic beverage   Any beverage that contains ethyl alcohol (ethanol), the intoxicating sedative-hypnotic in fermented and distilled liquors. Made synthetically or produced naturally by fermentation of fruits, vegetables, or grains, alcohol is the oldest and the most widely used social drug in the world.

Alcoholics Anonymous (AA)   A program of recovery from alcohol abuse open to anyone with a desire to stop drinking.

aliquot   A portion of a specimen used for testing.

alkaloid   Any of a diverse group of bitter compounds of plant origin that are usually physiologically or pharmacologically active. Examples include caffeine, morphine, and nicotine. The term is also used to describe a synthetic substance that has a structure similar to that of a plant alkaloid.

American Council on Marijuana and Other Psychoactive Drugs   A nonprofit organization established to help reverse national trends in drug abuse. The council is concerned about all abused psychoactive drugs but has especially targeted marijuana.

amphetamines   A family of stimulants whose medical use is currently limited to narcolepsy, attention deficit disorders in children, and obesity. They constitute a class of synthetic sympathomimetic amines that is similar in some ways to the body's own adrenaline (epinephrine) and that acts with a pronounced stimulant effect on the central nervous system.

analyte   In drug testing, the substance to be measured.

antibody   A blood serum protein produced by the body to destroy or inactivate a specific antigen (foreign substance).

antigen   A substance, usually a protein, that stimulates the body to produce an antibody against it. An antigen-antibody reaction is the process by which the immune system recognizes an antigen and calls for the production of antibodies to fight that antigen.

assay   A procedure for analyzing and quantifying the chemical components of a substance.

barbiturates   The largest and most common group of the synthetic sedative/hypnotics. Barbiturates are often used in combination with or as a substitute for other depressants, such as heroin, and are often taken alternately with amphetamines, as they tend to enhance the euphoric effects of amphetamines while calming the overwrought nervous states they produce. Although still considered indispensable in medicine, their medical applications have declined due primarily to the availability of other drugs with similar effects, such as the antianxiety tranquilizers and other nonbarbiturate sedative-hypnotics.

benzodiazepines   A family of depressants that relieves anxiety, tension, and muscle spasms, produces sedation, and prevents convulsions. They are marketed as anxiolytics (mild tranquilizers), sedatives, hypnotics, or anticonvulsants. Benzodiazepines currently sold in the U.S. include Xanax, Librium, Clonopin, Tranxene, Valium, Dalmane, Paxipam, Ativan, Serax, Centrax, Restoril, and Halcion.

bioassay A test, usually involving living organisms, of the effect or potency of a drug.

blank A biological specimen, such as urine, containing no detectable drugs. Blanks are routinely used in a laboratory's quality-assurance program to guard against false-positive test results.

blind sample Control material submitted to a laboratory analyst for the purpose of determining whether the analyst is producing accurate test results. For example, the blind sample might be urine spiked with a known amount of cocaine. The analyst would be expected to detect and correctly measure the cocaine in the sample.

blood alcohol concentration (BAC) The relative proportion of ethyl alcohol within the blood. BAC is usually expressed in one of two ways: as a percent of alcohol present in a volume of blood, or as the number of milligrams of alcohol per deciliter of blood.

blood alcohol tester An instrument for capturing and analyzing for alcohol content a deep lung breath sample. A tested typically has an energy source, calibrating controls, a readout, a chamber for holding a breath sample, and components for analyzing hydrocarbons that may be present in the deep lung breath.

blood alcohol zones Standards that are commonly used to measure a person's level of intoxication. In one common set of standards, the parts of alcohol per thousand parts of blood are expressed as a percentage. Three zones are used: Zone 1 includes blood alcohol values from 0.00 to 0.5 percent and is considered fairly good evidence that the person is sober. Zone 2 ranges from 0.5 to 0.15 percent and is inconclusive as to whether or not the person is under the influence. Zone 3 relates to findings above 0.15 percent. At this level a person is considered to be intoxicated.

breath alcohol test A test for determining BAC by analysis of a breath sample. A sample of deep lung breath is collected from the subject's air output and held captive in a device that measures hydrocarbons. Hydrocarbons will be present in the deep lung breath of a person who has recently consumed an alcoholic beverage. An exaggerated reading can occur if the subject consumed or regurgitated alcohol within 15 minutes of the test. Thus, a 15-minute waiting period prior to testing is recommended to guard against an exaggerated reading. A breath alcohol test is regarded as a screen that, if positive, should be immediately followed by a confirmation test using a more sensitive analytical technique.

cannabinoids The highly potent, rapid-acting psychoactive ingredients of cannabis products, such as marijuana and hashish.

certified urine Urine obtained from a subject under observation and certified to be from the subject and not adulterated in any way. Several techniques can be used at the point of collection to verify this. *See* direct observation technique; dry bathroom technique; modified dry bathroom technique; temperature check; pH check; specific gravity check.

chain of custody   1. A written record listing the persons who had custody of a specimen from the time of initial custody to final disposition. The custody record reflects the dates and reasons of custody. 2. The policies and procedures that govern collection, handling, storage, and testing of a specimen and dissemination of test results in a manner that ensures correct matching of the specimen with the donor. The purpose of chain of custody is to ensure that the specimen was not altered in any way from the moment it was collected until it was discarded.

chromatography   A method of drug testing in which the various components in a urine specimen are identified and measured by separating them according to their chromatographic properties. Several different types of techniques are used: thin-layer chromatography (TLC), gas chromatography (GC), and high-pressure liquid chromatography (HPLC). The combination of GC with mass spectrometry (GC/MS) provides the most accurate and reliable analytical tool currently used in urinalysis.

cocaine   An alkaloid refined from the coca plant that is a short-acting but powerful stimulant, pharmacologically similar to the amphetamines. Many of cocaine's therapeutic applications are now obsolete as the result of the development of safer anesthetics. Illicit cocaine is distributed as a white crystalline powder, often diluted by a variety of other ingredients, and is most commonly administered by "snorting" through the nasal passages. Less commonly, for heightened effect, the drug is injected directly into the bloodstream.

It is also smoked by a method called "freebasing" in which cocaine hydrochloride (the usual form in which it is sold) is converted to cocaine base.

A purified form of cocaine called crack is smoked by inhaling the vapors that are given off as the drug is heated. It is made by boiling cocaine to produce pea-sized crystalline chunks or rocks, which are smoked in cigarettes or a special pipe, usually made of glass. The drug gets its name from the sound it makes when heated.

collection site   A place where individuals present themselves for the purpose of providing body fluid or tissue samples to be analyzed for specified controlled substances. The site has all necessary personnel, materials, equipment, facilities, and supervision to provide for the collection, security, temporary storage, and transportation or shipment of the samples to a laboratory.

collection site person   A person who instructs and assists individuals at a collection site and who receives and makes an initial examination of the urine specimen provided by those individuals. A collection site person is usually required to have successfully completed training to carry out this function.

confirmatory (or confirmation) test   A second test by an alternate (different) and highly specific analytical method to identify a drug or metabolite. The principal purpose of confirmation testing is to eliminate any false-positive results obtained during screening (initial testing). At this time gas chromatography/mass spectrometry (GC/MS) is the only generally accepted confirmation method.

contamination   In drug testing, the addition of a foreign substance to a urine specimen, rendering it unsuitable for analysis. Contamination is most often the deliberate act of a donor seeking to mask the presence of a drug or to confuse the analytical procedures. Contaminants frequently include salt, sugar, vinegar, tea, bleach, and detergents.

Controlled Substances Act   The name given to Title II of the Comprehensive Drug Abuse and Prevention Act of 1970. This Act established five schedules or classifications of controlled substances according to their potential for abuse, physical and psychological dependence liability, and currently accepted medical use.

Schedule I, the most strictly controlled category, includes heroin, marijuana, and LSD, and other drugs considered to have high abuse potential and not recognized for medical use in the United States. These drugs can be obtained only for limited research purposes under special registration requirements.

Schedule II drugs (morphine, methadone, and amphetamines) are different from Schedule I drugs in that they have some currently accepted medical uses but they may lead an abuser to severe psychological and physical dependence. The manufacture and distribution of these drugs are controlled by production quotas, strict security regulations, import and export controls, and nonrefillable prescription requirements.

Schedule III substances have a potential for abuse that is less than that of the substances in Schedules I and II. They have currently accepted medical uses that may lead to moderate or low physical dependence or high physiological dependence.

Schedule IV substances have a low potential for abuse relative to the substances in Schedule III. They have currently accepted medical uses that may lead an abuser to limited physical or psychological dependence relative to the substances in Schedule III.

Schedule V substances have a low potential for abuse relative to the substances in Schedule IV. They have currently accepted medical uses that may lead an abuser to limited physical or psychological dependence relative to the substances in Schedule IV. Schedule V drugs are generally sold over the counter and are not subject to any refill limitations on prescriptions.

control material   In drug testing, a biological specimen (such as urine or blood) that contains certain drugs at specific concentrations. A laboratory analyst uses the control material to calibrate equipment and ensure that the routine procedures of the laboratory are operating within quality-control parameters.

cross-reacting substances   In drug testing with immunoassays, substances that give the appearance of a positive result.

cutoff level   A value that serves as a decision point for reporting a urine specimen as positive or negative. A cutoff level is an administrative mechanism for ensuring that a specimen containing a very small amount of a drug is not reported as positive. This procedure is designed to give the drug user the benefit of any doubt and to rule out the possibility of passive inhalation of marijuana smoke.

designer drugs   Synthetic drugs, chemically related to legitimate drugs, which are produced inexpensively and sold (sometimes legally) as substitutes for the legitimate products they imitate. The term was originally used to describe drugs designed to meet the tastes of particular clients.

direct observation technique   A technique for collecting urine specimens in which the voiding process is observed or closely monitored.

disposable alcohol screening device   A device used to conduct a one-time qualitative test of BAC. It typically consists of a small glass tube containing either a column or multiple bands of an alcohol-sensitive reagent and a breath-volume measuring device such as a balloon or plastic bag.

Drug Abuse Act of 1970   The name given to the Comprehensive Drug Abuse Prevention and Control Act of 1970, the first major federal drug legislation since the Harrison Narcotics Act of 1914. All the regulations advanced since the Harrison Act were repealed and replaced by this new statute. Possession penalties were generally reduced, but the act established strict import and export limitations, extended penalties for trafficking, and imposed new controls on previously unregulated psychoactive drugs. The Act was designed to create a comprehensive framework for the regulation of narcotic and nonnarcotic drugs. Title II of this act is known as the Controlled Substances Act.

drug education   Any program designed to provide information on the use of drugs and to change knowledge, attitudes, and/or behavior in a direction desired by the educator.

drug-free workplace   As used in the Drug-Free Workplace Act of 1988, a site for the performance of work done in connection with a specific grant or contract described in the act or an entity at which employees are prohibited from engaging in the unlawful manufacture, distribution, dispensation, possession, or use of a controlled substance in accordance with the requirements of the act.

drug testing   The scientific analysis of urine, blood, breath, saliva, hair, tissue, or other specimens of the human body for the purpose of detecting a drug or alcohol.

dry bathroom technique   A technique for collecting a urine specimen in which the subject disrobes or places out of reach any items that could be used to conceal a bogus specimen or adulterant. The subject voids, unwitnessed, in a room containing nothing that could be used to adulterate the specimen, including water.

dysfunctional drug use Drug use that results in physical, psychological, economic, legal, and/or social harm to the individual user or to others affected by the drug user's behavior.

employee assistance program (EAP) A program designed for early identification, referral, and treatment of employee problems such as drug and alcohol abuse, domestic strife, and mental instability.

enzyme immunoassay (EIA) An analysis of a body fluid for the purpose of detecting the presence of a drug or drug metabolite. The technique is based on the principle of competition between labeled and unlabeled antigens for binding sites on a specific antibody. An antibody is a protein substance to which a specific drug or drug metabolite will bind.

extended-care facility An institution that provides nursing, medical, and custodial care for a prolonged period, as in rehabilitation from drug abuse.

false positive/false negative Terms indicating that a test incorrectly identified or failed to identify the presence of a drug or drug metabolite. In urine testing, for example, a false positive means that the test indicated the presence of a drug when none was present, and a false negative means that the test failed to identify a drug that was present in the specimen analyzed.

flush the system To consume a large amount of fluid to wash drugs out of the body system or dilute drug concentrations that might be detected through urinalysis.

gas chromatography (GC) A laboratory technique for analyzing gas, liquid, and solid samples. The sample is converted to a gaseous state and injected into the gas chromatograph instrument, where it passes through a column of absorbent material. The gas is fractionated into compounds according to their chemical and physical properties. The compounds are portrayed as a pattern on a graph, which allows comparison with graphs of known samples.

gas chromatography/mass spectrometry (GC/MS) A laboratory technique that combines the separating power of gas chromatography with the high sensitivity and specificity of spectrometric detection. GC/MS is generally considered to be the most conclusive method of confirming the presence of a drug in urine.

high-performance liquid chromatography (HPLC) A laboratory technique that uses a column through which a specimen passes while undergoing equilibration between two liquid phases. The time it takes for the specimen to traverse the column at a given solvent flow rate is measured, and the speed of movement provides accurate indications as to the drug molecule in the specimen.

horizontal gaze nystagmus test (HGN) A test that measures the ability of the eye to maintain a fixation on objects moving out of the line of vision.

The test is based on the principle that the movement of the eyeball as it turns to the side may be aggravated by central nervous system depressants such as barbiturates and alcohol. By observing the onset and quantity of nystagmus (a rapid involuntary oscillation of the eyeball), a trained person may be able to estimate intoxication. The HGN test is used by some law enforcement agencies and employers as an on-scene sobriety test.

illegal drug   A term often used arbitrarily to denote chemical substances that the user (of the term) wishes for some purpose to prohibit. For example, an employer might use the term to describe substances that are not allowed in the employer's workplace. A commonly used definition for this purpose is: any drug that is not legally obtainable; any drug that is legally obtainable but has not been legally obtained; any prescribed drug not legally obtained; any prescribed drug not being used for the prescribed purpose; any over-the-counter drug being used at a dosage level different from that recommended by the manufacturer or being used for a purpose other than that intended by the manufacturer; and any drug being used for a purpose not in accordance with bona fide medical therapy. Examples of illegal drugs are Cannabis substances, cocaine, heroin, phencyclidine (PCP), and so-called designer drugs and look-alike drugs.

immunoassay   An analysis of a body fluid for the purpose of detecting the presence of a drug or drug metabolite. Two types of immunoassays are usually employed: enzyme immunoassay (EIA) and radioimmunoassay (RIA).

initial test   An immunoassay screen used to eliminate negative urine specimens from further consideration.

integrity check   In drug testing, any of several techniques for detecting contamination, dilution, substitution, or other attempts to render a urine specimen unsuitable for analysis. Integrity checks are usually performed at the point of specimen collection and include monitoring or direct observation of urination; not allowing the specimen donor to carry loose clothing and containers into the bathroom; removing from the bathroom soap, ashtrays, and other materials that can be used as contaminants; disconnecting the bathroom's faucets so that tap water cannot be used as a dilutant; and adding a dye to the toilet water. Integrity checks also include simple, out-of-laboratory tests involving measurement of specimen temperature, specific gravity, and pH content.

interfering substance   In drug testing, a substance other than the analyte (the drug being looked for) that gives a similar analytical response or alters the analytical result.

medical review officer   As used in the Mandatory Guidelines for Federal Workplace Drug Testing Programs, a licensed physician responsible for receiving laboratory results generated by an employer's drug-testing program. The physician must have knowledge of substance abuse disorders and appropriate medical training to interpret and evaluate an individual's positive test result together with his or her medical history and any other relevant biomedical information.

metabolite   A compound produced from chemical changes of a drug in the body; the biochemical by-product resulting from the metabolism of a substance; a substance taking part in metabolism, either as a product or as a substance of the metabolic process. A metabolite may produce a chemical effect that is altogether different from that of the original substance.

methadone   A synthetic opioid which prevents withdrawal symptoms and the craving to use opiates. This drug is largely used in the maintenance treatment of heroin dependency.

methaqualone   A nonbarbiturate sedative (hypnotic) that produces sleep for about 6 to 8 hours, originally marketed as an alternative to barbiturates. Since its introduction, methaqualone has become one of the most abused drugs in the United States.

modified bathroom technique   A technique for collecting a urine specimen in which all substances that can be used to contaminate a specimen are removed from the bathroom, the hot-water supply is disconnected, and the toilet water is dyed.

Narcotics Anonymous (NA)   A worldwide self-help fellowship for recovering drug abusers who give each other support to remain free of drugs. NA was formed in 1953 and has affiliated chapters throughout the United States. As its name suggests, NA has adopted the Alcoholics Anonymous (AA) model.

occupational alcoholism program   A type of program designed to identify and refer for treatment workers who have drinking problems.

on-site testing   Drug testing by an employer using paraprofessional staff and equipment provided by in-house resources.

opiates   A group of drugs, sometimes referred to as narcotics, used medically to relieve pain, but which also has a high potential for abuse. The term specifically refers to the two opium alkaloids morphine and codeine and to the semisynthetic drugs derived from them, such as heroin and hydromorphone.

pH   A measure of the acidity or alkalinity of a solution. A pH of 7 is neutral, below 7 acid, above 7 alkaline. A pH check is used to measure the balance between acidity and alkalinity in a urine specimen. When the balance is out of line, a presumption can be made that the specimen has been diluted or contaminated.

phencyclidine (PCP)   A synthetic depressant drug developed as an anesthetic agent that is now used medically only for veterinary purposes because of its severe adverse effects. It is illegally sold on the street as a hallucinogen.

proficiency (or performance) testing specimen   A biological specimen (such as urine or blood) having constituents that are known to an outside agency (such as a licensing agency) but unknown to the testing laboratory or analyst. Proficiency testing specimens are used to evaluate technical competency for purposes of certification and licensing.

qualitative test   A test that identifies the components of an unknown substance. In drug testing, for example, a qualitative test seeks to identify the specific drugs or metabolites of drugs. *See also* quantitative test.

quality assurance   In drug testing, practices and protocols designed and enforced to ensure accurate laboratory findings. Quality-assurance techniques include the use of blind samples, spiked samples, and proficiency or performance testing specimens.

quality control   In drug testing, those techniques used to monitor errors that can cause a deterioration in the quality of laboratory results. For example, a laboratory analyst will use a urine specimen containing specific drugs at precisely known concentrations. The specimen is analyzed using the laboratory's routine procedures and equipment. Any deviation from the expected findings indicates a need for an adjustment of the procedures or the equipment.

quantitative test   A test that determines the amounts or proportions of substances in a mixture. In drug testing, a quantitative test will measure the concentration of a drug in a specimen. *See also* qualitative test.

radioimmunoassay (RIA)   A method of determining the concentration of a protein in a serum by monitoring the reaction produced by the injection of a radioactive-labeled substance known to react in a particular way with the protein being studied.

reasonable belief   In the context of administering a workplace drug testing program, a belief based on objective facts sufficient to lead a prudent person to conclude that a particular employee is unable to perform his or her duties satisfactorily due to drug or alcohol impairment. Such inability to perform may include, but is not limited to, decreases in the quality or quantity of the employee's productivity, judgment, reasoning, concentration, and psychomotor control, as well as marked changes in behavior. Accidents, deviations from safe working practices, and erratic conduct indicative of impairment are examples of reasonable belief situations.

screen   In drug testing, a test or series of initial tests designed to determine whether a sample contains a drug or drugs at particular minimum concentrations. A positive finding on a screen is called a presumptive positive, that is, the sample requires further testing for confirmation or verification of the initial positive result.

screening test   *See* initial test.

selectivity   *See* specificity.

specific gravity check   A test of a urine specimen to determine its content of water. When the test reveals a high density or concentration of water, the specimen may have been diluted by the addition of a liquid or the ingestion of a large amount of liquid shortly before voiding.

specificity   In drug testing, the ability of a test method to identify a single chemical component in an unknown sample. This characteristic is a function of one or all of the processes of isolation, separation, and detection of a particular product in a biological matrix. Gas chromatography/mass spectrometry (GC/MS), the most specific urinalysis technique, permits highly efficient separation of components on the GC column, followed by extremely selective detection on the mass spectrometer. Also called selectivity.

specimen   A small sample of something; a part of a whole intended upon analysis to reveal characteristics of the whole, for example, a urine specimen used for urinalysis.

spectrophotometer   A laboratory instrument that analyzes an unknown substance according to the substance's capacity to absorb ultraviolet or infrared light. Since many substances of interest to an analyst (such as drugs) will absorb light at specific and unique wavelengths, the analyst compares the wavelengths of the unknown substance with those of the known substances. A finding by spectrophotometer analysis is usually cross-checked with a separate and more specific analytical technique.

split specimen   In drug testing, a specimen that is divided in half and submitted to the analyst as two separate specimens with different donor identifications. In some cases, the purpose is to evaluate the accuracy of work performed by the analyst.

standard   In drug testing, an authentic sample of a drug (the analyte) having a known purity or concentration.

temperature check   In drug testing, a test to determine whether the heat of a freshly collected urine specimen falls within a known range for such specimens. If the heat is outside the range, there is a suspicion that the donor is attempting to pass a bogus specimen.

turnaround time   The time that elapses between receipt of a specimen at the laboratory and the reporting of test results.

under the influence   A condition in which a person is affected by a drug or alcohol in any detectable manner. The symptoms of influence are not confined to those consistent with misbehavior or to obvious impairment of physical or mental ability, such as slurred speech, difficulty in maintaining balance, or the odor of alcohol. A determination of being under the influence can be established by a professional, a scientifically valid test such as urinalysis or blood analysis, and in some cases by a layperson.

under the influence of alcohol   Impairment of faculties due to alcohol consumption. A blood alcohol concentration of 0.10 grams of alcohol per 100 milliliters of blood or 210 liters of breath constitutes the legal presumption for intoxication under the laws of most jurisdictions.

urinalysis   1. Analysis of urine by physical, chemical, or microscopic means to reveal color; turbidity; pH; the possible presence of microorganisms, blood, pus, or crystals; or abnormal levels of ketones, proteins, sugar, or other compounds, including drugs. 2. In drug testing, an analytical technique for detecting the presence of illicit substances in urine.

Index

split specimens, 233, 359
suspect specimens, 229–230
temperature check, 229, 359
transfer to laboratory, 231
volume, 228–229
Specimen collection, sample materials for, 235–259
consent and waiver, 258–259
consent forms, 248–255
disclosure of medication and ingested substances, 256–257
urine specimen collection procedures, 235–247
Specimen storage, 279
Spectrophotometer, 359
Spiked specimen, 267, 281
Split specimen, 233, 359
Sponsoring organization, 79
Spot quiz for supervisor training, sample of, 167–169
Standard, defined, 359
Standards for drug-testing laboratories, 277–282
State and local legislation, 22–23
Statistical Manual of Disorders, 30
Steady-state level, 274–275
Stimulants, driving and, 145
Strabismus, 191
Substance abuser, defined, 30
Supervision, principles of, 152–154
Supervisor
drug-testing questions and answers for, 158–163
enabling, 176–178
intervention strategy of, 8–9, 173–182
postaccident testing and, 187
reasonable cause determination by, 9–11, 186
See also Training of supervisor
Supervisory follow-up, 181–182
Support for drug abuse education program, 114
Supreme Court, U.S., 301, 302
Survey, drug abuse, 32–33
sample, 36–45
Suspect specimens, 229–230
Symptoms of drug abuse, 173–176, 186, 359

Targeting the problems, 115
Technical error, 281
Temperature check on specimen, 229, 359
Testimony, preparing for, 18
Testing for drugs. *See* Drug test/testing
Test reports from certified laboratory, 280
Test results, circumstances warranting release of, 55
Tetrahydrocannabinol (THC), 144, 145, 272–275
Thin-layer chromatography (TLC), 16, 262–263, 264–265
Time-sensitive nature of urinalysis, 232–233
Title II of Comprehensive Drug Abuse and Prevention Act of 1970, 353
Tolerance, amphetamines use and, 141
Toluenes, 140
Topic preparation for education program, 119
Training
by federal employee assistance program, 288–289
of instructor for education program, 118
for reasonable cause testing, 10–11
Training of supervisor, 8–9, 147–171
body of knowledge for, 149–152
drug-testing questions and answers, 158–163
federal agency plans for, 285–286
methods of instruction, 154–155
nature of learning and, 147–148
objectives, 148–149
in principles of supervision, 152–154
process, 154–156
sample materials for, 164–171
transfer of knowledge in, 148–149
Transfer of knowledge, 148–149
Treatment
facilitating, 19–21
feedback on progress of, 181–182
knowing how to obtain, 153–154
modalities, 34–35
program, 9, 183–184
urinalysis as aid in, 13
Treatment benefits, 53
Troubled employee concept, 35
Trucking company, sample drug-testing policy for, 63–72